T0323640

Pandemic Ethics

Pandemic Ethics

From COVID-19 to Disease X

Edited by

DOMINIC WILKINSON AND
JULIAN SAVULESCU

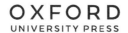

OXFORD
UNIVERSITY PRESS

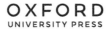

Great Clarendon Street, Oxford, OX2 6DP,
United Kingdom

Oxford University Press is a department of the University of Oxford.
It furthers the University's objective of excellence in research, scholarship,
and education by publishing worldwide. Oxford is a registered trade mark of
Oxford University Press in the UK and in certain other countries

© Oxford University Press 2023

The moral rights of the authors have been asserted

All rights reserved. No part of this publication may be reproduced, stored in
a retrieval system, or transmitted, in any form or by any means, without the
prior permission in writing of Oxford University Press, or as expressly permitted
by law, by licence or under terms agreed with the appropriate reprographics
rights organization. Enquiries concerning reproduction outside the scope of the
above should be sent to the Rights Department, Oxford University Press, at the
address above

You must not circulate this work in any other form
and you must impose this same condition on any acquirer

Published in the United States of America by Oxford University Press
198 Madison Avenue, New York, NY 10016, United States of America

British Library Cataloguing in Publication Data
Data available

Library of Congress Control Number: 2022950588

ISBN 978-0-19-287168-8

DOI: 10.1093/oso/9780192871688.001.0001

Printed and bound in the UK by
TJ Books Limited

Links to third party websites are provided by Oxford in good faith and
for information only. Oxford disclaims any responsibility for the materials
contained in any third party website referenced in this work.

Contents

II. LIBERTY

III. BALANCING ETHICAL VALUES

IV. PANDEMIC EQUALITY AND INEQUALITY

V. PANDEMIC X

Acknowledgement

The Editors would like to thank the Uehiro Foundation for Ethics and Education for their unfailing support of the development of this volume during the pandemic. Without the Foundation's generous support, this volume could not have been born. We would especially like to thank the Chairman, Mr Tetsuji Uehiro, for his inspiring leadership and vision for a brighter future beyond the COVID-19 pandemic and a better response to Pandemic X.

Dominic Wilkinson
Julian Savulescu

Foreword

The COVID-19 pandemic is the most significant global event of the twenty-first century, reaching every corner of the world, limiting the lives of millions, disrupting health systems, education, and business, and producing an economic shock that has increased inequality and poverty. The loss of life measured as excess deaths stands at more than 15 million, similar to that of the First World War of the twentieth century. While the global influenza outbreak of 1918 has long been the "model" for pandemic preparedness, there is no doubt that our experience of the COVID-19 pandemic, and our response to it, will be the major focus of academic study in the years ahead. So, how did we do?

I have had the privilege and, at times, the burden of sitting in the midst of the scientific, political, and media circus as a vaccine developer leading the clinical development of the Oxford–AstraZeneca COVID-19 vaccine in the UK, Brazil, and South Africa. I worked with some remarkable clinical and laboratory researchers, and more than 24,000 committed clinical trial participants across these nations, whose efforts led to the distribution of 3 billion doses of our vaccine to more than 180 countries, saving tens of millions from being hospitalized and sparing millions from death. So, one view is that, for vaccine development at least, we did well.... But there are very substantial scientific, regulatory, ethical, financial, and manufacturing challenges in vaccine development which have meant that it wasn't always so smooth. Indeed, of 349 COVID-19 vaccines being developed globally, only nine have so far been approved by the World Health Organization.

In Oxford, our ability to develop a vaccine rapidly was critically dependent on a twenty-year scientific backstory, which meant that we had a vaccine prototype ready to go as soon as the new virus was sequenced (11 January 2020), and had a pre-existing critical mass of expertise in the University to develop, manufacture, and test a vaccine ourselves. We don't have the same backstory for other potential pandemic threats, so we were lucky this time that it was a coronavirus. But we were also fortunate to be in the UK with the regulator, the Medicines and Healthcare products Regulatory Agency, ensuring speedy proportionate review (one week for the initial trial approval) and timely advice, which meant that we progressed as fast as could be done, knowing that any day lost meant another 10,000 people around the world would be dead. All documents and many amendments were ably reviewed by the national ethics committee who managed rapid review (four-day turnaround for the first trial submission) to ensure that speed of vaccine development was not curtailed by the ethical review process. These agencies provided insightful feedback in the development process, were careful guardians of the safety and integrity of the trials, and close partners in ensuring the pandemic was properly countered. Indeed, there are moments of desperate isolation when the world is watching your every move in a pandemic, and the strong regulatory systems around me provided great confidence and comfort that the path was right. The regulators in the three nations involved in the Oxford University trials, whilst fiercely maintaining their independence as regulators, shared our goal to support development of a vaccine for the world. The working relationship and dialogue with these regulators has had huge benefits for human health and very much enabled rapid progress, which they must retain for the future. It is no coincidence that MHRA in the UK was the first to approve the vaccine for emergency use, soon followed by ANVISA in Brazil. But not all regulatory systems were able to pivot to a way of working that expedited the approval process in the pandemic or were prepared to support developers with a common goal, and some took many months more to approve vaccines, or have still not done so. There is no doubt that lives have been lost because of the failure of some regulators to adapt to a pandemic. They ought to do better.

If the development of the AstraZeneca vaccine was a victory for research ethics, other elements of vaccine ethics have not fared so well. It has been very clear since early in the pandemic that older adults and individuals with health conditions (regardless of age) were most at risk of death in the pandemic and should be prioritized (with frontline health workers) for immunization once vaccines were available. This approach is also critical to relieving pressure on health systems to allow society and the economy to reopen. Strategies that focus on healthy young individuals whose risk of hospitalization or death is near to zero achieve neither an impact on mortality nor an end to the health systems crisis. Indeed, most countries took the approach in their own mass vaccination programmes of focusing on the elderly and those with other health conditions. However, despite the agreed position that global vaccine roll-out should follow this prioritized approach to save the most lives, high income countries (HICs) prioritized their own citizens, regardless of age, over those in other countries, only pledging most doses for low and middle income countries (LMICs) to arrive in 2022. This led, inevitably, to a large number of preventable deaths in 2021. It's obvious that you have to vaccinate before it's too late and your patient has died from the disease. The focus on vaccinating lower-risk members of populations in HICs before high-risk individuals in LMICs is one of the greatest tragedies of the pandemic, resulting in millions of preventable deaths. On the other hand, politicians are elected to protect their own populations, and the apparently immoral nationalistic approach, which is almost universal, is politically understandable. However, this approach does not make sense for global health security or recovery of the global economy. A major focus today must be on building the case for equitable distribution of future life-saving interventions by identifying the key political drivers, such as the study of macroeconomics, which led to the perverse approach to COVID-19. It may be that the poor in the future can only be protected by enshrining good global public health in international law.

Beyond vaccine policy, politicians, and the media response to them, have had a major role in promoting confidence in vaccines in the pandemic—some with great effect leading to high vaccine coverage and population protection. However, countries with politically divided opinion on vaccination, or limited public confidence in the government, have suffered from low vaccine uptake and resistance to other public health measures. Ill-advised comments by European politicians on vaccine efficacy or safety have sent shock waves far beyond Europe's borders. For example, the reports of the very rare side effects associated with RNA vaccines (myocarditis, which means heart inflammation) or viral vector vaccines (thrombosis with thrombocytopaenia, which is also known as rare blood clots) led to increased hesitancy at a time when there was a shortage of supply in many countries, and there is no doubt that some died from the much greater risk of COVID-19 because they remained unvaccinated. Of grave concern, some evidence also points to the risk of these side effects being deliberately amplified by malign states.

Whilst it is easy to blame politicians and the media, scientists have not always communicated well. Healthy scientific debate, in which we test evidence to get closer to the truth, does not play out well in the media when it is presented as a political debate by two scientists with differing ideological positions, leading to public uncertainty and vaccine hesitancy. A vital part of the review of our pandemic should be on political and scientific communications, and importantly on the communication of risk, to ensure that we don't make a pandemic worse than it needs to be.

Ethics is vital to public health and to management of infectious diseases. In this book, the authors expertly explore ethical issues that lie behind many aspects of the pandemic response, focused on Covid-19 and looking forward to the next pandemic. If politicians and their advisors had read this book in January 2020 and heard these perspectives, I have no doubt that we really would have done better for humanity. Hopefully they will read it before Pandemic X arrives.

Professor Sir Andrew Pollard

Director of the Oxford Vaccine Group
Professor of Paediatric Infection and Immunity
University of Oxford
2 June 2022

Preface

By any measure, the COVID-19 pandemic is a world-historic event. The two sponsoring organizations of this volume were born in similar moments of shock and loss. For this reason, we are especially keen to see that this global-scale tragedy leads not to chaos and despair but to the real possibility of a better future.

Carnegie Council for Ethics in International Affairs was founded in August 1914 to stop the slow-motion crisis that ignited World War I. The Uehiro Foundation on Ethics and Education was inspired by the life and work of Tetsuhiko Uehiro, a survivor of the atomic bomb. The COVID-19 pandemic is a generational calamity of similar magnitude that will forever be considered a "before and after" event.

This project was launched by the Oxford Uehiro Centre for Practical Ethics at the height of the crisis and concludes while many of its issues remain unresolved. It is useful to bear in mind that these chapters were written in the middle of real-time debates over the development and distribution of vaccines, lockdowns, and mask mandates, and skepticism of expert knowledge and advice.

Immediacy and direct engagement are critical to the purpose of this book. We hope it captures the contingencies and uncertainties of the times, when so much remains unknown and yet decisions cannot be avoided or delayed.

Practical ethics does its most important work when it addresses uncertainties, evaluates conflicting claims, and weighs competing values. As new facts become available, analyses evolve. Openness and self-correction are what separate ethics from power politics, ideology, and dogma—and this is why ethics is so important today.

The pandemic strikes at a time of particular political peril. Humanity has never been more connected yet more fractured. Global solidarity has collapsed at the very moment we are facing the potentially catastrophic effects of climate change, nuclear war, the migration of millions of refugees, and the COVID-19 pandemic.

The reality is stark. International institutions are mired in dysfunction. Nationalism is on the rise. Democracies are struggling for legitimacy. The situation has bred cynicism and despair, particularly among the youth. It has also bred political opportunism, demagoguery, conspiracy theories, and ubiquitous pundits who have become self-appointed experts on the lessons of this latest public policy crisis.

This project is our answer to this rather bleak assessment. The authors in this volume are experts in their fields, all working with empirical facts and according to professional standards of analysis and judgment. Work of this kind does not ensure wise or enlightened policy. But it is surely a required first step.

We empower ethics by recognizing that issues of exceptional complexity should be openly and rigorously debated—especially in times of stress and uncertainty. Only then can we build the trust necessary to mount collective responses to the global issues that affect us all.

Joel H. Rosenthal

President, Carnegie Council for Ethics in International Affairs
New York, NY
June 2022

List of Figures

Notes on Contributors

Matthew Adler is the Richard A. Horvitz Professor of Law and Professor of Economics, Philosophy and Public Policy at Duke University. Adler is the author of numerous articles and several monographs, including *New Foundations of Cost-Benefit Analysis* (Harvard, 2006; co-authored with Eric Posner); *Well-Being and Fair Distribution: Beyond Cost-Benefit Analysis*, which systematically discusses how to integrate considerations of fair distribution into policy analysis (Oxford, 2012); and *Measuring Social Welfare: An Introduction* (Oxford, 2019), an overview of the social-welfare-function methodology. With Marc Fleurbaey, he edited the *Oxford Handbook of Well-Being and Public Policy* (2016). Along with Ole Norheim, he is the co-founder of the Prioritarianism in Practice Research Network, whose work appears in an edited volume, *Prioritarianism in Practice* (Cambridge University Press, 2022).

Akira Akabayashi is Professor of the Department of Biomedical Ethics of the University of Tokyo Graduate School of Medicine, Adjunct Professor of New York University School of Medicine, and Affiliated professor of Department of Bioethics and Humanities, University of Washington (Seattle). His research interests span cross-cultural bioethics, global bioethics, medical/clinical ethics, and medical humanities. As an academic researcher, he has published more than 200 original articles and more than 20 books or chapters in English in addition to many Japanese publications.

Prof. Akabayashi established the first Bioethics Center (University of Tokyo Center of Biomedical Ethics and Law: CBEL) in Asia in 2003.

He wrote *Biomedical Ethics in Asia: A Casebook for Multicultural Learners* (McGraw-Hill, 2010). He also edited *The Future of Bioethics: International Dialogue* (Oxford University Press, 2014, 786 pages). His most recent book is *Bioethics Across the Globe: Rebirthing Bioethics (Springer Nature, 2020).*

Jennifer Blumenthal-Barby is the Cullen Professor of Medical Ethics and Associate Director of The Center for Medical Ethics and Health Policy at Baylor College of Medicine. She has published more than 150 academic articles on philosophical and ethical issues in decision science, medical decision-making, and neuroscience. She is the author of 'Good Ethics and Bad Choices: The Relevance of Behavioral Economics for Medical Ethics' (MIT Press, 2021). She is an Associate Editor of the Journal of Medical Ethics and The American Journal of Bioethics.

Richard Bradley is Professor of Philosophy in the Department of Philosophy, Logic and Scientific Method at the London School of Economics and a Fellow of the British Academy. His research is concentrated in decision theory, formal epistemology and the theory of social choice but he also works on conditionals and the nature of chance. His book *Decision Theory with a Human Face* (Cambridge University Press, 2017) gives an account of decision making under conditions of severe uncertainty suitable for rational but bounded agents. Recently he has been doing work on policy decision making under scientific uncertainty applied to climate change, natural catastrophes and pandemics.

Allen Buchanan is Laureate Professor of Philosophy and Research Professor at the Freedom Center, University of Arizona. His main research is in Political Philosophy, Philosophy of International Law, and Bioethics; and, most recently, in developing a normative theory of large-scale social-political change, including morally progressive change. He is the author of thirteen books and co-author of two books. His most recent book is Our Moral Fate: Evolution and the Escape From Tribalism. Buchanan's most recent articles are "The Fundamental Wrong of Colonialism," co-authored with Ritwik Agrawal and "Political Ideology and Revolution," co-authored with Alexander Motchoulski.

Maria Clara Dias is a Professor of Philosophy at the Federal University of Rio de Janeiro (UFRJ) and a Permanent Member of the university's Interinstitutional and Interdisciplinary Graduate Program in Bioethics, Applied Ethics and Public Health (PPGBIOS). She coordinates the Center of Social Inclusion (UFRJ) and the research group Nós: Dissidências feministas (CNPq). She is a research fellow of the Brazilian National Council for Scientific and Technological Development (CNPq) and of the Research Support Foundation of the State of Rio de Janeiro (FAPERJ).

She is the author and co-author of several books, including, About us: expanding the frontiers of morality, (Ape´Ku 2020); Fuctionings Approach: for a more inclusive point of view (Amazon 2014) and Bioethics: theoretical foundations and applications (Ape´Ku 2020), available for download on the website mariaclaradias.info. She was a Editor of the Diversitates International Journal of Medical Ethics from 2008–2014 and from 2018–2022.

Ezekiel Emanuel is the Vice Provost for Global Initiatives, the Diane v.S. Levy and Robert M. Levy University Professor, and Co-Director of the Healthcare Transformation Institute at the University of Pennsylvania. Dr. Emanuel received his M.D. from Harvard Medical School and his Ph.D. in political philosophy from Harvard University.

Ruth Faden is the founder of the Johns Hopkins Berman Institute of Bioethics, and its director from 1995 until 2016. She is also the Philip Franklin Wagley Professor of Biomedical Ethics. Her research focuses on structural injustice theory and public policy including national and global challenges in public health, food, agriculture and climate, women's health, health systems design and priority setting, and advances in science and technology. During the pandemic, Dr. Faden has worked at the intersection of structural justice and the COVID-19 response, primarily in vaccine allocation and prioritization, pregnancy, and K-12 education. Her latest book, with Madison Powers, is Structural Injustice: Power, Advantage, and Human Rights (September 2019; Oxford University Press).

Maddalena Ferranna is a Research Associate at the Harvard T.H. Chan School of Public Health. Her main research topics are welfare economics, global health and climate change economics. She is particularly interested in the development and application of methods to assess the equity implications of health and environmental interventions. She received a PhD in Economics from Toulouse School of Economics and was a Values and Public Policy Postdoctoral fellow at Princeton University.

Jessica Flanigan holds the Richard L. Morrill Chair in Ethics and Democratic Values at the University of Richmond, where she teaches Leadership Ethics, Ethical Decision-Making in Healthcare, and Critical Thinking. Her research addresses the ethics of public policy, medicine, and business. In Pharmaceutical Freedom (OUP 2017) she defends rights of self-medication. In Debating Sex Work (OUP 2019) she defends the decriminalization of sex work. Flanigan has also published in journals such as Philosophical Studies, The Journal of Business Ethics, Leadership, The Journal of Moral Philosophy, and the Journal of Political Philosophy.

Marc Fleurbaey is CNRS Senior Researcher, Professor at Paris School of Economics, and Associate Professor at ENS-Ulm, and up to 2020 was Robert E. Kuenne Professor at Princeton University. Author of *Beyond GDP* (with Didier Blanchet, OUP 2013), *A Theory of Fairness and Social Welfare* (with François Maniquet, CUP 2011), and *Fairness, Responsibility and Welfare* (OUP, 2008), he is a former editor of *Social Choice and Welfare* and *Economics and Philosophy* and is currently an associate editor of *Philosophy and Public Affairs* as well as *Politics, Philosophy and Economics*. He is one of the initiators of the International Panel on Social Progress, and lead author of its Manifesto for Social Progress (CUP 2018).

Larry Gostin is University Professor, Georgetown University, and Founding O'Neill Chair in Global Health Law. He directs the World Health Organization Center on National and Global Health Law. He is working with WHO on the global COVID-19 response, including impacts on the health workforce and international migration. He served on the WHO/Global Fund Blue Ribbon Expert Panel on Equitable Access in Global Health and co-chaired the *Lancet* Commission on Global Health Law. Prof. Gostin is Global Health editor, *Journal of the American Medical Association (JAMA)*. He's a Member of the National Academy of Medicine and sits on its Global Health Board. He also serves on the National Academies' Committee on the Analysis to Enhance the Effectiveness of the Federal Quarantine Station Network based on Lessons from the COVID-19 Pandemic. President Obama appointed Prof. Gostin to the President's National Cancer Advisory Board.

James Hammitt is professor of economics and decision sciences at the Harvard T.H. Chan School of Public Health and director of the Harvard Center for Risk Analysis. His research and teaching concern the development and application of benefit-cost, decision, and risk analysis to health and environmental policy. He holds degrees in applied mathematics and public policy from Harvard.

Jeffrey P. Kahn is the Andreas C. Dracopoulos Director of the Johns Hopkins Berman Institute of Bioethics, and the Levi Professor of Bioethics and Public Policy. He is also Professor in the Department of Health Policy and Management in the Johns Hopkins Bloomberg School of Public Health. His scholarly focus includes the ethics of research, ethics and public health, and ethics and emerging technologies. He speaks widely both in the U.S. and abroad, and has published six books, 140 articles and over 100 op-eds and commentaries. He is an elected member of the National Academy of Medicine and Fellow of the Hastings Center, and has chaired or served on policy committees for the National Institutes of Health, the Centers for Disease Control, and National Academies Sciences,

Engineering, and Medicine in the U.S., and Wellcome Trust and Royal Society internationally.

F.M. Kamm is the Henry Rutgers University Professor of Philosophy at Rutgers University and Distinguished Professor of Philosophy in the Department of Philosophy there. Kamm focuses on normative ethical theory and practical ethics in numerous articles and ten books, including *Morality, Mortality* vols. 1 and 2, *Intricate Ethics, The Trolley Problem Mysteries, Almost Over: Aging, Dying, Dead*, and most recently *Rights and Their Limits: In Theory, Cases, and Pandemics* (all from Oxford University Press). Kamm serves on the editorial board of *Philosophy & Public Affairs,* was a consultant to the WHO, and is a member of the American Academy of Arts and Sciences.

Nethanel Lipshitz is a Hecht-Levi Fellow at Johns Hopkins Berman Institute of Bioethics.

Eisuke Nakazawa, PhD, is a lecturer of Biomedical Ethics at School of Public Health, Faculty of Medicine, and the vice director of Bioethics Collaborative Research Organization, the University of Tokyo, Japan. He is also an affiliate instructor at School of Medicine, Department of Bioethics and Humanities, University of Washington. He received his doctorate in Philosophy of Science from the University of Tokyo. He has published more than 100 academic articles relating to biomedical ethics. His current research area is Biomedical Ethics, Public Health Ethics, Neuroethics and Philosophy of Science. His recent publications include Sadato N, Morita K, Kasai K, Fukushi T, Nakamura K, Nakazawa E, Okano H, Okabe S. 2019. Neuroethical issues of the Brain/MINDS project of Japan. Neuron 101:385–389; and Nakazawa E, Yamamoto K, Tachibana K, Toda S, Takimoto Y, Akabayashi A. 2016. Ethics of Decoded Neurofeedback in Clinical Research, Treatment, and Moral Enhancement. AJOB Neuroscience 7(2): 110–117.

Fabio A. G. Oliveira is Professor of Philosophy of Education at the Instituto do Noroeste Fluminense de Educação Superior, Universidade Federal Fluminense (UFF) and a Permanent Member in the Graduate Program of Bioethics, Applied Ethics and Public Health (PPGBIOS/UFF). He is also a coordinator of the Center for Environmental and Animal Ethics (LEA). Fabio has co-authored books include 'Ecofeminismos: fundamentos teóricos e praxis interseccionais' (Ape'Ku 2020) and 'Ética Animal: um novo tempo' (Ape'Ku, 2018). He was Editor and Associate Editor of the Diversitates International Journal of Medical Ethics from 2018–2022.

Kristina Orfali is a Professor of Bioethics (in Pediatrics) at Columbia University, a clinical ethicist, member of the New York- Presbyterian Morgan Stanley Children's Hospital Ethics Committee and a researcher at ISERP Columbia. K. Orfali has published numerous articles in *Social Science & Medicine, Sociology of Health & Illness, Journal of Clinical Ethics, American Journal of Bioethics, Hastings Report* and others, and co-edited several books, including *The View from Here: Bioethics and the Social Sciences* (2007), *Who is my Genetic Parent? Assisted Reproduction and Donor Anonymity: a cross- cultural perspective (2012), Families and End of Life. An international perspective (2013), The Female Body: A Journey through Law, Culture and Medicine (2014), Reproductive Technology and Changing Perceptions of Parenthood around the world (2014), Protecting the Human Body: Legal and Bioethical Perspectives around the World (2016)* and *The Reality of Human Dignity in Bioethics and Law: Comparative Perspectives (2018).*

Michael Parker is Professor of Bioethics and Director of the Ethox Centre at the University of Oxford. His main research interest is in global health bioethics. In 2012, together with colleagues in Kenya, Malawi, South Africa, Thailand, and Vietnam, he established the Global Health Bioethics Network, which conducts collaborative research on ethical questions in global health research, practice, and policy. From 2018–2020 Michael chaired a Nuffield Council on Bioethics International Working Group on the ethics of research conducted in global health emergencies. The Working Group's report was published in January 2020. From 2020 until 2022 Michael participated in the United Kingdom Government's Scientific Advisory Group on Emergencies (SAGE) and was a member of the WHO's Covid-19 Ethics and Governance Working Group.

Govind Persad is Assistant Professor at the University of Denver Sturm College of Law. He has published on ethical and legal issues related to COVID-19 in The Lancet, Science, the New England Journal of Medicine, JAMA, Annals of Internal Medicine, the Journal of Medical Ethics, and several law journals. He also has published op-eds on related topics in the New York Times, Washington Post, and elsewhere. He received the 2022 Baruch A. Brody Award in Bioethics and was a 2018–21 Greenwall Faculty Scholar in Bioethics.

Julian Savulescu was Director of the Oxford Uehiro Centre for Practical Ethics from 2002–2022 (including during the writing of this book). In August 2022, he took up the Chen Su Lan Centennial Professorship in Medical Ethics at the National University of Singapore, where he directs the Centre for Biomedical Ethics. An award-winning ethicist and moral philosopher, he trained in neuroscience, medicine, and philosophy.

He is Uehiro Chair in Practical Ethics at the University of Oxford, and co-directs the Wellcome Centre for Ethics and Humanities. He is Distinguished Visiting Professorial Fellow at Murdoch Children's Research institute and Melbourne Law School. He is a Fellow of the Australian Academy of Health and Medical Sciences and received an honorary doctorate from the University of Bucharest.

G. Owen Schaefer is an Assistant Professor at the Centre for Biomedical Ethics, Yong Loo Lin School of Medicine, National University of Singapore. He received his DPhil in Philosophy from Oxford University, and has completed fellowships at the National Institutes of Health's Department of Bioethics and the Oxford Centre for Neuroethics. His primary interests lie in the ethics of developing novel biomedical technologies. He has written on big data, research ethics, gene editing, human enhancement, precision medicine, vaccine allocation, assisted reproduction and in vitro meat.

S. Subramanian is a former Indian Council of Social Science Research National Fellow and a former professor of the Madras Institute of Development Studies. He is an elected Fellow of the Human Development and Capability Association. His research has been on measurement and other aspects of poverty, inequality, and demography, and on topics in collective choice theory, welfare economics, and development economics. His work has appeared in, among other publications, *Journal of Development Economics, Economics and Philosophy, Social Choice and Welfare, Theory and Decision, Mathematical Social Sciences*, and *Sankhya*. He is the author of *Social Values and Social Indicators* (Springer, 2021), among other books. He was a member (2015–16) of the World Bank-appointed Commission on Global Poverty.

John Tasioulas is Professor of Ethics and Legal Philosophy at the Faculty of Philosophy, University of Oxford, and Director of the Institute for Ethics in AI. He is also a Senior Research Fellow at Balliol College, Oxford. He was previously a Reader in Moral and Legal Philosophy at the University of Oxford and a Fellow of Corpus Christi College, Oxford, Quain Professor of Jurisprudence in the Faculty of Laws, University College London, and Yeoh Professor of Politics, Philosophy and Law at the Dickson Poon School of Law, King's College London. He has held visiting positions at the Australian National University, the University of Chicago, Harvard University, and the University of Melbourne. His writings focus on philosophical issues regarding punishment, human rights, international law, and artificial intelligence. He is the co-editor of *The Philosophy of International Law* (Oxford: Oxford University Press, 2010) and the editor of *The Cambridge Companion to the Philosophy of Law* (Cambridge: Cambridge University Press, 2020).

Rémi Turquier is a graduate student at Paris School of Economics and Ensae Paris. They have interned at the Swiss Tropical and Public Health institute, where they worked with a team of malaria modellers. Rémi also completed a traineeship at the European central bank. Their research focuses on global catastrophic risks like pandemics, and on the economics of the long term future more broadly.

Alex Voorhoeve is Professor and Head of Department of Philosophy, Logic and Scientific Method at the LSE. He studied economics and philosophy at Erasmus University, Cambridge University, and UCL and has held visiting positions at Harvard (2008–09), Princeton (2012–13), the National Institutes of Health, U.S. (2016–17) and Erasmus University Rotterdam (2017–21). He works on the theory and practice of distributive justice (especially as it relates to health), on rational choice theory, moral psychology and Epicureanism. He has acted as a consultant on justice in health to the World Health Organization, co-authoring its influential report *Making Fair Choices on the Path to Universal Health Coverage*. He is also a contributor to a forthcoming report by the World Bank and the Norwegian Institute of Public Health *Open and Inclusive: Fair Processes for Financing Universal Health Coverage*.

Dominic Wilkinson is Professor of Medical Ethics and Deputy Director of the Oxford Uehiro Centre for Practical Ethics, University of Oxford, a senior research fellow at Jesus College, Oxford and a consultant in newborn intensive care. Dominic has published more than 220 academic articles relating to ethical issues in intensive care for adults, children and newborn infants. Co-authored books include 'Medical Ethics and Law, third edition' (Elsevier 2019) and 'Ethics, Conflict and Medical treatment for children, from disagreement to dissensus' (Elsevier, 2018). He is also the author of 'Death or Disability? The 'Carmentis Machine' and decision-making for critically ill children' (Oxford University Press 2013). He was Editor and Associate Editor of the Journal of Medical Ethics from 2011–2018.

Introduction

The first reports of an undiagnosed severe respiratory illness in people working in or attending a street market in South East Asia attracted little international public attention. They caused barely a ripple amid the maelstrom of competing voices in mainstream and social media. The reports were read or shared by few, and the busy global news cycle rapidly moved on. After all, such reports have occurred many times before, and usually do not lead to anything. Comments by local public health officials were reassuring—investigations were underway, but they did not believe that there was any cause for alarm.

But the reports were noted by several international groups tasked with detecting and responding to possible pandemic threats. They were catalogued and classified by an automated early warning system, setting in motion preliminary steps to investigate the cause of the outbreak and assess the potential for wider spread. Real-time data from local hospital facilities, including the numbers of cases presenting, their clinical features, severity of illness, and apparent connections to the index cases were openly shared as part of a national and international surveillance network. International experts provided remote support for investigations into the organism causing the outbreak, including rapid genetic sequencing of the virus that had been obtained from some of those who were unwell. At the same time, automated monitoring of local social media accounts flagged the possibility of a wider group of patients with potential prodromal symptoms.

By the time results confirmed that this was a new variant of H7N9 avian influenza with human-to-human spread (bird flu), several pre-existing plans had been put in place. Stringent travel restrictions were implemented in the region of northern Thailand where the cases had been reported. Cross-border travel including most flights from regional and national airports were suspended. As previously rehearsed and planned, a snap lockdown was instituted in affected cities along with careful, thorough explanation to the community of the situation and rationale for the response. But there was also immediate release of a package of international financial support to Thailand to support the affected communities and work sectors. Medical and food supplies were released from regional stockpiles. Hospitals in Thailand implemented the first stages of triage plans to care for any affected patients as well as to prioritize access to intensive care. There was limited data initially to help identify which patients might be most likely to survive, but data from the first patients treated indicated that the virus had a high mortality among patients in

Introduction In: *Pandemic Ethics: From COVID-19 to Disease X.* Edited by: Dominic Wilkinson and Julian Savulescu, Oxford University Press. © Dominic Wilkinson and Julian Savulescu 2023. DOI: 10.1093/oso/9780192871688.003.0001

their early twenties without pre-existing illness. These results were fed into a national emergency triage plan that had been developed with input from national and international ethicists, community leaders, and the wider public. It was automatically enacted once the severity of the outbreak was recognized. At the same time, early experience was fed into the corresponding (but variable) triage plans that were in place internationally in the event that the outbreak spread further. mRNA vaccine hubs in Bangkok and in Vietnam had already started work on modified vaccines for the new strain of the virus. As part of an international agreement, vaccine trials and early access to the vaccine would prioritize regions with greatest disadvantage and highest rates of circulating virus.

In the event, the 2027 avian influenza epidemic remained largely confined to northern Thai cities. Variable lockdowns and travel restrictions remained in place for much of the next twelve months, while other cities in the region and elsewhere imposed brief snap lockdowns in response to cases of possible spread (but which fortunately turned out not to be). A generous package of support and investment meant that the Thai economy was not negatively affected overall, while individuals disadvantaged by the infection (or the response) were able to access compensation. The Thai government received high levels of political support nationally and internationally for their rapid proportionate response together with their commitment to transparent communication with the population. When the vaccine became available, priority access for Thailand and a rapid dissemination program meant that the Thai community had high levels of vaccination by mid 2028.

Pandemic experts around the world breathed a sigh of relief. It might have been so different…

The above fictional vision of a coordinated, carefully planned and executed, national and international response to a future deadly epidemic might appear frankly utopian, but it is clear from our recent experience that there are good and less good ways that we might respond to such a future threat.

The COVID-19 pandemic has been a defining event of the twenty-first century. Global estimates of excess mortality indicate that it has taken 15 million lives over 2020–1 (Knutson et al. 2022).[1] It has closed national borders, put whole populations into quarantine, and devastated economies. Almost half of workers in low or middle income countries lost a job or business due to the pandemic (Anonymous 2021).[2] The International Monetary Fund has estimated a global loss to the world economy of US$12 trillion by the end of 2021 (Bill and Melinda Gates Foundation 2020).[3] It led to a rise in rates of extreme poverty for the first

---

[1] Knutson, Victoria, et al. (2022), 'Estimating Global and Country-Specific Excess Mortality During the COVID-19 Pandemic', *arXiv e-print*, https://arxiv.org/abs/2205.09081.

[2] Anonymous (2021), 'Wellcome Global Monitor 2020: Covid-19' (updated 29 Nov. 2021), https://wellcome.org/reports/wellcome-global-monitor-covid-19/2020 (accessed 21 July 2022).

[3] Bill and Melinda Gates Foundation (2020), '2020 Goalkeepers Report: COVID-19 A global perspective' (updated September 2020), https://www.gatesfoundation.org/goalkeepers/report/2020-report/#GlobalPerspective (accessed 21 July 2022).

time in twenty-five years, with 37 million additional people experiencing this in 2020. The pandemic toll and the cost of measures taken to combat it—both effective and ineffective—have been paid in human lives, mental and physical suffering, and economic hardship. The costs will continue to be paid by individuals and societies for decades to come.

While the COVID-19 pandemic has been catastrophic, it is not unique. It is not as severe as Spanish influenza, estimated to have killed between 50 million and 100 million people. Recent MERS and SARS epidemics were more deadly to those infected, but less contagious. Future influenza pandemics, perhaps like the hypothetical example above, undoubtedly lie ahead. We await 'Disease X', the World Health Organization's placeholder name for "a serious international epidemic...caused by a pathogen currently unknown to cause human disease". In some ways, the COVID-19 pandemic has been a wake-up call. Children who have been home-schooled during the COVID pandemic will almost certainly face another pandemic in their lifetime—one at least as bad—and potentially much worse—than this one.

Responding to current or future pandemics requires action based on unresolved, fundamental, and controversial ethical issues. The defining feature of a pandemic is its scale—the simultaneous threat to millions or even billions of lives. That scale creates and necessitates awful choices since the wellbeing and lives of all cannot be simultaneously protected.

I.1 Choices

From allocating limited supplies of ventilators, treatments, vaccines, or personal protective equipment to policies of restricting movement and freedom, whose needs should be prioritized when not all can be? What ethical principle or principles should we use to make these decisions? Should society save the greatest number or use some other ethical approach?

Choices and trade-offs need to be made between those at higher risk and lower risk of becoming unwell. In the COVID pandemic, a key question has been about whether (and, if so, how much) it is acceptable to sacrifice the wellbeing of younger members of the community (i.e. children and young adults) for the sake of older, more medically vulnerable members. To frame the same question in the opposite way: how many premature deaths of older members of society would be acceptable to allow younger individuals to go about their normal lives? Future pandemics may have similar characteristics to COVID, or may (like the Spanish flu and the hypothetical Thai epidemic) be worse in the young, which may lead to different decisions.

In the face of extremely high demand, choices need to be made between patients who are already unwell. For example, that has led to questions about triage or prioritization decisions when there are more patients with severe COVID who need ventilators or admission to intensive care than there is available capacity. But there are also difficult choices between patients with pandemic-related illness and other non-pandemic health needs. And, of course, there are choices between resources, energy, and attention devoted to healthcare, and other needs in society (for example, education, policing, social welfare, and justice). These raise questions about what matters most, but also about commensurability—how (and whether) to compare different priorities.

There are also difficult questions about how to respond to the needs of people in different countries. That raises important issues of partiality and how much it is justified to prioritize the needs of those who are within one's own community over the needs of those living elsewhere. Some degree of partiality towards those who are close to us seems important. But the extreme national partiality adopted by some countries in the COVID pandemic is hard to ethically reconcile.

The difficult nature of these choices can lead to several tempting, but ultimately mistaken, responses. One such mistake is to attempt to avoid choosing. For example, many countries tried in the COVID pandemic to avoid having to make difficult triage decisions by rapidly expanding intensive care capacity through purchasing additional equipment, building field hospitals, etc. However, this strategy doesn't avoid difficult choices; it just displaces the impact. For example, in the UK, surgery and many forms of medical treatment were suspended in order to redirect resources to treatment of COVID patients. That led to harm to other patients, for example those who had delayed diagnosis or treatment for their cancer, and a massive ballooning of treatment waiting lists. Where additional resources were purchased, that has often required very considerable increases in national debt. That then displaces the harm onto future members of society, who will have to bear those costs in the form of increased taxation, reduced availability of services (or likely both). The mistake here is not the decisions themselves. They may have been the right ones (though not all agree on this). Rather, the mistake is to pretend that choices do not need to be made. Clearly choices *have* been made—often priori-tizing visible, immediate needs over the needs of other less visible individuals.

Another avoidance strategy is to conflate questions of relative benefit with absolute benefit. Where treatments are withheld in the setting of limited resources, it is sometimes claimed that the treatment would not work. On that basis, some elderly patients were not transferred to hospitals, masks were not recommended (at early stages), or vaccines were said to not be indicated for some groups. It is easier for health professionals or health systems to withhold a treat-ment on the grounds that it would be ineffective than to explain that another patient or individual needs the treatment more. But such a communication strat-egy obscures the value-based choices that underlie decisions and may threaten public trust in public health communication as well as prevent important debate.

A third strategy tries to avoid value judgements or choices by resorting to the fig leaf of scientific evidence. In the COVID pandemic, political leaders claimed to be "following the science". To be clear, the claim is not that science is not helpful in responding to a pandemic. On the contrary, it is absolutely vital to both gather and appraise scientific evidence to inform decisions. However, that evidence does not make decisions. For one thing, the nature of pandemics is that they always reflect novel infectious agents. (It is the absence of pre-existing immunity that gives them the potential to spread across the world and infect millions within a short space of time.) That means that there will always be a lag between the onset of a pandemic and evidence emerging about the best ways to respond to it. Although the COVID pandemic saw a completely unprecedented level of dedicated research effort (with more than 100,000 published articles by the end of 2020) (Else 2020),[4] much evidence emerged only after the initial waves had already passed. Especially in the initial phases of a pandemic (when rapid responses may be vital to minimize the total impact), there will always be significant uncertainty about the impact of different choices. We will need ethics to make decisions in the face of uncertainty. For example, when a new possible threat arises, as in the case example above, policymakers will need to decide whether to take pre-emptive actions (that might prove to be unnecessary), or risk responding too late to prevent wider spread of the pathogen. But importantly, even when there is good scientific evidence available, there is a need for value judgements to make decisions about which strategy to pursue.

Science alone can never tell us what we should do. It can tell us how to achieve a goal, but not what that goal should be. Decisions require not merely evidence but values. The identification and weighing of values are ethical tasks. For example, through the pandemic the public were presented with COVID death counts, or strictly deaths associated with COVID. The goal was to reduce COVID deaths. But that is only one value. It ignores the deaths or impacts on wellbeing of those who don't have COVID. In the UK, vaccines were rolled out to the oldest first, starting with those aged 90–100. This places a value equally on all lives, regardless of age. However, many people believe that younger lives should have priority over older lives. The outcome of the pandemic could have been in terms of years of life lost, or quality-adjusted life years (QALYs) lost. China chose to prioritize its working population for vaccination. These all illustrate different values. It is the job of ethics, not science, to adjudicate between competing values.

I.2 Freedom

Next, our response to pandemics intersects with some fundamental questions about basic human rights and liberties. That is because infectious diseases spread when humans interact. Our most powerful ways to diminish or stop the spread of

---

[4] Else, Holly (2020), 'How a torrent of COVID science changed research publishing—in seven charts', *Nature*, 588/7839: 553–4.

infections involve measures that reduce or stop human interactions. This was recognized in the fourteenth century when ships arriving in European ports were required to remain offshore for a period of forty days (from which derives the English term "quarantine") to reduce the risk of bringing plague ashore. But, of course, such measures have the obvious potential to conflict with individuals' freedom to move, to associate, and to go about their lives as they would otherwise wish to.

The vital question is how much restriction of liberty is justified in order to prevent transmission of infections. This might include those confirmed or suspected to have a pandemic infection. Yet it may be impossible to identify people carrying the infection in the early phases. (The most successful pandemic agents typically have a prodromal stage in which patients are infectious but unaware of this and thus do not know to modify their behaviour.) So potential measures to stop pandemic spread will often include many individuals who do not actually carry the infection, but are at risk of doing so.

One mistaken response to this problem is to assume that the benefits of preventing transmission can be achieved through voluntary measures. For example, some claim that equivalent effects on spread of COVID-19 could be achieved without mask mandates, work-from-home orders, or restrictions on social gathering. But it seems fairly indisputable that voluntary measures, in most circumstances, have a smaller impact on interactions and spread of infections than compulsory ones. In general, during the COVID-19 pandemic, those jurisdictions that imposed the fastest, most stringent restrictions on movement and travel had the greatest success in curtailing spread of the virus (at least in the early stages). That does not necessarily mean that these were the better options. It means that in a pandemic individual liberties have a price. The ethical question is how much of a price we are willing to pay to preserve liberties (or, to put it the other way, how many liberties we are willing to suspend in order to allay a pandemic threat).

Questions of individual liberty versus containing spread of a pandemic arise in a different way once vaccines become available. Then (as discussed in a number of chapters in this volume), individuals' freedom to decline a vaccine potentially comes into conflict with the good of controlling the contagion and permitting life to return to normal. During the COVID-19 pandemic, in debate about vaccines but also in many other issues, a further liberty became highly relevant—freedom of speech. That was because of the large amount of incorrect and misleading information being disseminated about the pandemic, pandemic responses, and choices. Such misinformation is enormously damaging to society's ability to gather and maintain support for appropriate responses to the pandemic. Once again, there are important questions to be asked about how to balance individuals' right to reach opinions and express their own views against the greater good. If there is acceptance that, in an emergency like a pandemic, some of our usual liberties may be permissibly curtailed, the question then becomes—by how much, and for how long?

I.3 Equality

Finally, pandemic ethics brings emerging ethical debates about the structure of society, its inequalities, and our experiences as groups to the foreground:

It is sometimes suggested that death is the great equalizer, since it befalls alike "the righteous and the wicked,…the good and the bad,…the clean and the unclean" (Ecclesiastes 9:2). Viruses do not respect national or class boundaries. However, while all are potentially susceptible to a new infectious threat, it does not follow that all are equally susceptible, nor (more importantly) do all have access to equal means to mitigate that threat. It has been abundantly clear that the experience of the COVID-19 pandemic has not been the same for all.

The pressure of the pandemic has pressed on society's weaknesses, turning cracks into fissures. Where inequalities exist, the pandemic has exacerbated them with deeply unequal distribution of both disease harms and lockdown burdens across different groups in society.

Within societies, some groups have been more vulnerable to serious complications of COVID-19 because of pre-existing medical illness or older age. Others (for example, healthcare workers, aged-care workers, police officers, teachers) have had high rates of infection related to their work. Still others have been at higher risk of infection or of critical illness and death because of belonging to certain socio-economic and racial groups. The cause of this risk is multifactorial, but it includes factors relating to underlying medical conditions (e.g. diabetes), type of work, household and living environment (e.g. living in large multigenerational households). It is also affected by access to healthcare, including measures to prevent transmission, and (at least in some places) by systematic or institutional discrimination.

Measures to respond to the pandemic have also fallen unequally. Some have been able to work from home throughout the pandemic. Others have had to continue to leave home to work (often thereby being exposed to the virus), or have lost their jobs. Some children and young people have had access to resources to facilitate online learning. Others (particularly from the most disadvantaged backgrounds) have missed out on essential periods of learning and will never catch up.

Despite the importance of equality, the solution cannot be simply to treat everyone equally. That is because it is impossible in a pandemic to provide the same treatment at the same time to all who might benefit. Second, strictly equal treatment creates unequal outcomes when people differ in their underlying health and health needs. We should potentially focus more on *equity of outcome* than equality of treatment. However, we must also recognize that strict equity is also going to be impossible. Whatever we do, some people are going to become seriously ill, while others will have only mild illness; some will live, while others will die. Some children will graduate from school with high marks, others with low. Third, as some of the chapters in this volume discuss, the value of equality/equity is only one of the ethical values that might underpin a pandemic response, and these principles often conflict. As noted above, choices will be inevitable. Fourth, responding in a way that is sensitive to social and other inequalities can be much more complicated and costly than a uniform approach. That will mean that some parts of the world find it easier or much harder to adopt this approach.

Inequality has been even more evident on a global scale. Some countries have fared much better than others. That has arisen partly as a function of geography. For example, some island countries have found it much easier to isolate their population. It has partly related to population differences (for example, in how closely people are living and in the age distribution). It has also arisen as a consequence of domestic political decision-making, meaning that some countries that were deemed prior to the pandemic to be well prepared for a global outbreak have fared extremely badly. But, as exemplified by the global distribution of vaccines, inequality in pre-existing resources and political power has led to enormous disparity in the ability of populations to access effective means of preventing infection. It is all too clear that the dissemination of key resources in a pandemic cannot be left to the free market. However, equally it is clear that existing international institutions (that in theory were supposed to be able to coordinate global responses such as vaccines) were not capable of overriding the competitive and self-protective instincts that drove wealthy countries to arrange unilateral vaccine deals. Pandemics (like other global threats such as climate change and antibiotic resistance) pose collective action problems that require careful coordinated solutions.

I.4 Pandemic X

The experience of COVID-19 means that medicine, epidemiology, and public health will potentially be better placed to face Disease X. This volume addresses the ethical and social lessons of the current pandemic. What lessons can we learn from the COVID-19 pandemic to prepare for future pandemics?

The international authors in this volume provide a range of different suggestions for such a future response. Here are some highlights:

In the first chapter, Larry Gostin suggests ways to make the response to Pandemic X more globally solidaristic: this might use versions of programmes that already exist (for example COVAX), but considerably strengthened, globally distributed, and resourced in advance. Other suggestions include new global pandemic treaties to support robust early detection programmes as well as financial support to facilitate pandemic responses. It will be important for responses internationally and nationally to be ethically transparent in order to engender and maintain public trust. Allen Buchanan echoes this call, arguing that global institutions need to be reconfigured (or ideally a new one created) to enshrine and enforce a 'duty to rescue' on countries—so that wealthy countries do not resile from their obligations and resort to extreme national partiality in the face of a future pandemic threat. John Tasioulas argues for a more fundamental conceptual shift—suggesting that clarifying the scope and content of human rights is vital for ethical debate and discourse in pandemics. He also notes (highly relevant given some of the responses to COVID-19) the relationship between political structures and human rights in a pandemic.

In Part II, authors examine some of the challenges of conflicts between rights and public health in a pandemic. Jennifer Blumenthal-Barby, Jessica Flanigan, and Frances Kamm, in their respective chapters, examine public debates relating to individual freedoms, harms, and choices in a pandemic. Blumenthal-Barby identifies some complexities in the arguments used to support vaccine mandates, and ways that they need to be more nuanced for Pandemic X. Flanigan is critical of the resort to prohibitions such as mandates and lockdowns for the sake of public health in pandemics. She suggests that there should be a presumption against such policies in future pandemics. Kamm, from an opposite perspective, dissects the libertarian arguments against social distancing, mask wearing, and vaccine requirements. She suggests that clear understanding of the nature of contagious threats would recast individual responsibilities in a pandemic—and mean that libertarians *should support* rather than oppose these various measures. One important question for future pandemics will be whether responses should be uniform or different for different groups. Govind Persad and Ezekiel Emanuel compare some debates in relation to public health policies during the COVID-19 pandemic to the mythological story of Procrustes. (According to the story, the figure of Procrustes attempted to fit travellers to a single-size bed [by either stretching them or cutting them to size].) They argue that the principle of the 'least restrictive alternative' means that, in future pandemics, even if universal restrictions (e.g. masks/social distancing) are initially justified, they should be selectively eased for members of the population who no longer pose a risk of transmitting the virus or overwhelming the health system. One of the editors of this volume (Julian Savulescu) extends this argument by providing a principled ethical rationale for unequal liberty restrictions in a pandemic. He argues that a dualist consequentialist approach (incorporating both equality along with utility) could provide a basis for deciding when lockdowns or other measures should apply to all or only part of the community.

The importance of developing sophisticated ethical approaches for future pandemics is taken up in Part III of the volume. Matthew Adler and colleagues examine the prospect for using a novel social welfare function as a way of quantifying the impact of different policy options and mathematically combining some of the competing ethical values. They illustrate the importance of modelling for identifying which policies are likely to be optimal (e.g. minimizing economic costs and maximizing welfare) and which values are most important to clarify. In Chapter 10, one of the editors (Dominic Wilkinson) also defends a pluralist ethical approach. He points out that conflicts between values are more of a problem for some choices and dilemmas than for others. At least in the coronavirus pandemic, vaccine allocation posed a simpler ethical choice since different principles potentially converged on similar policies (prioritizing the elderly and medically vulnerable). In other policy areas, there may not be a single correct way of reconciling conflicting ethical values, meaning that we should expect (and not regret) some differences in international approaches. Owen Schaefer examines one such challenge—how to distribute doses of vaccines between countries. He proposes a hybrid model that attempts to combine elements of a population-proportionate (egalitarian) model with one based on needs. Although he is motivated primarily by uncertainty in needs estimation, such a hybrid approach could also give some ethical weight to the value of equal access. Christina Orfali, in Chapter 12, examines a controversial question from early in the COVID-19 pandemic: she highlights the mixed experience of developing and implementing triage guidelines in the US and Europe. Whichever approach is taken to these difficult decisions for future pandemics, there are important lessons from COVID for how triage policies can be made transparent and accountable, and how public trust may be promoted.

As noted earlier in this Introduction, pandemics can deepen social inequality and injustice. Michael Parker points out one important element that is relevant even before the next pandemic arrives. The burden and potential harms of surveillance and pandemic early detection programmes (like those that detected the avian influenza outbreak in our example) will likely fall on some of the globe's most disadvantaged communities. There will need to be attention (and resources) devoted to meeting the world's obligations to those communities. Several authors catalogue and draw lessons from the unequal experiences of the COVID-19 pandemic. Sreenivasan Subramanian argues that preparation for pandemics needs to pay attention to basic needs of the population—nutrition, health, and education. Those states in India that had strong social safety nets fared much better in responding to the COVID-19 pandemic. Political responses to the pandemic should resist the temptation to go 'big'—e.g. draconian policies that look impressive. Simultaneously, they must pay attention to the small—to the needs of those who might otherwise be 'invisible'—the marginalized and poor. Clara Dias and Fabio Oliveira highlight the disproportionate impact of the pandemic on those with pre-existing disadvantage. This within-nation social inequality intersects with factors that mark and manifest disadvantage—gender, sexuality, race, and poverty. They provocatively argue that one of the most important steps that societies might take in preparation for the next pandemic is not directly pandemic-related at all—it is to recognize, take seriously, and urgently address structural injustice. But problems of inequality in a pandemic are not confined to low and middle income countries. Nakazawa and Akabayashi explore the unequal impacts of the pandemic in Japan. They suggest that future pandemic responses need to pay attention to those most vulnerable, not just to the infection, but also to the measures used to stop its spread, for example those suffering severe social isolation in a lockdown.

Finally, Lipshitz, Kahn, and Faden draw together some of the common strands of the volume. There are different voices included in this book, and areas of reasonable disagreement. But there are also important areas of consensus. Lipshitz and colleagues also highlight some areas that are crucial for thinking about future Pandemic X, but which do not feature prominently in this work—including the challenge to democracy posed by public health crises, public health governance, and the interests of children.

What will our response to Pandemic X look like? Some of the suggestions arising from this volume are included in the hypothetical avian influenza epidemic that begins this Introduction. But is it realistic to think that we could (within five years) get to a position where we could respond to an outbreak of novel influenza or some other pathogen in such a coordinated, calibrated, and sophisticated way? There are some reasons to be optimistic. Our recent experience has identified success stories as well as challenges. We have a reasonably clear idea of what we need to do differently for Pandemic X. The proposals summarized above and described in more detail throughout this book are achievable. Some people (you, for example) are interested enough in these problems to pick this volume up and engage seriously with these questions.

On the other hand, in a workshop that included most of the authors of this volume, our Japanese contributors noted the experience of severe earthquakes in Japan (for example, the severe Tohoku earthquake in Fukushima in 2011, and the Great Hanshin earthquake near Kobe in 1995). Although such earthquakes have occurred multiple times in modern history, when they occur anew, lessons appear not to have been learned. Our contributors attributed this to factors that may be relevant for thinking about Pandemic X. First, collective memories of tragic events (earthquakes, pandemics) fade with time, meaning that attention and motivation diminish if there is a long gap between events. We may be better off in some ways if the next pandemic threat arises in 2027 than if it does not come until 2047 (though, for purely selfish reasons, most readers, we suspect, would share our own preference for the latter!). Second, preparation for future disasters requires significant resources. It can be difficult to attain and maintain sufficient commitment to this when the timing and magnitude of future disasters is unknown. Third, when future outbreaks occur, they are likely to be different in important ways from those that occurred previously. Some of the responses that were important for COVID-19, and some of the lessons, may not be relevant or apply straightforwardly to the next pandemic when it comes.

So we must not underestimate the challenge we face. Pandemic X will test us, in ways that we can predict and in ways that we cannot. Moreover, preparing for Pandemic X will cost us. There will be things that we will have to forego to invest in the things that we need—whether those are equipment or food stockpiles, early detection systems, policies and processes for decision-making, global treaties, or institutional reform. But at least some of these will have spin-off benefits that will be valuable for our communities, even if the next pandemic does not arrive for fifty or a hundred years. Investing in our healthcare systems, addressing socio-economic disadvantage and inequality, and building global capacities in vaccine production (as well as global understanding of vaccination) are important general-purpose social goods. Developing ethical frameworks for public health interventions and resource allocation (drawing on engagement with the wider community as well as rigorous ethical analysis) will help us to be ready for other non-pandemic health crises that we are likely to face. Finally, if we can recognize that pandemics pose a globally shared problem and existential risk, if we can come together to develop pandemic treaties and collective response plans, that may help us to address some of the other great existential risks and collective problems of our age.

One element of preparation for Pandemic X is not necessarily highly costly. As the rest of this volume makes clear, ethical analysis, ethical reflection, and ethic-ally informed decision-making are vitally important to pandemic response. We need to take advantage of our recent experience and learn from the lessons of the COVID pandemic. In advance of another crisis, we need to publicly discuss and debate the values and the approaches that we should use, identifying what we are willing to sacrifice, and what we should prioritize. We need to educate our policy makers to recognize the ethical dimensions of their decisions, and build into our policymaking institutions expertise that can provide critical and constructive ethical advice.

We ignore these challenges, and these preparations, at our peril.

Dominic Wilkinson and Julian Savulescu

PART I

GLOBAL RESPONSE TO THE PANDEMIC

1

The Great Coronavirus Pandemic

An Unparalleled Collapse in Global Solidarity

Larry Gostin

The COVID-19 pandemic precipitated an unparalleled collapse in global solidarity at a crucial moment in human history when international cooperation was most needed. A novel coronavirus originating in Wuhan, China, exposed the world's shared vulnerability and deep interconnectedness (UNGA 2021a). As the virus devastated the globe in waves, it reminded us that no country acting alone can effectively respond to pandemic threats in a globalized world (Gostin et al. 2020a).

By virtually every measure, global solidarity failed—from nationalist leaders fuelling distrust in science to a weakened World Health Organization (WHO) and shockingly inequitable global distribution of life-saving medical resources. Even the most basic global health functions failed, including reporting of the initial Wuhan outbreak, ascertaining the origins of that outbreak, and complying with binding legal norms. Stepping back, the only constant was the gravitation to a "my nation first" mentality—the exact opposite of the global cooperation and coordination needed for an effective response.

This chapter describes important areas in which global health solidarity failed, with a timeline of pivotal events (Figure 1.1), the reasons for those failures, and reforms to advance global cooperation, mutual responsibilities, and equitable responses when the next novel outbreak occurs. Before exploring the multiple failures of international cooperation, I will briefly explain what I mean by solidarity, and why it matters.

1.1 Norms of Solidarity

Global solidarity aims to foster common understandings, shared values, and collaborative action in addressing global threats, irrespective of self- or national interests. Solidarity encourages mutual support within the community of nations, in recognition that we are all human beings with a shared responsibility toward one another. Key actors see themselves engaged in a common project to reduce overall harms, including preventing illness, saving lives, and maximizing wellbeing everywhere. Global solidarity requires more than international

Larry Gostin, *The Great Coronavirus Pandemic: An Unparalleled Collapse in Global Solidarity* In: *Pandemic Ethics: From COVID-19 to Disease X*. Edited by: Dominic Wilkinson and Julian Savulescu, Oxford University Press.
© Oxford University Press 2023. DOI: 10.1093/oso/9780192871688.003.0002

12/08/19 - First case of SARS-like illness, later confirmed as COVID-19, becomes ill.

12/26/19 - Chinese lab identifies SARS-like virus in samples.

12/30/19- Scientists report genome sequencing results as "highly suspicious of SARS". Dr. Li Wenliang notifies colleagues of SARS-like illness. Wuhan Municipal Health Commission issues an urgent notice to hospitals about cases linked to Huanan Market.

12/31/19- WHO becomes aware of novel pneumonia circulating in Wuhan via ProMED. WHO China Country Office notifies WPRO IHR Focal Point of Wuhan Municipal Health Commission bulletin, noting no IHR notification has been issued.

01 /01 /20 - Doctors questioned by Wuhan police. Huanan Market closes. WPRO IHR Focal Point requests information about cluster from Chinese National Focal Point. WHO asks Chinese National Health Commssion for information. WHO asks WPRO for verification.

01 /02/20 - WHO and GOARN hold teleconference, China CDC does not join. WHO urges National Health Commission and IHR National Focal Point to respond to information requests. Wuhan Institute of Virology decodes majority of virus genomic sequence.

01/03/20 - WPRO requests information from Chinese National Focal Point who confirms information issued by Wuhan Municipal Health Commission. Chinese officials confirm cluster of "viral pneumonia of unknown cause."

01/04/20 - WHO WPRO and WHO HQ tweet that China has reported a cluster of pneumonia cases in Wuhan with investigations underway.

01/05/20 - WHO reports 44 cases via Disease Outbreak News to Member States, states that there is "no evidence of significant human-to-human transmission" and advises countries to take precautions to reduce the risk of acute respiratory infections.

01 /07/20 - China CDC successfully isolates the first novel coronavirus strain.

01 /09/20 - WHO announces that China has identified a new coronavirus in Wuhan.

01 /11/20 - Chinese researchers publish a draft genome of the coronavirus on GenBank.

01/14/20 - WHO tweets: "Preliminary investigations conducted by the Chinese authorities have no clear evidence of human-to-human transmission of the novel coronavirus (2019-nCoV) identified in Wuhan, China".

01/21/20 - WPRO tweets "It is now very clear from the latest information that there is at least some human-to-human transmission of #nCoV2019. Infections among health care workers strengthen the evidence for this."

01/22/20 - WHO's mission in Wuhan reports evidence of community transmission, but notes "more investigation was needed." WHO IHR Emergency Committee holds first meeting on COVID-19. WHO reports 314 cases: 310 in China, 4 in 3 countries outside China.

01 /23/20 - WHO IHR Emergency Committee does not recommend COVID-19 outbreak be declared a PHEIC but urges countries to prepare for further spread. WHO reports 581 cases: 571 in China, 10 in 4 countries outside China. Wuhan inititiates a lockdown.

01 /29/20 - WHO DG extolls China's transparency, calling it "a model."

01/30/20 - WHO DG reconvenes IHR Emergency Committee. The DG declares a PHEIC. WHO reports 7,834 cases.

Figure 1.1 Timeline of the COVID-19 pandemic.

cooperation, charitable donations, and humanitarian assistance. It extends to equal partnerships and equitable sharing of benefits and burdens. Solidarity matters not only because it benefits lower-income nations and populations but also because it improves health outcomes worldwide.

National sovereignty and self-interest are often in tension with solidarity, as governments maximize domestic benefits, irrespective of harms imposed elsewhere. Sovereign leaders act primarily for the benefit of their own citizens—for example, hoarding medical resources, refusing to share scientific knowledge, and

02/07/20 - Dr. Li Wenliang dies from COVID-19.

03/03/20 - WHO calls on medical supplies manufacturers to ramp up production by 40%. WHO warns of global PPE shortages caused by "buying, hoarding, and misuse" leading to extreme price gouging.

03/11/20- WHO DG announces that COVID-19 is a pandemic.

04/03/20 - UN General Assembly resolution calls upon UN system to mobilize a coordinated global response to the pandemic and its social and economic impact.

04/14/20 - President Trump announces that the US will suspend funding for WHO.

05/18/20- 73rd World Health Assembly begins, with de minimus sessions held remotely May, 18- 19, 2020, resuming on November, 9- 14, 2020.

07/01/20 - UN Security Council adopts a resolution calling for a global ceasefire so the world can focus on fighting COVID-19.

07/02/20 - 239 scientists from 32 countries publish an open letter to WHO, citing evidence that smaller airborne particles could infect people with SARS-CoV-2.

09/11 /20- UN General Assembly resolution on COVID-19 calls for coordinated Member State action to contain, mitigate and overcome the pandemic and its consequences.

09/18/20 - CDC updates its guidelines to say that SARS-CoV-2 could be transmitted via aerosolized airborne particles. However, CDC removes that recommendation from its website, days later, on September 21, 2020.

01/01 /21 - China allows a WHO team of scientists to enter its sovereign territory to investigate the virus' origins.

01/20/21 - President Biden, on his first day in office, withdraws the US' intention to withdraw from WHO.

02/26/21 - UN Security Council resolution calls for, among other demands, unhindered humanitarian access to enable COVID-19 vaccination.

02/28/21 - WHO-China Global Study releases its joint report.

05/04/21 - WHO describes aerosolized transmission as a major risk.

05/14/21 - 18 European and North American scientists urge for a deeper investigation to as certain origins of SARS-CoV-2.

05/21/21 - The IPPPR releases its landmark report: "COVID-19: Make it the Last Pandemic."

05/26/21 - President Biden orders a full intelligence review of SARS-CoV-2 proximal origins.

08/24/21 - US intelligence releases a report stating it could not conclusively determine whether a natural zoonosis or laboratory leak was most probable for the source of COVID-19.

Figure 1.1 Continued.

closing borders. Yet global solidarity could reduce domestic harms by curbing threats elsewhere. More equitable vaccine allocation could help prevent viral mutations resulting in dangerous variants reseeding outbreaks anywhere. But powerful nations believe (with considerable historical support) that they can accrue more domestic health protection from self-interested nationalism than through altruistic globalism. And it is precisely for that reason that it is so hard to nurture a sense of mutual obligation. Next, I discuss critical failures of solidarity during the COVID-19 pandemic.

1.2 The International Health Regulations: Fracturing of the Global Instrument to Govern Pandemic Response

The International Health Regulations (IHR) were substantially reformed in 2005 in the aftermath of global failures in the SARS response. The IHR govern pandemic detection and response. With a remarkable 196 states parties, the IHR have near universal support in theory, but COVID-19 revealed a starkly different reality, as nations widely violated the Regulations' binding norms (WHO 2016). As a result of the IHR's failures during the global COVID-19 response, the World Health Assembly is considering targeted amendments to the Regulations, first proposed by the United States. The Assembly also created an Intergovernmental Negotiating Body (INB) to negotiate a new international pandemic instrument, often called a "Pandemic Treaty" (Gostin et al. 2021a).

1.2.1 Core Health System Capacities

The IHR require all states to build core health system capacities to detect, assess, notify, and report novel pathogen outbreaks, and respond to public health risks—including laboratories, surveillance, risk communication, and human resources (WHO 2016: IHR (2005) Art. 5, 13, Annex 1). Through national self-assessment, most countries reported that they had not attained required IHR health capacities. Moreover, the IHR require states parties to collaborate in ensuring robust health systems, including funding, technical assistance, and logistical support (WHO 2016: IHR (2005) Art. 44.1). However, the Independent Panel for Pandemic Preparedness and Response (IPPPR) found that national governments lacked effective preparedness plans and core public health capacities (IPPPR 2021: 18).

1.2.2 China's Delays in Reporting a Novel Coronavirus Outbreak

No IHR requirement is more basic than states' duties to report a novel outbreak to WHO within twenty-four hours, honestly and accurately. China, however, did anything but. Credible reports suggest that a novel SARS-like respiratory virus was circulating in Wuhan by mid to late December 2019, if not much earlier (Singh et al. 2021).

China did not just fail to report that outbreak to WHO promptly; it never reported it. The WHO first became aware of novel viral pneumonia circulating in Wuhan on December 31, 2019, using "unofficial" sources, including posts on the Wuhan Municipal Health Commission's website and on ProMED, a public global surveillance system (WHO 2021a). The WHO requested confirmation from

Chinese authorities on January 1, 2020, and wrote to the Chinese National Health Commission the following day. On January 3, Chinese officials finally confirmed a cluster of "viral pneumonia of unknown cause" (WHO 2021a). The WHO tweeted about the cluster on January 4 but did not officially share the data through the IHR Event Information System until the following day. On January 9 WHO announced that the clusters were caused by a novel coronavirus—a time lag, minimally, of nine days. It's unclear if prompt reporting would have changed the pandemic's trajectory. But it was the world's only chance. And WHO missed that opportunity.

1.2.3 WHO's Inability to Independently Verify State Reports

Not only was notification delayed but it was also inaccurate. In its January 4 tweet, WHO reported no community transmission or deaths. Ten days later, on January 14, WHO tweeted that China found "no clear evidence of human-to-human transmission" (WHO 2020a). Yet large numbers of circulating cases could not be traced back to the Huanan seafood market, including health worker infections and deaths.

As early as December 30, 2019, the Wuhan Municipal Health Commission issued emergency warnings to local hospitals. Epidemiological data strongly suggested widespread community transmission. It wasn't until January 21 that WHO's Western Pacific Regional Office (WPRO) tweeted about "at least some human-to-human transmission" (WHO 2020b). A day later, WHO's mission in Wuhan reported evidence of community transmission, but "more investigation was needed" (WHO 2020c).

Retrospective investigations also showed that Hubei Province officials suppressed information of growing case clusters (China Media Project 2020). Dr. Li Wenliang, an ophthalmologist at Wuhan Central Hospital, notified his colleagues of a SARS-like illness on December 30, but was censured by Chinese authorities for "spreading rumors" online (BBC News 2020). Dr. Li died from COVID-19 on February 6.

Western democracies harshly criticized WHO and its Director-General, Dr. Tedros Adhanom Ghebrcycsus, for these misleading WHO statements and for publicly praising Chinese President Xi Jinping. Dr. Tedros extolled China's transparency, calling it "a model" (Rauhala 2020). It's likely Dr. Tedros strategized that he could gain better cooperation from China by strong internal negotiations, while publicly lauding China's response. But whatever the public stance, the IHR didn't provide WHO with independent investigatory powers. Other than using unofficial data sources, WHO relied on truthful reporting through China's National Focal Point (Gilsinan 2020). As a fierce advocate of national sovereignty, China blocked WHO investigators at every turn.

1.2.4 Declarations of a Public Health Emergency of International Concern and Global Pandemic

Faced with a rapidly escalating global crisis, Dr. Tedros convened an IHR Emergency Committee (EC) consisting of fifteen experts on January 22 (Singh et al 2021: Appendix). By that time, COVID-19 cases were already pouring across borders. Under the IHR, China had a major role in that EC meeting as the source of the outbreak. Remarkably, the EC said it hadn't received crucial information from China and reconvened the next day. When it did, the EC did not recommend a declaration of a Public Health Emergency of International Concern (PHEIC). Dr. Tedros reconvened the EC on January 30. By that time, eighteen countries outside China had reported SARS-CoV-2 cases. The EC recommended a declaration of a PHEIC, which Dr. Tedros accepted (Singh et al. 2021: Appendix). Thus, it took a month from the initial outbreak before WHO declared an international emergency.

Then, on March 11, WHO declared the novel coronavirus a global pandemic. Dr. Tedros commented that cases outside China had increased thirteenfold and urged the world to "be more aggressive." Yet no international instrument, including WHO's Constitution and the IHR, grants WHO any such power. The declaration of the pandemic only created confusion and panic.

1.2.5 Travel Bans

More than 90% of the world's population lived in countries with travel restrictions during the initial COVID-19 wave (Connor 2020). The reflexive closing of borders contravened the IHR. Hindsight demonstrates that travel restrictions were partially effective in stemming the pandemic in certain countries (Gostin 2021b: 26). But even the greatest success stories like in China, Australia, New Zealand, and Vietnam did not prevent subsequent surges. Importantly, the world implemented restrictions without solid evidence of whether they work, which kind of restrictions, and at what time.

Most travel restrictions, moreover, were largely ineffective and impeded supplies of COVID-19 medical resources and humanitarian assistance. They also separated families, while disrupting trade, commerce, and tourism. The IHR permit countries to implement measures aimed at greater protection than recommended by WHO, but these must be proportional, scientifically validated, and not more restrictive of international traffic or invasive to persons than is needed for health protection. And states must inform WHO of their rationales and underlying scientific bases for such measures (WHO 2016: IHR (2005) Art. 43.28). But instead, virtually every country exceeded WHO's guidance on travel without clear scientific basis (Wilson et al. 2020). While nationalism may have encouraged nations to seal off their borders, border closures themselves likely contributed to nationalist sentiments.

Across the world, nations turned inward. The European Union (EU), ordinarily an open-border bloc, saw most of its members seal off their borders with dire consequences for border communities (Peyrony et al. 2021). Some feared that prolonged internal border closures would lead to a resurgence in nationalism among individual EU member states (Kirschbaum et al. 2020). In the US, then-president Trump was relatively quick to impose a travel ban from China. But it was not until mid-March that he imposed a ban on travel from Europe. Genetic sequencing later confirmed that travel from Europe was a key facilitator of the first catastrophic outbreak in New York City (Bushman et al. 2020).

Consistent with the prevailing narrative of the pandemic, travel bans hurt the world's poor the most. Border closures were particularly harsh for refugees and other migrants for whom international mobility is a necessity. In early 2020, new asylum applications fell by a third compared to the same period in 2019 (Benton et al. 2021). Global job losses affected migrant communities particularly severely. And when international mobility became a reality for only those with access to vaccines, the mobility gulf between rich and poor widened (International Organization for Migration 2021).

1.3 SARS-CoV-2 Proximal Origin

As the pandemic caused untold human and economic hardship, world leaders and public opinion grew intensely interested in discovering SARS-CoV-2's proximal origins. Again, WHO appeared impotent, as China blocked an impartial and rigorous investigation on Chinese soil, especially in Wuhan, the pandemic's epicenter, as well as in the bat caves of south China. In January 2021, a year after the outbreak had emerged, China finally allowed a WHO team of scientists to enter its sovereign territory to investigate the virus's origins, by which point critical evidence had been lost.

The WHO China Global Study—comprising many members from China or approved by the Chinese government—released its joint report on February 28, 2021 (WHO 2021b). The report said a naturally occurring zoonotic spillover was the most likely origin and discounted a leak from the Wuhan Institute of Virology, which we now believe was conducting gain-of-function research on novel coronaviruses. The report was roundly criticized, with several governments issuing a joint statement calling for a "transparent and independent analysis and evaluation, free from interference and undue influence" (US 2021). In a May 14 letter in *Science*, eighteen European and North American scientists urged deeper investigation to ascertain where SARS-CoV-2 came from, declining to rule out either the hypothesis that the virus spilled over from animals or that it was accidentally released from a laboratory (Offord 2021).

Dr. Tedros, in an unusually public rebuke to his own investigative committee, noted the difficulties the WHO team encountered in accessing raw data from China and expressed a hope that future studies "include more timely and comprehensive data sharing" (WHO 2021c). He would not rule out a laboratory leak.

The WHO has been pushed by both Western governments and scientists. President Biden ordered a full intelligence review of SARS-CoV-2 proximal origins. But even with all the covert resources available to United States intelligence agencies, the report could not conclusively determine whether a natural zoonosis or laboratory leak was most probable (National Intelligence Council 2021).

Faced with mounting criticism, WHO established a new Scientific Advisory Group for the Origins on Novel Pathogens (SAGO) (SAGO 2021). WHO's Health Emergencies Director called SAGO "our last chance" to determine the origins of the SARS-CoV-2 virus and urged China to provide data from early cases (WHO 2021d). Even still, global NGOs bemoaned conflicts of interest among SAGO members (Murray and Ruskin 2021). While zoonotic spillover events are the most likely culprit, it is unlikely that WHO and the world will ever unravel the mystery of SARS-CoV-2's proximal origins (Pekar et al. 2022). But SAGO remains important as an expert standing scientific committee that can be rapidly deployed at the first sign of a new future novel outbreak.

1.4 Failures in Risk Communication and Lost Public Trust in WHO and Public Health Agencies

A global pandemic, if anything, should solidify fidelity to science and trust in public health. COVID-19 did neither. Instead, at both the national and international level, politicians cast doubt about scientific findings and the public rapidly lost confidence in public health agencies, including WHO. Populist leaders like Donald Trump and Jair Bolsonaro underplayed the pandemic's severity and gave credence to unscientific products. Their support for medicines like hydroxychloroquine contradicted their own public health agencies. At one point, President Trump posited that chlorine dioxide could rid the body of COVID-19. Consequently, many Americans were harmed from drinking bleach. Trust in government officials and institutions was demonstrated to have statistically significant associations with lower population COVID-19 infection rates (Bollyky et al. 2022).

But public health agencies themselves contributed to plummeting confidence in science. The WHO at first rejected the use of masks as an effective mitigation measure. It also did not regard asymptomatic transmission as a major concern, and, as late as March 27, said that droplets were the prime mode of transmission, and there was little, or no, airborne spread (WHO 2020d). That turned out to be untrue, as were its early recommendations against masking. On July 4, 2020, 239 scientists from 32 countries published an open letter to WHO, providing evidence that smaller airborne particles could infect people (Mandavilli 2021). Yet WHO would not call aerosolized transmission a major risk until May 4, 2021, seventeen months after the initial outbreak.

The US Centers for Disease Control and Prevention (CDC) did little better than WHO in its risk communication. In September 2020, well before the WHO, CDC said SARS-CoV-2 could be transmitted via aerosolized airborne particles. But a few days later, CDC removed that statement from its website (Huang 2020). The CDC, like WHO, was late in recommending masks as well. But it was the agency's advice on risk mitigation measures for fully vaccinated Americans that was entirely confusing. On May 4, 2021, the agency said vaccinated Americans need not wear a mask indoors—a major faux pas (Gostin 2021a). Within the next eight weeks, the agency changed its guidance three times. Its subsequent guidance provided a case study in how *not* to do risk communication. Vaccinated Americans need not wear a mask indoors *unless* they were "in an area of substantial or high transmission" (CDC 2021a). Yet this could change rapidly. Washington, DC, for example, was not an area of high transmission on the day CDC issued its guidance. The day after, it was.

1.5 Failures in Scientific Cooperation

Failures in global solidarity were mirrored by failures in global scientific cooperation. On January 11, 2020, days after the initial WHO reports of COVID-19 in Wuhan, Chinese scientists released the genomic sequence of SARS-CoV-2 (Singh et al. 2021: Appendix). This kicked off a monumental global effort to develop diagnostics and vaccines in record time. WHO publicly praised China for its expediency, but behind the scenes WHO was growing frustrated with Chinese officials who had held back releasing the sequence; Chinese scientists had sequenced the genome over a week before it was published (Associated Press 2020). This delay stalled development of vital diagnostic tests to detect viral circulation. Chinese authorities tightly controlled other scientific information, including data on case numbers, preventing the global scientific community from assessing the basic reproduction number associated with the novel virus.

Importantly, China has not freely shared SARS-CoV-2 pathogen samples from different geographic regions and times. Such virus sharing is vital to study how the novel coronavirus mutates and evolves. The practice of member states withholding critical virus information is not new. China refused to freely share virus samples during the SARS pandemic. And in December 2006, Indonesia refused to share samples of avian influenza A (H5N1) with WHO's Global Influence Surveillance Network. Indonesia and other lower-income countries based their refusal on another treaty, the Nagoya Protocol on Access and Benefit Sharing (United Nations Environmenal Programme 2010; Gostin et al. 2014). Indonesia was conscious that it would be financially barred from reaping the rewards of such information sharing: therapeutics (Gostin 2021b: 159).

Following Indonesia's refusal, WHO brokered an international agreement for the sharing of influenza virus samples and access to benefits resulting from their sharing, culminating in the Pandemic Influenza Preparedness (PIP) Framework (WHO 2011). While the PIP Framework does not apply to non-influenza viruses like coronaviruses, the principles it espouses, like the importance of international scientific cooperation to stemming dangerous outbreaks, were critical to the early stages of the COVID-19 pandemic. Once the world had access to genomic sequencing data, international scientific cooperation accelerated, stimulating development of effective PCR tests and, eventually, vaccines. However, early failures in scientific cooperation cost time and lives.

1.6 Nationalism, Isolationism, and Science Denial

COVID-19 revealed the fragile state of global governance (Global Preparedness Monitoring Board 2020). Our world today looks utterly different than that which emerged from the rubble of World War II—a world nearly unified, committed to building a new world order based on political coordination and global solidarity. The most notable post-World War II reforms were the formation of the United Nations (UN) and its first specialized agency, the WHO. Nations coalesced around the Universal Declaration of Human Rights.

The COVID-19 pandemic revealed a much more fractured world, often characterized by nationalism, division, distrust of science, and stark global inequalities (Global Preparedness Monitoring Board 2021). Contrasting the vision of global solidarity promulgated by the UN and its organizations, nationalist governments implemented isolationist policies that undermined global coordination (Gostin et al. 2020a). After years of refusing to adequately finance WHO's emergency programming, nationalist leaders criticized the agency's leadership and weakened its authority at its time of greatest need (Gostin et al 2020a). Coordinated action by the UN Security Council was also undermined by conflict between nationalist governments. It was not until July, months after the Secretary-General's initial request, that the Security Council adopted a resolution calling for a global ceasefire so the world could focus on fighting COVID-19 (UNSC 2020).

In the years prior to the virus's emergence, a tide of populist nationalism swept parts of the globe, culminating in the election of leaders who rejected long-held values of international cooperation in favor of more inward-looking agendas (UNGA 2020b). These leaders and their parties promoted exclusionary nationalist policies in some of the world's largest nations. Success of the "America First" platform of Donald Trump in the US and the campaign for Brexit in the United Kingdom echoed that of the nationalism promoted by Narendra Modi in India,

Vladimir Putin in Russia, Andrés Manuel López Obrador in Mexico, and Jair Bolsonaro in Brazil. Authoritarian leaders also asserted absolute power and fierce national sovereignty, including Viktor Orbán in Hungary, Recep Tayyip Erdoğan in Turkey, and Alexander Lukashenko in Belarus.

While nationalist populism has taken many different forms, common themes often emerged, including a distrust in scientific 'experts' and public health institutions, and the demonization of the 'elite'. The political mainstreaming of these ideas would soon prove catastrophic to effective national and global responses to COVID-19.

Against this backdrop, it was no surprise that many countries with the worst response to COVID-19 had populist leaders (UCSF Institute for Global Health Sciences 2021). I'll discuss several particularly characteristic examples—Brazil, Mexico, Russia, and the US.

By November 2021, Brazil had lost over 610,000 lives to COVID-19, a major undercount (Felter 2021). President Bolsonaro publicly downplayed the virus's threat, blocked a centrally coordinated response, and refused to implement evidence-based mitigation measures like mask mandates and physical distancing. Following then-president Trump in the US, Bolsonaro promoted hydroxychloroquine among other unproven treatments, while spreading harmful misinformation about vaccines. A Brazilian congressional panel would recommend charges against Bolsonaro for crimes against humanity for allowing the virus to wash over the nation.

Similarly, in Mexico a populist leader downplayed the virus and spread misinformation. Mexico was second only to Brazil in Latin America in its COVID-19 death toll (Our World in Data 2021), but the real toll is probably much higher due to low levels of testing (Knaul et al. 2021). President Andrés Manuel López Obrador ignored scientific advice and failed to acquire personal protective equipment (PPE) or expand testing and trace capacities (Verdugo 2021).

Rejection of science played out elsewhere. By late October 2021, Russia was experiencing a devastating fourth wave, setting records in daily COVID-19 cases and deaths (Dixon 2021). However, excess mortality rates paint an even grimmer picture of the country's loss due to COVID-19, and contrast the figures provided by the Kremlin (Dixon 2021). The Kremlin blamed the fourth surge on the country's low levels of vaccination, despite availability of the Sputnik vaccine. But the Kremlin's own propaganda machine had spread distrust of science and vaccines long before the pandemic (Maynes 2021).

These dangerous patterns were replicated in the US by then-president Trump. In his early press briefings, Trump compared the virus to a flu, suggested that it would go away naturally, and dismissed the expertise of his public health advisors. By July 2020, Trump was pressuring states to reopen their economies, despite dire predictions from the CDC that cases and deaths would skyrocket if states relaxed restrictions too quickly (Gostin 2021b). Cases and hospitalizations exploded that summer, largely in states that raced to reopen on the president's request. Trump fired public health experts who contradicted him and promoted unproven treatments for COVID-19 to the chagrin of medical professionals nationwide.

Metrics to measure countries' pandemic preparedness like WHO's Joint External Evaluation (JEE) and the Global Health Security Index do not consider the impact of populism and accompanying lack of trust in institutions in their assessments, to catastrophic effect (IPPPR 2021; Global Health Security Index 2021).While the US scored highest on the Global Index, it recorded the most deaths from the virus. And despite having a surplus of approved vaccines by November 2022, the US ranked 52nd in the world in vaccination rates (Holder 2021), largely due to hesitancy in groups supportive of the former president and his anti-vaccination rhetoric (Kates et al. 2021).

1.7 WHO Caught in the Middle of Two Political Superpowers

The WHO became a major casualty in the geopolitical jousting of the world's largest superpowers. President Trump, eager to deflect attention away from his administration's domestic failings, criticized WHO for its "China-centric" response and fueled anti-Asian sentiment (Gostin 2021b: 133). China, without evidence, countered that a US military installation leaked the novel coronavirus. On April 14, 2020, Trump announced that the US would suspend funding for WHO, accusing it of bias towards China, of declining to support travel restrictions from China, and parroting the Chinese government's claims that there was no evidence of human-to-human transmission (White House Office of the Press Secretary 2020).

The 73rd World Health Assembly took place virtually in May 2020 for the first time in the body's history (Gostin 2021b: 7). President Trump was notably absent, but instead wrote a letter to Director-General Tedros threatening to withdraw funding and US WHO membership if WHO did not commit to making unspecified "substantive improvements" (LeBlanc 2020). President Trump formally notified WHO that the US would withdraw from the agency on July 6, 2021 (Rogers and Mandavilli 2021). This notification coincided with new records in daily infections in the US and globally (Gostin et al. 2020b). The US's departure from WHO would have been disastrous for global health and solidarity. Not only would it have stripped the agency of substantial funding as it faced a once-in-a-century health emergency, but it would also have signaled to the world that the US had retreated from its role as a leader in global governance for health—a role it had proudly occupied for decades. President Biden, on his first day in office, withdrew the US's decision to withdraw from WHO (Morales 2021).

1.8 Exacerbating the Global Narrative of Deep Inequities

The world was experiencing vast health inequities even before COVID-19. By one measure, global inequities are responsible for 16 million deaths every year (Garay et al. 2021). Life expectancy in Europe is twenty years higher than in sub-Saharan Africa (World Bank 2021), and the maternal mortality rate is over 100 times greater in sub-Saharan Africa than in Europe (UNICEF 2019).

Immense health inequities also existed within countries before COVID-19. Relatively high levels of women with at least a secondary education have access to skilled birth attendants in Ethiopia and Guatemala, 85% and 92% respectively, but only 22% and 42% of women without any formal education do (WHO 2021i). There is over a twenty-year life expectancy difference between several low-income neighborhoods in Washington, DC, with largely Black residents and several afflu-ent white neighborhoods (Kimelman and Chiwaya 2019). That disparity likely grew during COVID-19. While overall life expectancy in the US for whites fell by 0.68 years in 2020, it fell by 2.10 years for Blacks—and 3.05 years for Latinx (Miller 2021).

Pre-existing vulnerabilities and marginalization—less access to healthcare, crowded housing, underlying health conditions, living paycheck to paycheck—meant that COVID-19 caused the most harm to already marginalized popula-tions. Native Americans, Latinx, and Black Americans were two or more times likely to die from COVID-19 as white Americans, and well over twice—and in the case of Native Americans, more than three times—as likely to be infected (CDC 2021b). In the UK, ethnic minorities and Black Britons experienced far worse outcomes than white Britons. Such disparities were echoed the world over. As in the US, Indigenous communities were among the hardest hit, including First Nations people in Australia (Yashadhana et al. 2020) and Indigenous com-munities in Brazil, with the latter experiencing infection rates four times higher than white Brazilians during Brazil's first wave of COVID-19 (Henderson 2020). Migrants (Yaya et al. 2020; Illmer 2020), people with disabilities (Hakim 2020), people who are incarcerated (Carlisle and Bates 2020; Levenson 2020), and people who are homeless (Perri et al. 2020) were among other marginalized populations who experienced heightened levels of infection and death.

Levels of excess mortality paint a far different picture of the global death toll than that officially reported. By April 2022, while more than 6.2 million COVID-19 deaths were registered worldwide (WHO 2022a), the reality was likely closer to 18 million dead by the end of 2021 alone (Adam 2022). India likely had the high-est toll, with as many as 3 million deaths by 2021's end, while Latin America had very high numbers of deaths (Jha et al. 2022). While vaccinations blunted the toll from the Delta variant in Europe and the US, many low- and middle-income countries saw deaths surge over the summer of 2021. COVID-19 had likely killed

10,000 Zambians in 2020 and the first half of 2021, but from June through August 2021 it killed 20,000 more (Institute for Health Metrics and Evaluation 2021); however, recent studies have estimated the real toll to be significantly higher (Kreier 2022). Then, as 2022 began, the highly transmissible Omicron variant and subvariants caused record infections and large fatalities in mainland China, Hong Kong, and European countries like Germany and the UK.

Meanwhile, diseases and health risks that have long fallen primarily on people in lower-income countries worsened due to health service disruptions, ending years of continuous improvements. Tuberculosis deaths increased from 1.2 million in 2019 to 1.3 million in 2020 (WHO 2021e), maternal mortality deaths increased (Chmielewska et al. 2021), and malaria deaths were expected to increase as well (Al Jazeera 2020). Meanwhile, the number of people experiencing hunger increased from 135 million to 270 million from 2019 to 2020 due to COVID-19, along with conflict and the climate crisis (World Food Programme 2021).

COVID-19 is leading to a more unequal future. The World Bank estimated that 97 million more people were thrust into poverty in 2020 (Mahler et al. 2021). On top of this are the untold tens, if not hundreds, of millions of people pushed into less extreme poverty. Education disruptions may have the most severe consequences in lower-income countries, where governments have the fewest resources to help children catch up, and where hundreds of millions of children could not access remote learning, with children in sub-Saharan Africa most affected (New York Times 2020). And increases in unemployment and severe economic downturns—lasting longest in countries where vaccines were slow to arrive, and governments lack finances to stimulate the economy and mitigate harm—threaten longer-term development.

The pandemic highlighted and exacerbated existing inequities. High-income countries were directly responsible for many of these disparities. Here are several ways that inequities were amplified.

1.8.1 Hoarding of Medical Equipment and Public Health Tools

In the early months of the pandemic, a global shortage of hospital gowns, gloves, goggles, medical masks, and respirators caused world leaders to panic. When COVID-19 first hit China, the country increased imports and decreased exports of PPE, eliminating substantial quantities from the global market (Bown 2021). The US and EU responded with their own export controls, reserving supplies for their own populations. On March 3, 2020, WHO warned that PPE shortages on the global market—caused by "buying, hoarding, and misuse"—were leading to extreme price gouging (WHO 2020e). Surgical masks cost six times their typical price, the cost of N95 respirators doubled, and the cost of hospital gowns tripled (WHO 2020e). Low-income countries were unable to compete in global bidding wars for scant medical supplies, crippling their capacity to prepare for COVID-19 surges just beginning to manifest.

Healthcare workers and their patients suffered the most from supply shortages. Many doctors, nurses, and other frontline workers went to work "dangerously ill-equipped to care for COVID-19 patients" (WHO 2020e). As the pandemic progressed, supply shortages extended to ventilators, hospital beds, and COVID-19 diagnostic tests. Supply chains for medicines and therapeutics for non-COVID conditions were disrupted, too.

Even wealthy countries like the US saw their stockpiles of emergency medical equipment depleted. Failures to invest in preparedness and replenish the Strategic National Stockpile proved dire—both for the US and other countries that lost out when the US reacted with export controls and bought up global supplies (Handfield 2020).

In March 2020, WHO called on manufacturers of medical supplies to ramp up production by 40%, and urged governments to develop industry incentives, such as easing restrictions on exports and facilitating distribution channels (WHO 2020e). But instead of directing resources to regions most in need, rich countries exerted their control over global supply chains to prioritize their own needs. By April 2020, eighty countries had banned or limited the export of PPE and other goods (Shalal 2020). Though such restrictions would typically violate international trade law, there are exceptions to prevent critical country shortages. And while the G20 called on countries to take only "targeted, proportionate, transparent and temporary measures," the hoarding of medical supplies by rich nations would continue throughout the pandemic, with this nationalistic mindset most obvious with the emergence of COVID-19 vaccines (WTO 2020a).

1.8.2 Vaccine Nationalism

In January 2020, the first vaccine candidates were ready for testing just weeks after the release of the virus's genetic sequence. Thanks to years of prior research in mRNA vaccinology, and with funding and political will galvanized by the pandemic, vaccine candidates proceeded at record pace through the regulatory phases of clinical trials, a process that typically takes years to complete (Ball 2020).

Before 2020 ended, stringent regulatory authorities in the US, Canada, and UK, and WHO, had approved safe and effective COVID-19 vaccines for emergency use. Countries rolled out plans to vaccinate their populations, beginning with vulnerable groups like healthcare workers, the immunocompromised, and the elderly.

Countries' access to COVID-19 vaccines was a factor of wealth, not need. Wealthy countries contracted with manufacturers to vaccinate their populations many times over, while poorer countries could not vaccinate even their most vulnerable (Randall et al. 2021). The failure to direct vaccines to the hardest-hit zones proved detrimental. As COVID-19 continued raging in regions of low vaccination coverage, the virus would mutate into even deadlier and more contagious variants like Delta and Omicron.

1.8.3   Failure to Back the ACT Accelerator and COVAX

Amidst the terror of the early months of the pandemic, a bold approach emerged: what if we put the best minds and the greatest resources behind the development and distribution of COVID-19 tests, treatments, and vaccines? The WHO's Access to COVID-19 Tools (ACT) Accelerator brought together governments, scientists, businesses, civil society, philanthropists, and global health organizations to support the development and equitable distribution of the resources needed to quell COVID-19 cases and deaths, and restore social and economic life (WHO 2021f).

A momentous aspect of the ACT Accelerator was the COVAX Facility, a global initiative to support equitable access to COVID-19 vaccines, led by Gavi, the Vaccine Alliance; the Coalition for Epidemic Preparedness and Innovation (CEPI); and WHO. At a time of high uncertainty, COVAX attracted high-income countries to buy into the initiative to pool their risk, and then use group purchasing power to make cost-effective deals with vaccine manufacturers (Eccleston-Turner and Upton 2021). Additional donations would help cover the cost of providing vaccines to low-income countries. Its initial goal was to provide 2 billion doses by the end of 2021, equitably shared so that participating countries could vaccinate 20% of their populations (Berkley 2020).

Yet, as time would prove, COVAX would fall short of reaching this goal. By September 2021, COVAX had delivered a little over 240 million doses to 139 countries—a monumental effort but far off target, and far from achieving the equity it aimed for. Delivery ramped up and COVAX would eventually deliver 1.43 billion doses to 145 countries by April 2022, but those doses came too late for so many. By April 2022 African countries had on average vaccinated and boosted just over 15% and 1% of their populations respectively, compared to the large majority of high-income countries, which had offered third and even fourth doses to their populations (Africa CDC 2022).

These shortcomings were caused by the same concerns that COVAX was launched to evade: "vaccine nationalism, self-interest, unequal access to limited supply" (Ducharme 2021). COVAX grappled to secure financing and vaccine doses as high-income countries turned inward (Mueller and Robbins 2021). The US and China initially opted out of COVAX altogether. By the time President Biden took office in 2021, pledging to support COVAX with funding and donated doses, the inequities were irreversible. It would take years for low-income countries to achieve the same vaccination levels that high-income countries had reached in months.

Despite its flaws, the launch of COVAX was an historic achievement, and it mustn't take until the next pandemic to fix it. Wealthy countries are unlikely to commit the funding to help vaccinate poorer countries during a global outbreak; the funding must be secured far ahead of time. The distribution channels for vaccines must also be strengthened, so that vaccines can be properly stored, transported, and administered to any area, with no doses going to waste.

1.8.4 Wealthy Countries Hoard Vaccine Supplies

By early 2021, there were 137 bilateral agreements between governments and vaccine companies, putting nearly 10 billion vaccine doses under contract (Randall et al. 2021). There was little global manufacturing capacity left for countries that lacked the finances to enter pre-purchase agreements, and instead relied on COVAX.

Aside from pre-purchase agreements, export controls were a major tool for wealthy countries to hoard vaccines (Ibrahim 2021). The US and the EU, which together account for half the world's total exports of key vaccine ingredients, temporarily restricted exportation of critical raw materials, derailing efforts to produce vaccines in other parts of the world (Peters and Prabhakar 2021). In April 2021, India prohibited the export of COVID-19 vaccines as the country's own case and death rates skyrocketed (Arora and Das 2021). Home to the Serum Institute, a major vaccine producer that had contracted to provide hundreds of thousands of doses to COVAX, India's decision was a key factor in COVAX's inability to reach its targets.

As COVID-19 demonstrated, pre-purchase agreements and export controls remain tempting tools for rich countries to prioritize their own populations. But tighter protections must be in place so that the world's wealthiest cannot turn their backs on the world's poorest, especially during times of greatest need.

1.8.5 Vaccine Diplomacy from the World's Largest Dictatorships

Where countries did donate or make vaccines affordable to lower-income countries, it was often for politically motivated reasons, or "vaccine diplomacy," especially when such vaccine sharing occurred outside of COVAX. China and Russia, the world's two largest dictatorships, both produced their own COVID-19 vaccines and shared them with countries desperate for aid across Latin America, Africa, South Asia, and parts of Europe (Cullinan and Nakkazi 2021). This vaccine sharing was politically strategic. China provided vaccine doses to numerous Latin American countries, yet refused to give any to Paraguay, which recognizes

Taiwan as its own country (Alhmidi 2021). In Brazil, receiving Chinese vaccines was reportedly conditional on allowing a Chinese telecommunication company, Huawei, to enter the auction in creating Brazil's new 5G wireless network (Londoño and Casado 2021). Russia focused on sharing its Sputnik V vaccine with countries whose leaders were agreeable to Putin's policies, such as Hungary and Slovakia (Alhmidi 2021).

There are clear political ramifications when leaders take advantage of countries' desperation to gain soft power within a region. But there are health impacts, too. Both of China's vaccines (CoronaVac and Sinopharm) were used widely around the world before being approved by WHO (Mallapaty 2021). And WHO delayed approval of Russia's Sputnik V indefinitely, due to incomplete data on its effectiveness (Al Jazeera 2021) and Russia's invasion of Ukraine in February 2022 (Hassan 2022). While over seventy countries administering Russia's vaccine had granted it emergency approval, these regulatory authorities are far less stringent than WHO's. There is enormous potential for harm when poor countries are forced to take political and health risks for a chance to gain control over a raging epidemic.

Preventing harmful vaccine diplomacy falls in large part on the shoulders of wealthy countries that could have helped prevent poorer countries' desperation in the first place. If countries like the US had provided significant early funding and political backing to COVAX, low- and middle-income countries wouldn't have had to rely so heavily on outside sources. China and Russia's COVID-19 vaccine diplomacy should provide a lesson to the US on the dangers of failing to serve as a reliable global partner.

1.9 A Failure of Imagination of Global Bodies

Echoing states' failure to prioritize global solidarity over national interests, collective action through global political bodies was tragically limited.

The UN General Assembly's September 2020 COVID-19 resolution was full of critical demands, including for international solidarity, respecting, protecting, and fulfilling human rights, countering discrimination, and ensuring equal access for all countries to needed medical technologies (UNGA 2020c). Separate resolutions sought to focus global attention on the rights of women and girls (UNGA 2020d; UNGA 2020e). But the resolutions lacked binding legal force and accountability and fell on often unreceptive ears. Secretary-General Guterres's calls for an immediate global ceasefire (Guterres 2020a), treating the COVID-19 vaccine as a global public good, collective action (United Nations 2020), and mobilizing funding to "build forward better" were similarly ignored (Guterres 2020b). The Security Council, acting through a narrow peace and security lens, twice demanded all parties to hostilities to respect the Secretary-General's call for an immediate global ceasefire, to no discernible effect. Its second resolution also called for unhindered humanitarian access to enable COVID-19 vaccination (UNSC 2020; UNSC 2021).

A short, earlier General Assembly resolution called upon the UN system to mobilize a coordinated global response to the pandemic and its social and economic impact (UNGA 2020a). Here is where the UN shined: calling out human rights concerns, working to protect refugees and asylum seekers, and providing food to the hungry, culminating in the World Food Programme receiving the 2020 Nobel Peace Prize.

Likewise, WHO's Secretariat, in collaboration with the civil servants of other UN organizations and additional partners, established the COVID-19 Supply Chain Task Force and Supply Chain System, which has used purchasing consortia to procure PPE, diagnostics, oxygen concentrators, and ventilators to make them more affordable for countries that could otherwise not afford them (WHO 2020f). This mechanism did increase access—purchases topped $1 billion from February 2020 through December 2020, with low-income and lower-middle-income countries receiving 61% of the supplies (WHO 2021g). Still, countries' available funding was an obstacle, and this system couldn't compensate for wealthy countries' ability to pay premium prices to gain priority access to supplies in short supply (WHO 2021g).

Small, powerful groups of nations—the G7 and G20—did take several useful actions, but nowhere near commensurate with the scale or scope that a once-in-a-generation crisis demanded. The G20 established the Debt Service Suspension Initiative, suspending bilateral government-to-government debt service payments from the world's poorest countries through June 2021, with seventy-three countries eligible, and urging private creditors to follow suit. China limited its impact, however, by classifying its state-owned institutions as private creditors, not bound by the agreement. The leaders also launched a Common Framework to extend the debt suspension to private creditors and assist eligible countries restructure their debt and manage issues with insolvency and protracted liquidity, but implementation was slow, and as of December 2021 very few countries had used the Framework for debt relief (Georgieva and Pazarbasioglu 2021). The most significant G7 action was a June 2021 commitment to donate a total of 870 million vaccine doses through COVAX to countries in need over the next year (G20 Research Group 2021).

1.10 How to Solidify Global Cooperation and Equity

We can imagine how different the response would have been in a world where countries were committed to equity and global solidarity. Yet, while a genuine commitment to global solidarity could have made an immense difference, an equitable global response cannot rely on goodwill alone. Rather, mechanisms to facilitate and require global cooperation can and must be developed.

One key mechanism would be a permanent, but enhanced, COVAX. Building on an IPPPR recommendation, such a mechanism would have universal participation—which could be required through a pandemic treaty—and encompass equitable and needs-based distribution of vaccines as well as diagnostics, therapies, and other supplies (IPPPR 2021; Gostin et al. 2021b). Countries would be prohibited from bilateral pre-purchase agreements, and funding could come from additional WHO mandatory assessments, which could cover not only the costs of these health technologies but also delivery and administration costs in lower-income countries, including education and social mobilization (Haynes et al. 2021). As with COVAX, advanced market commitments could incentivize production.

Such a global sharing mechanism does not solve the problem of possible supply shortages, and non-compliance could remain a reality, potentially yielding many of the same access inequities experienced during COVID-19. Expanded manufacturing capacities, spread across all regions, would go a long way towards addressing these concerns. Going further, and in line with a proposed Pandemic Open Vaccine Access Accelerator, the mechanism could require countries to share, and require companies over which they have authority to share, data, knowledge such as key ingredients, methods, and sourcing, and technology related to pandemic-related health technologies. This open access would enable more manufacturers worldwide to produce these technologies, greatly reducing supply bottlenecks (Basu et al. 2021). This could be required through a pandemic treaty and reinforced by a waiver for health emergencies through the World Trade Organization (WTO), as proposed by South Africa and India for COVID-19-related technologies, leading to lengthy negotiations at WTO (Haynes et al. 2021; WTO 2020b; WTO 2021).[1]

To further enable robust global capacity and supply, two steps are needed now. First, building on the WHO-backed mRNA vaccine hub in South Africa, every region of the world should have hubs for mRNA vaccines and other pandemic-related technologies and equipment. Relevant manufacturing capacity would no longer be concentrated in a few countries, including for COVID-19 vaccines, whose production is now primarily in higher-income countries, enabling them to exert control over the world's supplies. Wealthier nations should provide financial backing. And some combination of a WTO waiver and state requirements, such as through agreements that provide for public funding and legislation like

---

[1] World Trade Organization members agreed in June 2022 to grant a limited waiver for COVID-19 vaccines, but did not agree at that time on a waiver for other COVID-19-related technologies including treatments and tests, instead deferring that decision to the end of 2022: World Trade Organization (2022), 'Ministerial Decision on the TRIPS Agreement' (June 22, 2022), WT/MIN(22)/30, WT/L/1141.

the Defense Production Act in the US—and ultimately pandemic treaty requirements—would provide access to needed know-how. The benefits would be twofold: not only would low-income countries have greater access to vaccines and other technologies, these new hubs would also create employment and economic opportunities in these countries, foreseeably countering the economic harms from the pandemic. Second, countries should gradually build up a robust, regionally disbursed global stockpile of pandemic-related technologies and equipment, such as existing vaccines and personal protective equipment (Dave 2020).

Such measures should enable rapid, equitable, needs-based disbursements of health technologies to respond to pandemics. Yet global, equity-focused actions must also attend to inequities in other aspects of pandemic response and to factors that enable emerging and novel infections to become pandemics in the first place. A well-funded International Pandemic Financing Facility, as the IPPPR proposed (IPPPR 2021), should be developed to fund early outbreak through to pandemic responses with a mandate that encompasses mitigating the social and economic impacts of health emergencies (Gostin et al. 2021b).[2]

Furthermore, all countries need robust public health systems to detect and respond to outbreaks—as the IHR require. Funding could come through phased increases in mandatory WHO assessments, a mechanism through the pandemic treaty, or a separate agreement (WHO 2022b). A pandemic treaty could also expand the narrow scope of required public health system capacities.[3]

The UN could have done more. The Security Council could have imposed arms embargoes and other sanctions on all parties to hostilities that disregarded UN calls for a ceasefire and its demand to allow humanitarian access for vaccination. And the UN could have organized a health worker exchange program more expansive than WHO's Emergency Medical Team initiative, which saw limited use during COVID-19 despite extreme need (WHO 2021h). Such a program could have sought volunteers worldwide, with teams travelling where COVID-19 surges occurred.

Much as the global community could have stood with people in the world's poorest countries in these ways, it could have stood with the poorest and most marginalized people in every country. A pandemic treaty could require countries to develop domestic pandemic preparedness strategies that incorporate equity, systematically covering poor and marginalized populations and requiring their participation in developing the strategies (Friedman et al 2021). This participation

---

[2] A World Bank-hosted Financial Intermediary Fund for Pandemics was officially established in September 2022: World Bank (2022), 'The Pandemic Fund: Overview' https://www.worldbank.org/en/programs/financial-intermediary-fund-for-pandemic-prevention-preparedness-and-response-ppr-fif/overview, (accessed Nov. 26, 2022).

[3] In May 2022, the World Health Assembly agreed to phased increases in mandatory WHO assessments: World Health Organization (2022), 'World Health Assembly Agrees Historic Decision to Sustainably Finance WHO' (May 24, 2022) https://www.who.int/news/item/24-05-2022-world-health-assembly-agrees-historic-decision-to-sustainably-finance-who, (accessed Nov. 26, 2022).

could also build trust, critical for adherence to socio-behavioral mitigation measures and vaccine uptake. Alternatively, such strategies could be required to benefit from a permanent equitable distribution mechanism. An independent or JEE process to ensure the implementation and quality of these strategies could provide a measure of accountability.

1.11 A Thought Experiment: Pandemic X

If leaders and societies learn from the lessons of COVID-19 and implement the types of mechanisms described above, it would make a world of difference when the next pathogen of pandemic potential emerges—which I refer to here as Pandemic X. COVID-19 demonstrated how a country could violate the IHR to conceal an early outbreak with scant repercussions under the Regulations, but with enormous repercussions to people's health in that country and around the world. An independent inspectorate empowered to investigate pandemic-related matters could help identify Pandemic X, and alert the world while it is still in a manageable phase. Yet even if Pandemic X spreads around the globe, we could still prevent the levels of severe suffering, death, and economic devastation that we have experienced with COVID-19 (Gostin 2021b).

With global stockpiles and widespread production capacities (including in LMICs), health workers everywhere could sufficiently protect themselves from infection. Diagnostics could be scaled up rapidly and distributed widely and equitably. Greater testing would result in better surveillance, facilitating more targeted national responses and enhancing the effectiveness of isolation and quarantine. Perhaps there would be enough N95, or KN95, respirators not only for health workers but also for essential workers and others in high-risk settings or with heightened risk of severe illness and death.

Because of all of this, global infections and deaths would be significantly lower, as would the level of hospital surges, enabling better care for those who are hospitalized. If health systems were not overwhelmed, countries could ensure routine services such as childhood vaccinations, prevention of chronic diseases, injury prevention, and tobacco and alcohol control. Perhaps variants of concern would evolve less often due to fewer infections. Or they may emerge but with fewer dangerous mutations, mitigating their harm.

More funding for the socioeconomic consequences of Pandemic X and its reduced spread, and consequentially the need for lockdowns, would limit increases in poverty, hunger, and similar virus-related harms. A Security Council resolution with teeth might not only save lives but also limit the number of people suffering from acute hunger (with not only COVID-19 but also conflict and climate change the sources of 2020's hunger spike), and enable vaccination in areas that may otherwise be unreachable.

The most dramatic difference would be in vaccination. With far greater manufacturing capacity and equitable, needs-based vaccine rollouts, health workers and other vulnerable or most at-risk populations would be quickly vaccinated, with countries experiencing surges, whether rich or poor, being the first in line, thus saving the most lives. The expanded manufacturing capacity and funding for vaccine delivery and administration would enable rapid and widespread global vaccination, quite possibly near universal vaccination within the first year after vaccines gain regulatory approval. Even if Pandemic X ultimately becomes endemic (much would depend on the ability of countries to counter vaccine hesitancy, while developing a robust vaccine-delivery infrastructure), its levels and death toll would be far lower than we have experienced during the COVID-19 pandemic. And with pandemic preparedness and a robust response, human beings everywhere would be able to return to their normal lives far sooner.

Bibliography

Adam, David (2022), 'COVID's True Death Toll: Much Higher than Official Records', *Nature*, March 10, 2022, https://doi.org/10.1038/d41586-022-00708-0.

Africa CDC (2022), 'COVID-19 Vaccination', https://africacdc.org/covid-19-vaccination/ (accessed Apr. 27, 2022).

Alhmidi, Maan (2021), 'China, Russia Using Their COVID-19 Vaccines to Gain Political Influence, Experts Say', *CTV News*, April 17, 2021, https://www.ctvnews.ca/health/coronavirus/china-russia-using-their-covid-19-vaccines-to-gain-political-influence-experts-say-1.5391422.

Al Jazeera (2020), 'Malaria Gains at Risk from COVID-19 Pandemic: WHO', November 30, 2020, https://www.aljazeera.com/news/2020/11/30/malaria-gains-at-risk-from-covid-19-pandemic-who.

Al Jazeera (2021), 'WHO Says Approval for Russia's Sputnik V Vaccine 'Still on Hold'', October 13, 2021, https://www.aljazeera.com/news/2021/10/13/who-says-approval-for-russias-sputnik-v-vaccine-still-on-hold.

Arora, Neha, and Krishna N. Das, (2121), 'India to Restart COVID Vaccine Exports to COVAX, Neighbours', *Reuters*, September 20, 2021, https://www.reuters.com/world/india/india-resume-covid-vaccine-exports-next-quarter-2021-09-20/.

Associated Press (2020), 'China delayed releasing coronavirus info, frustrating WHO', June 2, 2020, https://apnews.com/article/united-nations-health-ap-top-news-virus-outbreak-public-health-3c061794970661042b18d5aeaaed9fae.

Ball, Philip (2020), 'The Lightning-Fast Quest for COVID Vaccines – and What It Means For Other Diseases', *Nature*, December 18, 2020, https://www.nature.com/articles/d41586-020-03626-1.

Basu, Kaushik, Lawrence O. Gostin, and Nicole Hassoun (2021), 'Pandemic Preparedness and Response: Beyond the WHO's Access to COVID-19 Tools

Accelerator', *Brookings*, April 28, 2021. https://www.brookings.edu/research/pandemic-preparedness-and-response-beyond-the-whos-access-to-covid-19-tools-accelerator/.

BBC News (2020), 'Li Wenliang: Coronavirus kills Chinese Whistleblower Doctor', February 7, 2020, https://www.bbc.com/news/world-asia-china-51403795.

Benton, Meghan, Jeanne Batalova, Samuel Davidoff-Gore, and Timo Schmidt (2021), 'COVID-19 and the State of Global Mobility in 2020', Migration Policy Institute and International Organization for Migration, https://publications.iom.int/system/files/pdf/covid-19-and-the-state-of-global.pdf.

Berkley, Seth (2020), 'COVAX Explained', *Gavi*, September 3, 2020, https://www.gavi.org/vaccineswork/covax-explained.

Bollyky, Thomas J., Erin N Hulland, Ryan M Barber, et al. (2022), 'Pandemic Preparedness and COVID-19: An Exploratory Analysis of Infection and Fatality Rates, and Contextual Factors Associated with Preparedness in 177 Countries, from Jan 1, 2020, to Sept 30, 2021', *The Lancet* 399/10334: 1489–512.

Bown, Chad P. (2021), 'How COVID-19 Medical Supply Shortages Led to Extraordinary Trade and Industrial Policy', Peterson Institute for International Economics, July 2021, https://www.piie.com/sites/default/files/documents/wp21-11.pdf.

Bushman, Dena, Karen A. Alroy, Sharon K. Greene, et al. (2020), 'Detection and Genetic Characterization of Community-Based SARS-CoV-2 Infections – New York City, March 2020', *MMWR Morbidity and Mortality Weekly Report (MMWR)* 69/28 (July 2020): 918–22, http://dx.doi.org/10.15585/mmwr.mm6928a5.

Carlisle, Madeleine, and Josiah Bates (2020), 'With Over 275,000 Infections and 1,700 Deaths, COVID-19 Has Devastated the U.S. Prison and Jail Population', *Time*, December 28, 2020, https://time.com/5924211/coronavirus-outbreaks-prisons-jails-vaccines/.

CDC (2021a), 'Use and Care of Masks', October 25, 2021, https://www.cdc.gov/coronavirus/2019-ncov/prevent-getting-sick/about-face-coverings.html.

CDC (2021b), 'Risk for COVID-19 Infection, Hospitalization, and Death by Race/Ethnicity', September 9, 2021. https://www.cdc.gov/coronavirus/2019-ncov/covid-data/investigations-discovery/hospitalization-death-by-race-ethnicity.html.

China Media Project (2020), 'The Truth About 'Dramatic Action'', *China Media Project*, January 27, 2020, https://chinamediaproject.org/2020/01/27/dramatic-actions/.

Chmielewska, Barbara, Imogen Barratt, Rosemary Townsend, et al. (2021), 'Effects of the COVID-19 Pandemic on Maternal and Perinatal Outcomes: A Systematic Review and Meta-Analysis', *The Lancet Global Health* 9/6 (June 2021): e759–72, https://doi.org/10.1016/S2214-109X(21)00079-6.

Connor, Phillip (2020), 'More Than Nine-in-Ten People Worldwide Live in Countries with Travel Restrictions amid COVID-19', Pew Research Center, April 1, 2020, https://www.pewresearch.org/fact-tank/2020/04/01/more-than-nine-in-ten-people-worldwide-live-in-countries-with-travel-restrictions-amid-covid-19/.

Cullinan, Kerry, and Esther Nakkazi (2021), 'Russian And Chinese Bilateral Vaccine Deals & Donations Outmaneuver Europe & United States - Health Policy Watch', April 3, 2021, https://healthpolicy-watch.news/russia-and-chinas-bilateral-vaccine/.

Dave, R. K. (2020), 'COVID-19: 'Global Stockpile for Health Emergency Response (GSHER)' – A Conceptual Framework', April 4, 2020, https://www.academia.edu/42645401/COVID_19_Global_Stockpile_for_Health_Emergency_Response_GSHER_A_conceptual_Framework.

Dixon, Robyn (2021), 'In Russia, Experts Are Challenging Official Pandemic Figures as Too Low. They Refuse To Be Silenced', *Washington Post*, October 17, 2021, https://www.washingtonpost.com/world/europe/russia-covid-count-fake-statistics/2021/10/16/b9d47058-277f-11ec-8739-5cb6aba30a30_story.html.

Ducharme, Jamie (2021), 'What Went Wrong with COVAX, the Global Vaccine Hub', *Time*, September 9, 2021, https://time.com/6096172/covax-vaccines-what-went-wrong/.

Eccleston-Turner, Mark, and Harry Upton (2021), 'International Collaboration to Ensure Equitable Access to Vaccines for COVID-19: The ACT-Accelerator and the COVAX Facility', *Milbank Quarterly* 99/2 (June 2021): 426–49, doi:10.1111/1468-0009.12503.

Felter, Claire (2021), 'By How Much Are Countries Underreporting COVID-19 Cases and Deaths?' *Council of Foreign Relations*, May 10, 2021, https://www.cfr.org/in-brief/how-much-are-countries-underreporting-covid-19-cases-and-deaths.

Friedman, Eric A., Kelly E. Perry, and Luiz Galvão (2021), 'An International Treaty Enshrining the Right to Health Should Be Part of Post-Covid Reforms', *BMJ Opinion*, June 24, 2021, https://blogs.bmj.com/bmj/2021/06/24/an-international-treaty-that-enshrines-the-right-to-health-should-be-part-of-post-covid-reforms/.

G20 Research Group (2021), 'Carbis Bay G7 Summit Communiqué: Our Shared Agenda for Global Action to Build Back Better', University of Toronto, June 13, 2021, http://www.g8.utoronto.ca/summit/2021cornwall/210613-communique.html.

Garay, Juan, Nefer Kelley, David Chiriboga, and Adam Garay (2021), 'Global Health Inequity 1960–2020: Equity vs. Equality, Dignity vs. Poverty, Equitable and Sustainable Wellbeing vs. Human Development Index', Policies for Equitable Access to Health, April 21, 2021, http://www.peah.it/2021/04/9658/.

Georgieva, Kristalina, and Ceyla Pazarbasioglu (2021), 'The G20 Common Framework for Debt Treatments Must Be Stepped Up', *IMF Blog*, December 2, 2021, https://blogs.imf.org/2021/12/02/the-g20-common-framework-for-debt-treatments-must-be-stepped-up/.

Gilsinan, Kathy (2020), 'How China Deceived the WHO', *The Atlantic*, April 12, 2020, https://www.theatlantic.com/politics/archive/2020/04/world-health-organization-blame-pandemic-coronavirus/609820/.

Global Health Security Index (2021), '2019 GHS Index Country Profile for United States', https://www.ghsindex.org/country/united-states/, (accessed Nov. 16, 2021).

Global Preparedness Monitoring Board (2020), 'A World in Disorder: GPMB 2020 Annual Report', September 14, 2020, https://www.gpmb.org/annual-reports/overview/item/2020-a-world-in-disorder.

Global Preparedness Monitoring Board (2021), 'From Worlds Apart to a World Prepared: GPMB 2021 Annual Report', October 26, 2021, https://www.gpmb.org/annual-reports/overview/item/from-worlds-apart-to-a-world-prepared.

Gostin, Lawrence O. (2021a), 'Op-Ed: What Was CDC Thinking With Its New Mask Guidance?' *MedPage Today*, May 14, 2021, https://www.medpagetoday.com/infectiousdisease/covid19/92596?trw=no.

Gostin, Lawrence O. (2021b), *Global Health Security: A Blueprint for the Future* (Cambridge, MA, Harvard University Press).

Gostin, Lawrence O., Alexandra Phelan, Michael A. Stoto, John D. Kraemer, and K. Srinath Reddy (2014), 'Virus Sharing, Genetic Sequencing, and Global Health Security', *Science* 345/6202 (September 2014): 1295–6, doi: 10.1126/science.1257622.

Gostin, Lawrence O., Suerie Moon, and Benjamin Mason Meier (2020a), 'Reimagining Global Health Governance in the Age of COVID-19', *American Journal of Public Health* 110/11 (October 2020): 1615–19, doi: 10.2105/AJPH.2020.305933.

Gostin, Lawrence O., Harold Hongju Koh, Michelle Williams, et al. (2020b), 'US Withdrawal from WHO Is Unlawful and Threatens Global and US Health and Security', *The Lancet* 396/10247 (July 2020): 293–5, https://doi.org/10.1016/S0140-6736(20)31527-0.

Gostin, Lawrence O., Sam F. Halabi, and Kevin A. Klock (2021a), 'An International Agreement on Pandemic Prevention and Preparedness', *JAMA* 326/13 (2021): 1257–8, doi:10.1001/jama.2021.16104.

Gostin, Lawrence O., Sarah Wetter, and Eric Friedman (2021b), 'This Investigation Lays Out What the World Needs to Fight the Next Pandemic', *Forbes*, May 20, 2021, https://www.forbes.com/sites/coronavirusfrontlines/2021/05/20/this-investigation-lays-out-what-the-world-needs-to-fight-the-next-pandemic/?sh=4b9a36743d44.

Guterres, António (2020a), 'Remarks to the Security Council on the COVID-19 Pandemic', *United Nations*, April 9, 2020, https://www.un.org/sg/en/content/sg/speeches/2020-04-09/remarks-security-council-covid-19-pandemic.

Guterres, António (2020b), 'Remarks at the G20 Riyadh Summit', *United Nations*, November 22, 2020, https://www.un.org/sg/en/content/sg/speeches/2020-11-22/remarks-g20-riyadh-summit.

Hakim, Danny (2020), ''It's Hit Our Front Door': Homes for the Disabled See a Surge of COVID-19', *New York Times*, April 17, 2020, https://www.nytimes.com/2020/04/08/nyregion/coronavirus-disabilities-group-homes.html.

Handfield, Robert, Daniel Joseph Finkenstadt, Eugene S. Schneller, A. Blanton Godfrey, and Peter Guinto (2020), 'A Commons for a Supply Chain in the Post-COVID-19 Era: The Case for a Reformed Strategic National Stockpile', *Milbank Quarterly* 98/4 (November 2020): 1058–90, https://doi.org/10.1111/1468-0009.12485.

Hassan, Adeel (2022), 'W.H.O. Delays Assessing Russia's Sputnik Vaccine Over Ukraine War', *New York Times,* March 16, 2022.

Haynes, Leigh Kamore, Eric A. Friedman, Adam Bertscher, Jingyi Xu, and Luiz Galvão (2021), 'Addressing Inequity and Advancing the Right to Health to Strengthen Pandemic Prevention, Preparedness, and Response', Global Health Centre, November 5, 2021, https://www.graduateinstitute.ch/sites/internet/files/2021-11/FCGH-v2.pdf.

Henderson, Emily (2020), 'Brazil Becomes Global Hotspot for COVID-19 Pandemic', *News Medical Life Sciences,* September 24, 2020, https://www.news-medical.net/news/20200924/Brazil-becomes-global-hotspot-for-COVID-19-pandemic.aspx.

Holder, Josh (2021), 'Tracking Coronavirus Vaccinations Around the World', *New York Times,* November 16, 2021, https://www.nytimes.com/interactive/2021/world/covid-vaccinations-tracker.html.

Huang, Pien. (2020), 'CDC Takes Down Its Guidance on Aerosol Transmission on the Coronavirus', *NPR,* September 21, 2020, https://www.npr.org/2020/09/21/915381480/cdc-takes-down-its-guidance-on-aerosol-transmission-on-the-coronavirus.

Ibrahim, Imad Antoine (2021), 'Overview of Export Restrictions on COVID-19 Vaccines and Their Components', *American Society of International Law* 25/10 (June 2021), https://www.asil.org/insights/volume/25/issue/10.

Illmer, Andreas (2020), 'COVID-19: Singapore Migrant Workers Infections Were Three Times Higher', *BBC News,* December 16, 2020, https://www.bbc.com/news/world-asia-55314862.

Institute for Health Metrics and Evaluation (2021), 'Cumulative Deaths', https://covid19.healthdata.org/global?view=cumulative-deaths&tab=trend (accessed Nov. 16, 2021).

International Organization for Migration (2021), 'First Comprehensive Global Analysis of COVID-19 Travel Restrictions, Border Closures Weighs Future Impacts on Mobility', April 8, 2021, https://www.iom.int/news/first-comprehensive-global-analysis-covid-19-travel-restrictions-border-closures-weighs-future-impacts-mobility.

IPPPR (The Independent Panel for Pandemic Preparedness and Response) (2021), 'COVID-19: Make it the Last Pandemic', May 2021, https://theindependentpanel.org/wp-content/uploads/2021/05/COVID-19-Make-it-the-Last-Pandemic_final.pdf.

Jha, Prabhat, Yashwant Deshmukh, Chinmay Tumbe, et al. (2022), 'COVID Mortality in India: National Survey Data and Health Facility Deaths', *Science* vol. 375 (2022): 667–71, https://doi.org/10.1126/science.abm5154.

Kates, Jennifer, Jennifer Tolbert, and Kendal Orgera (2021), 'The Red/Blue Divide in COVID-19 Vaccination Rates', Kaiser Family Foundation, September 14, 2021, https://www.kff.org/policy-watch/the-red-blue-divide-in-covid-19-vaccination-rates/.

Kimelman, Jeremia, and Nigel Chiwaya (2019), 'MAP: How Long People in Your City Are Expected To Live', *NBC News*, April 14, 2019, https://www.nbcnews.com/news/us-news/map-neighborhood-life-expectancy-united-states-n979141.

Kirschbaum, Erik, Laura King, and Meg Bernhard (2020), 'Nationalism Rears Its Head as Europe Battles Coronavirus with Border Controls', *Los Angeles Times*, March 19, 2020, https://www.latimes.com/world-nation/story/2020-03-19/nationalism-could-rear-its-head-as-europe-battles-coronavirus.

Knaul, Felicia Marie, Michael Touchton, HéctorArreola-Ornelas, et al (2021), 'Punt Politics as Failure of Health System Stewardship: Evidence from the COVID-19 Pandemic Response in Brazil in Mexico' *The Lancet Regional Health—Americas* 4, no. 100086 (December 2021), https://doi.org/10.1016/j.lana.2021.100086.

Kreier, Freda (2022), 'Morgue Data Hint at COVID's True Toll in Africa', *Nature* 603/7903 (2022): 778–9, https://doi.org/10.1038/d41586-022-00842-9.

LeBlanc, Paul (2020), 'Trump Threatens to Permanently Pull Funding from WHO and 'Reconsider' US Membership', *CNN*, May 19, 2020, https://www.cnn.com/2020/05/18/politics/trump-world-health-organization-coronavirus/index.html.

Levenson, Eric (2020), 'Prison Inmates Are Twice as Likely to Die of COVID-19 Than Those on the Outside, New Report Finds', *CNN*, September 3, 2020, https://www.cnn.com/2020/09/02/us/prison-coronavirus-clusters-report/index.html.

Londoño, Ernesto, and Letícia Casado (2021), 'Brazil Needs Vaccines. China is Benefiting', *New York Times*, March 15, 2021, https://www.nytimes.com/2021/03/15/world/americas/brazil-vaccine-china.html.

Mahler, Daniel Gerszon, Nishant Yonzan, Christoph Lakner, R. Andres Castaneda Aguilar, and Haoyu Wu (2021), 'Updated Estimates of the Impact of COVID-19 on Global Poverty: Turning the Corner on the Pandemic in 2021?' *World Bank Blog*, June 24, 2021, https://blogs.worldbank.org/opendata/updated-estimates-impact-covid-19-global-poverty-turning-corner-pandemic-2021.

Mallapaty, Smriti (2021), 'WHO Approval of Chinese CoronaVac COVID Vaccine Will Be Crucial to Curbing Pandemic', *Nature*, June 4, 2021, https://www.nature.com/articles/d41586-021-01497-8.

Mandavilli, Apoorva (2021), '239 Experts with One Big Claim: The Coronavirus Is Airborne', *New York Times*, October 1, 2021, https://www.nytimes.com/2020/07/04/health/239-experts-with-one-big-claim-the-coronavirus-is-airborne.html.

Maynes, Charles (2021), 'With Record-High Deaths, Moscow and Other Parts of Russia Enter a Partial Lockdown', *NPR*, October 28, 2021, https://www.npr.org/2021/10/28/1049976625/moscow-russia-covid-deaths-lockdown.

Miller, Jenesse (2021), 'COVID-19 Reduced U.S. Life Expectancy, Especially Among Black and Latino Populations', *USC News*, January 14, 2021, https://news.usc.edu/180718/covid-19-american-life-expectancy-black-latino-populations-usc-research/.

Morales, Christina (2021), 'Biden Restores Ties with the World Health Organization That Were Cut by Trump', *New York Times*, January 20, 2021, https://www.nytimes.com/2021/01/20/world/biden-restores-who-ties.html.

Mueller, Benjamin, and Rebecca Robbins (2021), 'Where a Vast Global Vaccination Program Went Wrong', *New York Times*, October 7, 2021, https://www.nytimes.com/2021/08/02/world/europe/covax-covid-vaccine-problems-africa.html.

Murray, Shannon, and Gary Ruskin (2021), 'Letter from U.S. Right to Know to WHO Regarding Public Comments on SAGO Members', U.S. Right to Know, October 26, 2021, https://usrtk.org/wp-content/uploads/2021/10/USRTK_WHO-SAGO1.pdf.

National Intelligence Council (2021), 'Updated Assessment on COVID-19 Origins', Office of the Director of National Intelligence, https://www.dni.gov/files/ODNI/documents/assessments/Declassified-Assessment-on-COVID-19-Origins.pdf (accessed Nov.16, 2021).

New York Times (2020), 'Almost 500 Million Children Are Cut Off From School in Pandemic, Report Says', August 28, 2020, https://www.nytimes.com/2020/08/26/world/covid-19-coronavirus.html.

Offord, Catherine (2021), 'COVID-19's Origins Need Further Investigation, Say Scientists', *The Scientist*, May 14, 2021, https://www.the-scientist.com/news-opinion/covid-19-s-origins-need-further-investigation-say-scientists-68770.

Our World in Data (2021), 'Mexico: Coronavirus Pandemic Country Profile', https://ourworldindata.org/coronavirus/country/mexico (accessed Nov. 16, 2021).

Pekar, Jonathan E., Andrew Magee, Edyth Parker, et al. (2022), 'SARS-CoV-2 Emergence Very Likely Resulted from at Least Two Zoonotic Events', *Zenodo*, February 26, 2022, https://zenodo.org/record/6291628#.Yn1IgBPMJTY.

Perri, Melissa, Naheed Dosani, and Stephen W. Hwang (2020), 'COVID-19 and People Experiencing Homelessness: Challenges and Mitigation Strategies', *Canadian Medical Association Journal* 192/26 (June 2020): E716–19, https://doi.org/10.1503/cmaj.200834.

Peters, Ralf, and Divya Prabhakar (2021), 'Export Restrictions Do Not Help Fight COVID-19', UNCTAD, June 11, 2021, https://unctad.org/news/export-restrictions-do-not-help-fight-covid-19.

Peyrony, Jean, Jean Rubio, and Raffaele Viaggi (2021), 'The Effects of COVID-19 Induced Border Closures on Cross-Border Regions: An Empirical Report Covering the Period March to June 2020', European Commission, February 3, 2021, https://op.europa.eu/en/publication-detail/-/publication/46250564-669a-11eb-aeb5-01aa75ed71a1/language-en.

Randall, Tom, Cedric Sam, Andre Tartar, and Christopher Cannon (2021), 'Covid-19 Deals Tracker: 9.6 Billion Doses Under Contract', Bloomberg, March 9, 2021, https://www.bloomberg.com/graphics/covid-vaccine-tracker-global-distribution/contracts-purchasing-agreements.html.

Rauhala, Emily (2020), 'Chinese Officials Note Serious Problems in Coronavirus Response. The World Health Organization Keeps Praising Them', *Washington Post*, February 8, 2020, https://www.washingtonpost.com/world/asia_pacific/chinese-officials-note-serious-problems-in-coronavirus-response-the-world-health-organization-keeps-praising-them/2020/02/08/b663dd7c-4834-11ea-91ab-ce439aa5c7c1_story.html.

Rogers, Katie, and Apoorva Mandavilli (2021), 'Trump Administration Signals Formal Withdrawal from W.H.O', *New York Times*, September 22, 2021, https://www.nytimes.com/2020/07/07/us/politics/coronavirus-trump-who.html.

Scientific Advisory Group for the Origins of Novel Pathogens (2021), 'Terms of Reference', August 20, 2021, https://cdn.who.int/media/docs/default-source/scientific-advisory-group-on-the-origins-of-novel-pathogens/sago-tors-final-20-aug-21_-(002).pdf?sfvrsn=b3b54576_5.

Shalal, Andrea (2020), 'WTO Reports Says 80 Countries Limiting Exports of Face Masks, Other Goods', *Reuters*, April 23, 2020, https://www.reuters.com/article/us-health-coronavirus-trade-wto/wto-report-says-80-countries-limiting-exports-of-face-masks-other-goods-idUSKCN2253IX.

Singh, Sudhvir, Christine McNab, Rose McKeon Olson, et al. (2021), 'How an Outbreak Became a Pandemic: A Chronological Analysis of Crucial Junctures and International Obligations in the Early Months of the COVID-19 Pandemic', *The Lancet*, November 8, 2021: Supplementary Appendix, https://doi.org/10.1016/S0140-6736(21)01897-3.

UCSF (Institute for Global Health Sciences) (2021), 'Mexico's Response to COVID-19: A Case Study', April 12, 2021, https://globalhealthsciences.ucsf.edu/sites/global-healthsciences.ucsf.edu/files/mexico-covid-19-case-study-english.pdf.

UNGA (United Nations General Assembly) (2020a), 'Global Solidarity to Fight the Coronavirus Disease 2019 (COVID-19)', UNGA 74th Session (April 3, 2020), UN Doc. A/RES/74/270.

UNGA (United Nations General Assembly) (2020b), 'Human Rights and International Solidarity', UNGA 75th Session (July 20, 2020), UN Doc A/75/180.

UNGA (United Nations General Assembly) (2020c), 'Integrated and Coordinated Implementation of and Follow-Up to the Outcomes of the Major United Nations Conferences and Summits in the Economic, Social and Related Fields', UNGA 74th Session (September 15, 2020), UN Doc A/RES/74/306.

UNGA (United Nations General Assembly) (2020d), 'Strengthening National and International Rapid Response to the Impact of the Coronavirus Disease (COVID-19) on Women and Girls', UNGA 75th Session (December 23, 2020), UN Doc A/RES/75/156.

UNGA (United Nations General Assembly) (2020e), 'Women and Girls and the Response to the Coronavirus Disease (COVID-19)', UNGA 75th Session (December 23, 2020), UN Doc A/RES/75/157.

UNGA (United Nations General Assembly) (2021a), 'International Solidarity in Aid of the Realization of Human Rights During and After the Coronavirus Disease (COVID-19) Pandemic — Report of the Independent Expert on Human Rights and International Solidarity, Obiora Chinedu Okafor', UN Doc. A/HRC/47/31.

UNICEF (2019), 'Maternal Mortality Declined by 38 Per Cent Between 2000 and 2017', September 2019, https://data.unicef.org/topic/maternal-health/maternal-mortality/.

United Nations (2020), 'Secretary-General's Video Message for the World Health Summit', October 25, 2020, https://www.un.org/sg/en/content/sg/statement/2020-10-25/secretary-generals-video-message-for-the-world-health-summit.

United Nations Environmental Programme (2010), 'The Nagoya Protocol on Access to Genetic Resources and the Fair and Equitable Sharing of Benefits Arising from Their Utilization to the Convention on Biological Diversity', October 29, 2010, UN Doc. UNEP/CBD/COP/DEC/X/1.

United States Department of State (2021), 'Joint Statement on the WHO-Convened COVID-19 Origins Study', March 30, 2021, https://www.state.gov/joint-statement-on-the-who-convened-covid-19-origins-study/.

UNSC (UN Security Council) (2020), Res. 2532 (July 1, 2020), UN Doc S/RES/2532.

UNSC (UN Security Council) (2021), Res. 2565 (February 26, 2021), UN Doc S/RES/2565.

Verdugo, Eduardo (2021), 'Report: Mexico's COVID-19 Policies Cost Huge Number of Lives', *Associated Press*, April 14, 2021, https://apnews.com/article/science-pandemics-mexico-coronavirus-pandemic-california-cec1db095e2e447bd86ec66912d064fa.

White House, Office of the Press Secretary, 'President Donald J. Trump Is Demanding Accountability from the World Health Organization', U.S. Department of State – Global Public Affairs, April 15, 2020, https://2017-2021-translations.state.gov/2020/04/15/president-donald-j-trump-is-demanding-accountability-from-the-world-health-organization/index.html.

WHO (World Health Organization) (2016), *International Health Regulations (2005)*, 3rd ed. (Geneva: World Health Organization, 2016).

WHO (World Health Organization) (2011), *Pandemic Influenza Preparedness Framework—for the Sharing of Influenza Viruses and Access to Vaccines and Other Benefits*, 2nd ed. (Geneva: World Health Organization, 2011).

WHO (World Health Organization) (2020a), January 14, 2020, https://twitter.com/WHO/status/1217043229427761152.

WHO (World Health Organization) (2020b), Western Pacific. January 20, 2020, https://twitter.com/WHOWPRO/status/1219478544041930752.

WHO (World Health Organization) (2020c), 'Mission Summary: WHO Field Visit to Wuhan, China 20-21 January 2020', January 22, 2020, https://www.who.int/china/news/detail/22-01-2020-field-visit-wuhan-china-jan-2020.

WHO (World Health Organization) (2020d), 'Modes of Transmission of Virus Causing COVID-19: Implications for IPC Precaution Recommendations', March 29, 2020, https://www.who.int/news-room/commentaries/detail/modes-of-transmission-of-virus-causing-covid-19-implications-for-ipc-precaution-recommendations.

WHO (World Health Organization) (2020e), 'Shortage of Personal Protective Equipment Endangering Health Workers Worldwide', March 2020, https://www.who.int/news/item/03-03-2020-shortage-of-personal-protective-equipment-endangering-health-workers-worldwide.

WHO (World Health Organization) (2020f), 'COVID-19 Supply Chain System: Requesting and Receiving Supplies', April 30, 2020, https://www.who.int/publications/m/item/covid-19-supply-chain-system-requesting-and-receiving-supplies.

WHO (World Health Organization) (2021a), 'Listings of WHO's Response to COVID-19', January 29, 2021, https://www.who.int/news/item/29-06-2020-covidtimeline.

WHO (World Health Organization) (2021b), 'WHO-Convened Global Study of Origins of SARS-CoV-2: China Part', March 30, 2021, https://www.who.int/publications/i/item/who-convened-global-study-of-origins-of-sars-cov-2-china-part.

WHO (World Health Organization) (2021c), 'WHO Director-General's Remarks at the Member State Briefing on the Report of the International Team Studying the Origins of SARS-CoV-2', March 30, 2021, https://www.who.int/director-general/speeches/detail/who-director-general-s-remarks-at-the-member-state-briefing-on-the-report-of-the-international-team-studying-the-origins-of-sars-cov-2convened-global-study-of-origins-of-sars-cov-2-china-part.

WHO (World Health Organization) (2021d), 'COVID-19 Virtual Press Conference Transcript – 13 October 2021', October 13, 2021, https://www.who.int/publications/m/item/covid-19-virtual-press-conference-transcript---13-october-2021.

WHO (World Health Organization) (2021e), '1. COVID-19 pandemic and TB Global Tuberculosis' in *Global Tuberculosis Report 2021*, October 14, 2021, https://www.who.int/publications/digital/global-tuberculosis-report-2021/covid-19.

WHO (World Health Organization) (2021f), 'What is the Act Accelerator', https://www.who.int/initiatives/act-accelerator/about (accessed Nov. 16, 2021).

WHO (World Health Organization) (2021g), 'Assessment of the COVID-19 Supply Chain System: Full Report', April 30, 2021, https://www.who.int/publications/m/item/assessment-of-the-covid-19-supply-chain-system-report.

WHO (World Health Organization) (2021h), Emergency Medical Teams Initiative, 'News', https://extranet.who.int/emt/covid-19 (accessed Nov. 16, 2021).

WHO (World Health Organization) (2021i), 'Health Equity Monitor: Births Attended by Skilled Health Personnel (in the Two or Three Years Preceding the Survey) (%)', The Global Health Observatory, August 27, 2021, https://www.who.int/data/gho/data/indicators/indicator-details/GHO/hem-births-attended-by-skilled-health-personnel-(in-the-two-or-three-years-preceding-the-survey)-(-).

WHO (World Health Organization) (2022a), 'WHO Coronavirus (COVID-19) Dashboard', https://covid19.who.int/ (accessed Apr. 26, 2022).

WHO (World Health Organization) (2022b), 'Sustainable financing: Report of the Working Group', January 10, 2022, WHO Doc EB150/30.

Wilson, Kumanan, Sam Halabi, and Lawrence O. Gostin (2020), 'The International Health Regulations (2005), The Threat of Populism and the COVID-19 Pandemic', *Globalization and Health* 16/70 (2020), https://doi.org/10.1186/s12992-020-00600-4.

World Bank (2021), 'Life Expectancy at Birth, Total (Years)', https://data.worldbank.org/indicator/SP.DYN.LE00.IN (accessed Nov. 16, 2021).

World Food Programme (2021), 'WFP Urges Billionaires to Support 42 Million People on the Edge of Famine', November 3, 2021, https://www.wfp.org/stories/assisting-42-million-people-edge-famine.

WTO (World Trade Organization) (2020a), 'DDG Wolff Urges G20 Trade Ministers to Step Up Engagement on WTO Reform', September 22, 2020, https://www.wto.org/english/news_e/news20_e/igo_22sep20_e.htm.

WTO (World Trade Organization) (2020b), 'Members to Continue Discussion on Proposal for Temporary IP Waiver in Response to COVID-19', December 10, 2020, https://www.wto.org/english/news_e/news20_e/trip_10dec20_e.htm.

WTO (World Trade Organization) (2021), 'TRIPS Waiver: India Engaging WTO Members', November 16, 2021, https://timesofindia.indiatimes.com/business/india-business/trips-waiver-india-engaging-wto-members/articleshow/87728107.cms.

Yashadhana, Aryati, Nellie Pollard-Wharton, AnthonyB. Zwi, and Brett Biles (2020), 'Indigenous Australians at Increased Risk of COVID-19 Due to Existing Health and Socioeconomic Inequities', The Lancet Regional Health—Western Pacific 1, no. 100007 (July 2020), https://doi.org/10.1016/j.lanwpc.2020.100007.

Yaya, San, Helena Yeboah, Carlo Handy Charles, Akaninyene Otu, and Ronald Labonte (2020), 'Ethnic and Racial Disparities in COVID-19-Related Deaths: Counting the Trees, Hiding the Forest', BMJ Global Health 5, no. 6 (June 2020): p. ej002913, http://dx.doi.org/10.1136/bmjgh-2020-002913.

2

Institutionalizing the Duty to Rescue in a Global Health Emergency

Allen Buchanan

It is generally thought that the COVID-19 pandemic is a global health emergency. Emergencies have these characteristics: there is a serious threat of imminent dire harm, the occurrence of the threat was unpredictable, and averting the harm requires rapid action. To the extent that it makes sense to characterize the pandemic as an emergency, it is reasonable to consider whether and, if so, how the duty to rescue is applicable. That is because emergencies typically put people in a position in which they are in need of rescue: without prompt aid from others they will suffer great harm.[1] Timely provision of ventilators, for example, could count as rescue in the context of a pandemic, as could the provision of intensive care specialists and life-saving therapeutics.

My suggestion is not that the duty to rescue is the only relevant basic duty implicated in a global pandemic. There is also a duty to prevent foreseeable harms due to a pandemic when these harms are not imminent, as they are in rescue situations. Although I will focus on the duty to rescue, much of what I say will apply as well to the duty to prevent serious harms.

My aim in this chapter is to show that, in the context of a pandemic that constitutes an emergency, fulfilling the duty to rescue requires institutional innovation. My investigation might be framed using the notion of the duty of Samaritanism rather than that of rescue: both convey the idea of an individual or collective being in a position to render aid needed to avert imminent serious harm.

I will argue that, in preparation for another global health emergency (for example Pandemic X), governments, civil society organizations, and pharmaceutical companies have a duty of justice to work together to create a treaty-based institution that will perfect imperfect duties to rescue. Before I can make the case for this institutional innovation, it will first be necessary to develop an account of the duty to rescue. Having done that, I will then show how two polar political

---

[1] I have argued elsewhere that the emergency framing is perilous unless one is careful to do two things: ask what the scope of the emergency is (who exactly is at high risk for serious harm), and re-evaluate overtime whether the emergency exists and, if so, whether its scope has changed ("Learning from Flawed Responses to the Covid-19 Pandemic," *Social Philosophy & Policy*, forthcoming).

Allen Buchanan, *Institutionalizing the Duty to Rescue in a Global Health Emergency* In: *Pandemic Ethics: From COVID-19 to Disease X*. Edited by: Dominic Wilkinson and Julian Savulescu, Oxford University Press.
© Oxford University Press 2023. DOI: 10.1093/oso/9780192871688.003.0003

views, extreme cosmopolitanism and extreme nationalism, understand the duty to rescue. I will then argue that neither provides a plausible answer to a fundamental question: what are the proper scope and limits of national partiality in a global health emergency? Articulating the flaws of these two views will take us some distance toward understanding the contours of the duties that are in need of being perfected by institutionalization.

Moral cosmopolitans have an expansive conception of the duty to rescue; moral nationalists have a highly constrained conception of it. Moral cosmopolitans of the most extreme sort believe that all institutions, including national ones—and even under emergency conditions—should treat all persons as being worthy of equal consideration. Extreme moral nationalists, in contrast, believe that national institutions are morally permitted to show exclusive concern for a country's own citizens, at least when it comes to positive duties, including duties of rescue. (Even the most extreme moral nationalists, at least if they are in the broadly liberal camp, acknowledge that national partiality is limited by negative duties toward foreigners, including duties not to kill them, enslave them, or expropriate their territories.)

Thomas Pogge is a highly influential moral cosmopolitan (Pogge, 2008); David Miller (Miller, 2012) is in my judgment the most articulate representative of the moral nationalist view. Shortly, I will explore the implications of their respective positions for how the duty to rescue bears on the question of the proper scope and limits of national partiality in a global health emergency such as the current COVID-19 pandemic. First, it is necessary to clarify the duty to rescue in a way that is neutral as to the differences between moral cosmopolitans and moral nationalists.

Philosophers usually discuss the duty to rescue by focusing on a highly simplified, extreme case—a case of easy rescue of one victim by one rescuer. You see a child drowning in a shallow pond. You alone can save the child's life and you can do so without excessive cost to yourself. Moral cosmopolitans like Pogge and moral nationalists like Miller both hold that you have a duty to save the child and that that it is a duty of justice—that you owe the duty to the child or, to put the same point differently, that she has a right to your aid and will be wronged by you if you fail to provide it.

Further, both cosmopolitans and nationalists can acknowledge that the duty to rescue applies more broadly; that it is not limited to cases where the potential rescuer is in close physical proximity to the person in peril. Yet there is a difference as to how the two camps understand the duty in such cases. Cosmopolitans believe that we have duties *of justice* to render aid to persons in severely disadvantaged or perilous circumstances, even if they are far away, are not our fellow citizens, and we have no special relationship to them. Moral nationalists deny that we have duties *of justice* to rescue distant people who are not our fellow citizens and with whom we have no special relationship; instead, they believe we only have duties of beneficence. To appreciate the significance of these contrasting characterizations of the duty to rescue distant strangers, we need to get clear on the distinction between duties of justice and duties of charity or beneficence or humanity.

Duties of justice are traditionally said to be perfect duties, which means that they are directed duties, owed to someone; and that they have determinate content, that they specify clearly what the duty-bearer must do to fulfill the duty. Duties of beneficence, in contrast, are imperfect duties: they are not owed to anyone in particular and they are indeterminate in the sense of allowing the duty-bearer discretion as to whom to aid, when to provide aid, and what form of aid to render. Further, duties of justice are thought to be enforceable; duties of beneficence are not.

2.1 Extreme Nationalism

Let us first consider Miller's view, exploring its implications for the scope and limits of national partiality in a global health emergency. According to Miller, we have a perfect duty of rescue, a duty of justice, a determinate duty owed to the person in peril, only when the following three conditions are satisfied—and it so happens that they are typically only satisfied in cases where the potential rescuer is in close physical proximity to the person in peril.

First, I must be uniquely positioned to save you; second we must encounter each other in such a way that there is a mutual recognition that your safety depends uniquely on me; and third, the encounter must be within the bounds of my "personal space," a physical domain in which I can exercise considerable control and therefore within which I have significant responsibilities. Since Miller thinks these conditions are generally satisfied only when the potential rescuer and the one in need of rescue are in close proximity, he is committed to the view that we do not have duties of justice to citizens of other countries to help them avoid death and serious injury due to a global pandemic.

This is where Miller leaves us: with only imperfect duties to help foreigners in peril. Where he leaves us is, in my opinion, a morally untenable location. That is because imperfect duties have a number of imperfections.

First, the discretion that characterized imperfect duties permits moral laxity. One is morally lax if, over an extended period of time, one fails to take serious steps toward achieving a moral goal one views oneself as morally committed to. In the case of an imperfect duty to rescue, one may be tempted to rationalize doing nothing by consoling oneself with the thought, "Well, I'll do something at some point, for some of those people in peril—and there will always be plenty of such people." Second, due to their inherent vagueness as to how much aid to provide to whom and in what form, imperfect duties are subject to disagreement among those who acknowledge that they have the duty, and such disagreement has two unfortunate consequences: it will be difficult to achieve any consensus on how to evaluate the behavior of the relevant agents and therefore difficult for them to hold each other accountable. Third, even if agents do not succumb to moral laxity and strive to fulfill their duties in the absence of accountability, their efforts are likely to be uncoordinated, with the result that there will be both gaps and redundancies in aid. Fourth, where duties are imperfect, agents may rationalize not acting because they lack assurance that others will act appropriately: they may be unwilling to bear the costs of providing aid if they think others similarly situated are not bearing those costs. This is a feature of lack of enforceability and, more broadly, lack of accountability due to the indeterminacy of the duties. Fifth, where effective aid requires contributions by many parties, the free-rider problem may undercut successful collective action. Each party may reason that either enough others will contribute to achieve success in achieving some particular goal or they will not, regardless of whether she contributes. She may tell herself that it will be better, morally, if she only provides aid independently, not as part of a collective effort. Enforcement can solve such collective action problems, but if imperfect duties are unenforceable that option is not available. The point is that, in some cases, effective aid can only be rendered through a collective effort, because it depends on some threshold of contributions being reached that is beyond the resources of any particular individual. If individuals, because of either the free-rider problem or the assurance problem, do not contribute to such collective aid projects and engage only in independent aid provision, the result may be extremely inefficient.

In brief, in the real world, when it comes to quite imperfect creatures like us, relying solely on imperfect duties to rescue distant strangers in peril is predictably suboptimal from a moral point of view: moral underperformance is virtually guaranteed.

My main worry about Miller's view is that he ends his analysis with an implicit acceptance of a defective moral status quo and fails to consider how a better situation might be achieved. In brief, he fails to consider the fact that *we can work together to create institutions that perfect imperfect duties*—and that failure to do so is a moral fault. Or, to put it differently, he does not consider the possibility that there is a duty to prevent the predictable failures that result from relying only on imperfect duties to rescue distant foreigners. I will first argue that we do have such a duty and then argue that it is a duty of justice.

How can institutions perfect imperfect duties? They can (1) identify specific duty-bearers and right-holders, (2) in such a way as to distribute the costs of rescuing large numbers of people in a fair manner, and (3) can include mechanisms for compliance with the duties they specify, either through the threat of penalties for noncompliance or through rewards for compliance. Effective measures for compliance can prevent both the free-rider and assurance problems from stymying concerted efforts to provide aid, and they can prevent moral laxness.

Because they are both determinate and enforceable, perfect duties facilitate accountability: agents can be evaluated and either rewarded or penalized for failing to act on their professed moral commitments. The vagueness of imperfect duties, in contrast, makes accountability extremely difficult, if not impossible.

This is not merely a possibility; it actually occurs. The modern welfare state is a prime example of an institution that improves our moral situation by perfecting imperfect duties. There are in fact many cases where institutions improve moral performance relative to the noninstitutional situation. They do this by changing incentives and more specifically by providing incentives that counteract moral underperformance. For example, where there are clear, justiciable, and well-enforced property rights, with determinate correlative duties, people are better able to respect other individuals' claims to various objects, and opportunities for wrongful takings will be reduced. Where the law approximates key elements of the rule of law, unscrupulous government officials are less able to abuse the power of the law. The general point is that institutions can better enable us to act on our moral commitments; the particular point is that this applies to the commitment to the well-being of others that underpins the duty to rescue in the context of a pandemic.

If we have good moral reasons to rescue people in peril, then we ought to ensure that we are effective in rendering aid. Being committed to their safety means that we should not accept a situation in which aid will either not be forthcoming, or will be inadequate, or will be so seriously uncoordinated that some aid is wasted by being superfluous and some people in need will not receive it. If we can improve the moral status quo by working together to create institutions that, by perfecting imperfect duties of rescue, will better achieve the goal of preventing imminent serious harms, we ought morally to do so.

An analogy may help drive this basic point home. Suppose that I regularly encounter children drowning in a pond near my home, but am not able to rescue many of them because the pond is deep, they are typically far from the shore, and I am not a strong swimmer. I am able to save some of them, the ones that happen to be near to shore, but not most. So, I direct my efforts only to those who are close enough to shore that I can reach them, given my limited skills as a swimmer.

But now suppose that I have in my possession simple instructions for building a boat that will enable me to rescue any child in peril, and suppose also that I have all the necessary materials or can easily get them. I also have neighbors I can call upon to help me build the rescue boat. Surely, if I really care about saving lives, I will not rest content with a situation where my rescue efforts are so far from optimal. Instead, I will rightly feel obligated to increase the efficacy of my efforts by cooperating with my neighbors to construct a rescue boat.

Similarly, if we can construct institutions that will greatly increase the efficacy of our efforts to help foreigners imperiled by a pandemic, and we can do so without excessive costs to ourselves, we ought to do so. Moral consistency—indeed, integrity—requires that we do so. Notice that this conclusion applies not only to rescue, where harm is imminent, but also to prevention, where it is not.

2.2 The Moral Necessity of Institutionalizing Duties of Justice, not Just Duties of Beneficence

My strategy has been to begin to make the case for institutional innovation in preparation for the next pandemic by starting with a premise that even the most extreme anti-cosmopolitans can accept: that there is a duty of beneficence to prevent and mitigate serious harms to distant strangers. I will now show that the need for institutional innovation also applies if one assumes there is a duty of justice to prevent and mitigate serious harms to distant strangers.

This conclusion will seem counter-intuitive if one assumes that all duties of justice are perfect duties, where this means that they are all *both* undirected *and* determinate in content, that is, specific with respect to what is required of the duty-bearer. But that assumption, I will show, is unwarranted. Some duties of justice, including the duty of wealthy countries to prevent and mitigate serious harms to persons in poor countries, have one of the two features that are said to characterize imperfect duties, namely, indeterminacy of content. The more general point is that some duties of justice are quite unlike the duty to fulfill a promise, which is perfect in both respects, that is, directed and determinate in content. The failure to appreciate this fact may be due to taking the case of promising as paradigmatic of duties of justice.

In the case of the duty to prevent and mitigate serious harms due to a pandemic, there are several sources of indeterminacy as to exactly what is required of the duty-bearers. First, the duty by itself sets no priorities, yet even the resources of wealthy countries are limited and may not allow for helping all of those in peril. One needs to know whom to help first and who should get the most aid. Second, although whatever actions are to be taken to avert serious harms to those in poor countries may be constrained by some degree of partiality toward co-nationals, there is much honest disagreement about how robust this constraint is. Third, the duty to prevent and mitigate serious harms is presumably subject to a "no excessive cost" proviso; but what counts as an excessive cost may depend in part on what cost others are bearing. For example, one country bearing disproportionately greater costs because others were not acting appropriately either might be unfair in itself or might put the more generous country at a competitive disadvantage vis-à-vis those bearing lesser costs. In the absence of institutions to distribute costs fairly, duty-bearers may not be able to determine what counts as excessive costs; and until they know that, they will not know what exactly is required of them. Finally, without an institution to coordinate efforts on the basis of the best information available, even conscientious government officials may not know how to provide aid in a reasonably effective and efficient manner.

So, even if duties of justice are unlike imperfect duties of beneficence in that they are directed, they can in some cases share the other feature of imperfect duties, indeterminacy of content. One can know that one ought to, as a matter of justice, help prevent and mitigate serious harms to distant strangers, but not know exactly how to proceed in order to fulfill the duty in a reasonable and responsible manner.

This indeterminacy of content in the case of the duty to prevent serious harms, even when it is considered to be a duty of justice, facilitates the moral underperformance we encountered earlier in the world in which only the duty of beneficence existed. It encourages moral laxity, bias in the provision of aid, and inefficient discoordination. To rest content with these deficiencies when they can be reduced or eliminated is itself a moral fault.

It seems clear then that, under circumstances like those we now find ourselves in in the midst of a global pandemic, we have a duty to work together to construct institutions that will enable us to act more effectively on our moral commitments by perfecting imperfect duties of rescue. The only question is the status of that duty: is it a duty of justice, a perfect duty; or is it a duty of beneficence or charity or humanity, an imperfect duty? If we fail to work together to construct the needed institutions, do we wrong those who will perish because we failed to do so? Can they rightly say that we wronged them?

Here Rawls's notion of a natural duty of justice is helpful. The highly plausible claim is that, out of recognition of the basic moral equality of all persons, that is, to show proper respect and concern for all persons, we ought to cooperate to create conditions in which they will enjoy the benefits of justice. This is not a new idea. Kant thought that there is a fundamental duty to create conditions in which we can relate to others in a just way. For Hobbes the worst thing about the state of nature is that there is no justice.

It is a commonplace that justice means giving each person her due. Following Kant, Hobbes, and Rawls, my suggestion is that giving each person her due means, inter alia, establishing conditions in which there are clear duties of justice, if doing that is what is needed to secure their fundamental interests, including their interests in survival. In other words, I think the duty to work together to create institutions that perfect imperfect duties is a duty of justice. I think we wrong people if we fail to try to construct institutions that will perfect imperfect duties when doing so is vital for their very survival and we can do this without excessive cost to ourselves. I think that resting content with imperfect duties in such cases exhibits such a serious disregard for the welfare of those in peril as to constitute a failure to acknowledge their basic equal moral status as persons, and that this is to wrong them, to fail to accord them what is their due.

At this juncture, one might think that the same line of reasoning shows that the duty to rescue distant strangers is itself a duty of justice, even though, in the absence of institutionalization, it lacks sufficient determinacy to provide adequate practical guidance. In reply it could be said that, absent institutionalization, this duty is so indeterminate in content that one cannot say that any individual is wronged if they are not rescued, but that this need not be the case with the duty to create the relevant institution.

If the duty to construct institutions to perfect imperfect duties were too abstract and indeterminate, it would not qualify as a perfect duty and hence could not be a duty of justice.

I would argue that at present that is not so. We have good reason to believe there will be another pandemic and we cannot be confident that it will only occur so far in the future that we need do nothing now to prepare for it. Consequently, there is something very specific that wealthier countries, pharmas, and health-related civil society organizations ought to do *now*: namely, begin the process of building an institution to create a fair distribution of effectively incentivized, directed duties to ensure that those most endangered by the next global health crisis receive relief. Because it is unclear how long it will take to build the needed institutions, it is imperative to start now. One cannot plausibly say, "Oh, well, we'll do something, sometime." This would be like saying, "Oh, well, someday I'll build a boat to rescue children farther out in the pond," when a child may be drowning in the middle of the lake tomorrow.

In the current pandemic, we have seen the moral failures that result from the lack of institutions that would perfect imperfect duties—institutions that would identify duty-bearers, direct their duties toward specific recipients of aid, fairly distribute the duties so that no one bears unacceptably high or disproportionate costs in fulfilling their duties, and provide effective incentives for compliance with the assigned duties. Governments of wealthy countries and leaders of pharmaceutical companies have for the most part acknowledged that they ought to do *something* to ensure that poor countries have access to vaccines and other medical resources, but little has been done.

When duties are left imperfect, it is all but impossible to hold governments or pharmaceutical companies to account. Imperfect duties are too indeterminate and allow the duty-bearer too much discretion to make accountability feasible. Matters change dramatically when we can point to determinate, directed duties and ask whether they are being fulfilled.

Whether institutions that can perfect duties of rescue in a global pandemic can be constructed will depend crucially on the cooperation of governments and pharmaceutical companies. The public ought to mobilize to hold them accountable for helping to create conditions in which they can be held accountable. Acting alone, members of the public may have little power, but civil society organizations can mobilize and focus public opinion in ways that governments and pharmas may find it difficult to ignore.

2.3 A Dynamic Conception of Morality

My criticism of Miller can now be recast in general terms that have broad implications for moral philosophy. I reject his implicit and insupportable assumption
that the boundaries of justice are fixed and more specifically that the duty to rescue, as a duty of justice, cannot extend to rescuing distant strangers. If, as his
analysis implies, under present conditions there are only imperfect duties, not
duties of justice to prevent massive imminent harms to foreigners when we can
do so without serious cost to ourselves, then the proper response is not to acqui-
esce in this morally deficient situation, but rather to change it. I have argued that
the duty to perfect imperfect duties in this case is a duty of justice. Whether that
is so or not is irrelevant, however, to my dissatisfaction with where Miller's analysis leaves us. He takes the moral landscape as fixed, not recognizing that we can
and ought to change it.

Unfortunately, I think this static view of morality—in this case the assumption
that the boundary between justice, on the one hand, and beneficence (or charity
or humanity) on the other, is forever fixed—is all too common in contemporary
moral philosophy.[2] The problem with the static view is that it underestimates the
power of human beings to transform their moral predicament and thereby erects
an obstacle to moral progress. If we assume the static viewpoint, we can only
wring one's hands in response to some of the worst deficiencies of responses to
the current pandemic; we will not be in a position to see that we can do better
next time around.

I conclude, then, that Miller has not vindicated an extreme moral nationalist
position; he has given us no good reason to think that the duty of rescue cannot
be invoked to ground a policy of restricting national partiality for the sake of rescuing distant strangers, as a matter of justice. More specifically, he has not shown
that rich countries suffering relatively low mortality and little serious morbidity
from the pandemic have no obligations of justice to provide aid to countries
where the pandemic is much more lethal and that lack the resources for limiting
its lethality. My aim, however, is not to criticize Miller, but to expose the shortcomings of any extreme nationalist view on duties of rescue in a pandemic.

2.4 Extreme Cosmopolitanism

I now turn to an analysis of Pogge's view, as perhaps the most developed and
prominent instance of an extreme cosmopolitan view that has clear implications
for how we ought to frame our response to a global pandemic. He argues that

---

[2] For an argument to show that the boundaries of justice are not fixed, see Allen Buchanan, "Justice
and Charity," *Ethics*, Vol. 97, No. 3 (1987), 558–75.

citizens of wealthy countries have duties of justice to combat poverty and disease in poor countries, not just in the special case of pandemics but on an ongoing basis, because they are morally responsible for the disadvantaged positions the people of those countries occupy and which make them especially vulnerable to disease. Pogge thinks we are responsible for their disadvantaged position and its negative health consequences because we have caused the harms they suffer by participating in (and benefitting from) an unjust international order. Pogge does not frame his argument in terms of the duty to rescue. Nonetheless, it will be fruitful to construe it that way, since his approach to helping the world's most disadvantaged people can accommodate the idea that in some cases their plight is so dire that the notion of rescue applies.

In the case at hand, Pogge might well argue that most if not all countries that cannot afford vaccines are in this predicament because their economic development has been impeded by certain features of the international order, features that facilitate destructive, exploitive behavior on the part of both their own governments and powerful states and corporations. Instead of relying on a duty of rescue understood as a positive duty or, more generally, on a duty to prevent dire harm, whether imminent or not, Pogge opts for the idea of a duty of justice to mitigate harms for which we are responsible because we have caused them.

I find this approach to be both problematic and unnecessarily indirect. Pogge develops it because he thinks it is less controversial to argue for relieving the plight of the world's worst-off people from the premise that there is a duty not to harm, a negative duty, than from the premise that there is a positive duty, more specifically a duty to prevent harms one has not caused and is not in any way responsible for. Whether Pogge is right in assuming that more people will in fact acknowledge a negative rather than a positive duty is an empirical matter on which I choose not to speculate. But I think it is clear that Pogge's argument for why those in wealthier countries have a duty of justice to repair the damage of the international system they supposedly support and are causally implicated in is dubious. Opting for a duty not to harm in this case turns out to be a lot more costly in terms of argumentative cogency than Pogge assumes.

Pogge's approach is problematic for at least two reasons: first, it is far from clear that by merely acquiescing and/or benefitting from the unjust international order one is causing the harm it produces or is for some other reason responsible for that harm. Even if it could be established that you and I are making some causal contribution, it is presumably so miniscule as to be incapable of grounding any significant obligation. Second, Pogge overestimates the power of ordinary citizens to control their countries' policies—in this case, to achieve reform of the unjust international order or, failing that, to facilitate a massive transfer of resources from the rich to the poor. Further, if we lack this control, then it is all the more implausible to say either that we are causing the harms inflicted by that order or that we are responsible for them.

In addition, Pogge's approach is unnecessarily indirect because it assumes that one must first establish responsibility for a harm in order to show that one has a duty of justice to prevent that harm. That, in effect, is simply to deny that any duty of rescue is a duty of justice, including the duty to save the child in the pond. That is an extremely implausible view. One needn't show that a person is responsible for the child being in the pond in order to show that that person has a duty of justice to rescue the child.

My framing of the need to act in a global emergency avoids both the drawbacks of Pogge's view and the disturbing complacency of Miller's. My argument for why, as a matter of justice, we ought to work together to create institutions that will extend the domain of justice and not rest content with imperfect duties does not assume, as Pogge's argument does, that we are obligated, as a matter of justice, only for mitigating those harms we ourselves cause. On my view, it is not necessary to show that we are responsible in any way, either directly or indirectly, for the harms we have a duty of justice to prevent.

2.5 A Positive Cosmopolitan Duty

Given the problems of Pogge's brand of cosmopolitanism, it is worth considering whether a cosmopolitan account of the duty to rescue might be developed on the basis of a positive duty to aid, more specifically a duty to prevent imminent serious harms. The straightforward idea here would be that it is unnecessary to show that the better-off have somehow caused the special vulnerability of the worst-off to the damage due to a pandemic. Instead, they have a duty to rescue the latter from serious, pandemic-caused harms simply as a matter of recognizing the equal worth of all persons. In its extreme form, this cosmopolitan view denies that any national partiality is justified: aid should be rendered on the basis of need, regardless of boundaries.

I will assess this version of cosmopolitanism indirectly, by considering the limitations of three arguments for national partiality. The upshot of my analysis will be that, while these three arguments do not vindicate extreme nationalism, they do suffice to discredit extreme cosmopolitanism, including versions of that view that, unlike Pogge's account, rely on a positive duty. One advantage of this strategy is that my assessments will apply to both the duty to rescue and the duty to prevent pandemic-caused harms.

The three arguments for national priority are (1) the argument from the division of labor, (2) the argument from special obligations, and (3) the argument from local knowledge. Let us consider each in turn.

It is a fact about our world that there is no world government and that if justice and welfare are to be achieved it will be largely within and partly through the efforts of states. Given the lack of a world government and the greater resources and capacities of states relative to other institutions, it makes sense to acknow-ledge a division of labor, with states having the chief responsibility for the free-dom and welfare of those within their jurisdiction. But if states are to fulfill this role, it is proper that they should show partiality to their own citizens—after all, the responsibility for securing the freedom and welfare of those people rests on the shoulders of their state.

This first argument suffices to show that states may show some partiality to their own citizens in a global emergency such as the current pandemic. But it falls short of justifying the extreme partiality that the wealthier countries have in fact exhibited. That is because the argument is subject to two important limitations. The first and most obvious is that not all countries have the resources or the gov-ernment leadership to discharge the burden of securing the welfare and freedom of their citizens without external help. This simple fact is of extreme importance in the current pandemic because it is well documented that pandemics are most damaging in poorer countries. Such countries have more vulnerable populations due to poor medical care, nutrition, sanitation, and housing prior to the pan-demic, and because they have fewer resources for mitigating the damage caused by the pandemic.

The second limitation on the division of labor argument for national partiality is that wealthy countries have surplus capacity when it comes to responding effectively to a pandemic like the one we are now experiencing. They can reduce the risk of the pandemic to their own citizens to reasonable levels, compatible with their fiduciary duties to them, and still have resources to bestow on coun-tries that will suffer much greater harm if they do not receive external aid. When one combines the fact that some countries cannot achieve a reasonable response to the pandemic on their own with the fact that some countries have surplus capacity and resources, the inescapable conclusion is that the division of labor argument does not establish the conclusion that countries may exercise unre-strained partiality.

To drive home this point it is necessary to explain what counts as surplus capacity and resources. Surplus here means in excess of what is adequate, not what is optimal from the standpoint of reducing COVID-19 infection or medical or economic damage due to infections. To assume the latter would be to make the fundamental errors noted earlier: to ignore the marginal costs of risk reduction—including the costs to others who will be deprived of resources used for additional increments of risk reduction—and to think that the proper goal is to reduce the risk to as near to zero as possible.[3]

---

[3] Unfortunately, some public health experts seem to have convinced government leaders in the US that the goal is to stop or reduce as much as possible the spread of COVID-19—without regard to the economic, psychosocial, and other costs of doing so. I have argued elsewhere that this goal is morally untenable for two reasons: first, even from the standpoint of an exclusive focus on the well-being of Americans, it is wrong to ignore the costs of reducing the harms caused by COVID-19; second,

As noted earlier, in the early stages of global health threat, when there is great uncertainty as to just how bad things may get, state leaders, in honoring their special fiduciary obligations to their own citizens are permitted act with extreme partiality. In other words, under these conditions it is appropriate for leaders and the public to employ the emergency framing and to act on the assumption that national partiality is permitted. But once it becomes clear that the situation for those in wealthy countries is not so dire—and indeed that it is no longer right to call it an emergency—such extreme partiality is no longer justified.

In my judgment, it became clear quite some time ago that the risks posed to citizens of most of the wealthier countries was not so severe, relative to the resources those countries possess, that their leaders should disregard the far greater needs of people who don't happen to be their fellow citizens. And, as I also suggested earlier, it is simply incredible to assume that we are still in an emergency if morbidity and mortality from COVID-19 reach levels close to that of a normal or even somewhat unusually severe flu season.

The key point here is that, once we have gotten past the extreme uncertainty of the initial situation, what a country regards as an acceptable level of resource expenditure to protect its own citizens should not only avoid the hysteria of trying to reduce harm to zero but should also take into account the proportion between the harm to its own citizens that can be averted by additional risk reduction measures and the harm that foreigners will suffer if they do not have access to those resources.

Let me hasten to add that I am not advocating significant limitations on national partiality in all circumstances. I am willing to take seriously the possibility that if we faced a pandemic that was both more easily transmitted than COVID-19 and also had a much, much greater case morbidity rate—say 40%—it would be a kind of lifeboat ethics situation in which extreme, virtually unlimited national partiality would be justified. Or, I should say, such extreme partiality would be justified until the emergency had subsided. In other words, in a much more lethal pandemic than the one we are now experiencing, national partiality might trump the triage principle and negate the duty to rescue foreigners. The point is simply that we in the wealthier countries are nowhere near that extreme situation now, though our leaders are acting as if we were.

It is also worth pointing out that the argument from the division of labor features a gaping logical gap: from the premise that there is no world government it does not follow that each country should be responsible for the health needs of its

---

continuing to pursue the goal of stopping the spread of the virus beyond the point at which the risk caused by infection to Americans is tolerable is most likely to result in this wealthy country not doing enough to help people in greater need in poorer countries. There is one more negative consequence of the obsession with stopping the spread of the virus: it obscures a hard moral question, namely, how much cost should the vast majority who are not at risk of death or serious damage from COVID-19 bear to try to protect a tiny minority at high risk?

citizens. That is because the only alternatives are not a world government or exclusive reliance on self-help. A third alternative is to develop specific international institutions to convert imperfect duties of rescue to perfect duties of justice. Further, the institutional innovation could be quite specific and limited: its mission could be restricted to responding equitably and effectively to global pandemics.

Once we understand the flaws of the division of labor argument, it becomes clear that we should not succumb to the following fallacy: justifying refusal to cooperate to construct international institutions to create a duty to rescue as a duty of justice on the grounds that it conflicts with national partiality, and then justifying national partiality on the grounds that each nation must look out for itself exclusively because of the lack of international institutions.

The second argument for national partiality is simple: on the whole, the citizens of a country are in ongoing relationships of interdependence that are denser than their relations with foreigners. Special relationships generate special obligations here (as they do in families and friendships). The state, as the agent of the people, should facilitate the fulfillment of those obligations. Among those obligations are those of aid in times of danger. So, because of the special relationships among co-nationals and the special obligations they generate, it is appropriate for the state to exhibit national partiality in the face of a pandemic.

The problem with this second argument is that, like the argument from the division of labor, it only shows that some partiality, in some circumstances, is warranted, without either acknowledging or illuminating the moral limits of partiality. This becomes clear when we probe the analogy that proponents of the argument almost invariably use: that of the family or a friendship. If I am a wealthy person and there are many people who are not my friends or family who are in desperate need, then I can show proper partiality to those near and dear to me and still do something significant for the worst-off. Showing proper partiality to my son doesn't mean giving him a Mercedes rather than a Chevrolet, especially if the difference between what a Mercedes costs and a Chevrolet costs would save the life of someone who doesn't happen to be my son. Similarly, proper partiality toward American citizens does not mean spending all the money that might reduce the risk of COVID-19 infection for all of them, rather focusing on the most vulnerable of them.

The third argument for national partiality is even flimsier than the preceding two—if considered as an argument for extreme, virtually unlimited partiality.

Yes, it is true that local knowledge is often superior. But that is not always true when it comes to public health knowledge. Some countries are so poor that they lack not only a decent medical infrastructure but also decent information infrastructure, especially for information relevant to responding effectively to a pandemic. But even where local knowledge is superior, this does not rule out external aid; it only rules out external aid that ignores rather than partners with people on the ground.

An assessment of the three arguments for national partiality yields this conclusion, then: at best they show that some national partiality is justified in some circumstances and that consequently extreme cosmopolitanism, which denies the permissibility of any national partiality whatsoever, is untenable. But they do not establish extreme national partiality. This means that the duties that are to be institutionalized will reflect a rejection of both extreme cosmopolitanism and extreme nationalism. In this chapter I do not have the space to say more about the contours of the duties to be institutionalized, but instead will now proceed to outline what the institution should look like. Doing so will, I hope, help start the process of developing a moral coordination point that can lend sufficient determinacy to the duty to create the institution so as to vindicate my claim that there is such a duty and that it is already or soon could be determinate enough to be taken seriously.

2.6 Institutional Design

My chief conclusion in this chapter has been that there is a need for institutional innovation, aimed at ensuring a more effective, efficient, and ethical response to a future Pandemic X than was seen in the COVID pandemic. We need such innovation regardless of whether the duty to rescue distant strangers is (as cosmopolitans think) a duty of justice or (as nationalists think) a duty of beneficence. I have also argued that the duty to help create the needed institution will itself remain unhelpfully indeterminate without a normative coordination point, at least an outline of the main features the institution should possess. In this section, I begin the task of supplying that.

2.6.1 Creation or modification?

Should it be a new institution or a modification of an existing one? There are existing three candidates for modification: WHO, Gavi, and COVAX. In my judgment, each is sufficiently problematic that building on it would be inadvisable.

WHO (the World Health Organization) has suffered a loss of sociological legitimacy that will make it difficult for it to take on the more ambitious mission of perfecting imperfect duties of rescue in a pandemic. In particular, it has proved unable to stand up to China, in demanding timely information concerning the origins and early spread of COVID-19 and more generally is unable to act effectively in the face of political pressure from member states, especially the most powerful of these. It has also been unable or unwilling to work well with pharmas.

Gavi (formerly, the Global Alliance for Vaccines and Immunization) has operated with a seriously defective rationing system that ignores differences in need among vaccine recipient countries. In addition, its policies are unduly influenced by the preferences of one major donor, the Gates Foundation.

COVAX (COVID-19 Vaccines Global Access) has not achieved its vaccine distribution goal (only 5% of the projected 2 billion doses), and what distribution it has achieved has been grossly inequitable (90% to the richest G20 countries). In addition, there have been justifiable complaints of lack of transparency.

Given these problems, there is much to be said for creating a new institution, one that will not inherit the credibility deficits that would be entailed by building on any or all three of these entities. So let us now consider, in broad outline, what a new institution should look like.

2.6.2 Key moral desiderata

First, there is a need for principles and mechanisms for the distribution to poorer countries of vaccines and other medical supplies needed in a pandemic, compatible with fair rationing of these resources within countries. Second, the institution should at least approximate a fair distribution of the costs of providing aid, in part by a progressive schedule of contributions, with richer countries paying more. Third, the institution should be structured in such a way as to guarantee meaningful participation by the beneficiaries of aid, especially with regard to measures for accountability.

2.6.3 Structural-Procedural Desiderata

(1) The design of the institution should exemplify incentive compatibility with regard to joining, continued participation, and general institutional functioning.

(2) The institution should also be designed and presented to publics in such a fashion as to achieve sociological legitimacy, without which it will be unlikely to function successfully.

(3) The more important operations of the institution should be reasonably transparent, where this means, inter alia, that the institution should facilitate access to its operations on the part of credible external epistemic communities (such as non-governmental organizations), both for purposes of achieving sociological legitimacy and for effective accountability mechanisms.

(4) The institution should be engineered for adaptability in the face of changing challenges over time.

(5) There should be a clear delineation of the terms of accountability, including
   (i) specification of the key criteria for evaluating institutional performance,
   (ii) identification of the primary accountability-holders (those who are

tasked with applying the criteria for evaluation), and (iii) measures to impose costs on relevant institutional agents in the event of a negative evaluation by the primary accountability-holders.

2.6.4 Formal or Informal?

The institution should be treaty-based for three reasons: (1) legally binding commitments are, other things being equal, more effective in preventing free-rider and assurance problems and preventing shirking; (2) international treaty law provides procedures for creating institutions that help them achieve sociological legitimacy, which is important for effectiveness, and (3) legal obligations provide clear, public moral coordination points for mobilizing public pressure on governments and pharmas.

2.6.5 The Big Question: Why Should Rich Countries Ratify such a Treaty?

I remain unconvinced that self-interest on the part of the government leaders of wealthy countries will suffice. They may quite reasonably conclude that they can deal effectively enough with a future pandemic within their countries' borders to sustain their own power while indulging in excessive national partiality. I think it most probable that they will only participate sincerely in the needed institution if prompted to do so by sustained, focused public pressure. I think it is also highly likely that such pressure will not be achieved unless there is a clear moral coordination point: a reasonably detailed outline of what the needed institution would look like along with an understandable explanation of why it is needed. In the last section of this chapter, I have pointed the way toward achieving this first step on the path to institutional innovation.

Bibliography

Miller, David (2012), *National Responsibility and Global Justice* (Oxford: Oxford University Press).

Pogge, Thomas (2008), *World Poverty and Human Rights* (Cambridge: Polity).

3

The Uneasy Relationship between Human Rights and Public Health

Lessons from COVID-19

John Tasioulas

3.1 Introduction

In October 2019, the Global Health Security Index published its ranking of countries' preparedness for a health crisis, a mere two months before China informed the World Health Organization (WHO) of the outbreak of an acute respiratory illness in Wuhan—the new type of coronavirus now known as COVID-19 (see Global Health Security Index 2019: 20). In the ranking, the United States was placed top and the United Kingdom was runner-up. But these were two countries that, in fact, experienced great difficulty in controlling the effects of COVID-19, at least prior to the large-scale availability of vaccines. Meanwhile, countries that responded to the pandemic much more effectively, such as Singapore and New Zealand, were ranked twenty-eighth and fifty-fourth, respectively. These facts underline not only how poorly prepared some wealthy democratic states were to deal with a devastating health crisis but also how limited our ability is to measure preparedness for a health crisis in advance of its occurrence. The issue of preparedness, of course, goes beyond the narrow focus on individual states, and extends to the question of whether international law and international organizations, such as the WHO itself, are focused on appropriate health priorities and have at their disposal effective means—including requisite levels of cooperation from states—to achieve them.

Of course, preparedness for a health crisis has multiple dimensions. These include adequate stockpiling of personal protective equipment (PPE), ensuring the ability to overcome the problems of disrupted global supply chains, establishing clear lines of authority among regionally and institutionally dispersed decision-makers, and so on. But in this chapter I wish to focus on another kind of preparedness that the COVID-19 pandemic has made salient. This is preparedness with respect to the basic ethical categories we invoke in addressing major health crises of this magnitude. An essential part of such preparedness consists in

John Tasioulas, *The Uneasy Relationship between Human Rights and Public Health: Lessons from COVID-19*
In: *Pandemic Ethics: From COVID-19 to Disease X*. Edited by: Dominic Wilkinson and Julian Savulescu,
Oxford University Press. © Oxford University Press 2023. DOI: 10.1093/oso/9780192871688.003.0004

clear, defensible, and widely understood articulations of the relevant values governing health policy, including the goals it should be focused on, their interrelations, and how those goals may best be pursued.

The need for preparedness in our ethical repertoire is often obscured by politicians' and policymakers' desire to avoid being perceived as making life-and-death decisions based on controversial value judgments. Consequent avoidance tactics often take the form of portraying the relevant objectives of health policy as obvious to all and therefore not in need of either articulation or defence, or else the related form of treating health policy as a value-free technocratic exercise. In the United Kingdom, for example, the government studiously reiterated the mantra that it was "following the science" in responding to the COVID-19 pandemic. But this attempt to present a series of political value judgments—judgments about the proper objectives of health policy in response to the pandemic and the appropriate means for their realization—as fundamentally matters of scientific expertise, is, of course, conceptually obtuse, and ultimately an evasion of political responsibility. Sadly, in the United Kingdom and elsewhere, the attempt to pass the buck on to scientists for liberty-restricting measures such as lockdown led to ugly threats and attacks on scientists with advisory roles in the formation of pandemic policy (see Sridhar 2022: 154ff.).

There is no question of simply "following the science" when it comes to public health policy, because while science offers guidance for our beliefs about the world, it does not by itself instruct us as to how we should act in that world. In order to address the latter issue, we need to conjoin our most reliable scientific beliefs with a clear and defensible conception of our values. Epidemiologists inform us about the relative effectiveness of lockdowns or regimes of contact tracing in stemming the spread of COVID-19, and economists give us a picture of the economic cost of adopting such measures. But neither set of experts is equipped, simply in virtue of disciplinary competence, to make the multiple judgments needed in discerning which policy best realizes the values in play—saving lives, promoting health, respecting rights, mitigating inequality, and ensuring the ongoing economic prosperity needed to do all these things. The issue I wish to address in this chapter is that of our intellectual preparedness to deal with the COVID-19 pandemic in terms of our grasp of the relevant values, their interrelations, and their practical implications. Philosophers, I believe, can make valuable contributions to improving our preparedness to deal with health crises like COVID-19 by interrogating some of the key ideas we bring to bear when thinking through the challenges such crises pose.

Now, an easy way for me to establish my thesis of a lack of ethical preparedness would be to target the predominance of utilitarian and economistic modes of thought—both variants of a more general consequentialist stance—in public health policy. These modes of thought are often presented under the ubiquitous and seemingly commonsensical guise of 'cost-benefit analysis'. Despite their prominence—attributable in large part to the borrowed aura of scientific object-ivity and mathematical prevision that surrounds them—these approaches tend to suffer from two large defects. The first is a tendency to reduce values to what is subjectively *valued*—and often, indeed, valued in terms of the crude economistic measure of what one is actually willing and able to pay for. Second, they are com-mitted to forms of optimization across persons that threaten to lose sight of the inherent dignity of each individual human being. This dignity—which should largely, but not exclusively, be articulated by means of the notion of individual rights—erects powerful barriers to sacrificing individuals on the altar of the aggregate good of society as a whole. Various forms of this second objection were, I believe, at the root of the popular dismay at the United Kingdom government's apparent initial policy—based on a strategy initially developed for tackling swine flu and influenza—of promoting 'herd immunity' through the natural spread of COVID-19, rather than through mass vaccination (Sridhar 2022: 1371–147).

Instead of this comparatively easy target, however, I am going to focus on an entrenched public health discourse that *does* claim to uphold the dignity of each individual human being. This is the discourse of human rights in its application to public health policy. Although it embodies a very laudable ideal, I believe that much of our contemporary thinking about human rights, especially in the health context, is in poor shape, and that this contributes in no small measure to our lack of intellectual preparedness for dealing with a health crisis of societal and global proportions like the COVID-19 pandemic. Indeed, much of this discourse consists of little more than a thin rhetorical veneer, in which slogans about dig-nity and rights serve to mask the stubborn persistence of utilitarian and conse-quentialist modes of thinking in driving policy formation.

Failures to understand human rights, and how they relate to other values, ham-per us in fashioning public health policies that can win the intelligent support of our fellow citizens. Here, I am going to discuss two kinds of endemic errors about human rights: (1) errors regarding both the *scope* and *content* of human rights, and (2) errors about human rights' relation to certain other important values, i.e. *common goods* and *democracy*. In discussing human rights, I shall take as my main example the human right to health, both because of its obvious relevance in the present context and because the dominant understandings of it starkly illus-trate the two errors I have mentioned. Indeed, it is arguable that the standard understanding of the right to health in international human rights discourse is especially flawed, even in comparison with other human rights. This is partly because the discourse of socio-economic ('second generation') rights is historic-ally less developed than that of civil and political ('first generation') rights, but it is also partly owing to distinctive pathologies afflicting the interpretation of the right to health in particular.

The human right to health is listed in many key international human rights instruments—e.g. Article 25 of the Universal Declaration of Human Rights

(1948), and Article 1 of the International Covenant of Economic, Social, and Cultural Rights (1966), which refers to "the right of everyone to the enjoyment of the highest attainable standard of physical and mental health". This formulation, especially in referring to the "highest attainable standard", is open to various objections relating to its feasibility. But I shall assume that it is amenable to an interpretation that enables it to be affirmed as giving effect to a human right, by which I mean a moral right possessed by all human beings simply in virtue of their humanity. Now, much of the human rights discourse that I shall criticize in this chapter relates to international human rights law. However, I believe there is an important connection between the moral conception of human rights and this body of law, since the formative aim of the latter is to give expression and effect to the former to the extent that it is appropriate to do so through giving all human beings individual rights under international law (see Tasioulas 2017a). Therefore, any acceptable understanding of the right to health in human rights law must be defensible as an appropriate legalization of background moral rights, including the moral right to health.

3.2 Scope

The first worry I am going to address concerns the scope of the right to health. By scope, I mean the abstract subject matter or topic that the duties associated with the right are concerned with. It is natural to think that some human rights obligations with a given subject matter properly come within the scope of a given right, whereas other such obligations come within the scope of different rights. Positive duties to prevent people from suffering hunger come within the scope of the right to food (or, perhaps more broadly, the right to an adequate standard of living, under which the right to food can be subsumed as a component), not the right to freedom of religion or a fair trial. This is so despite the fact that it is unlikely that someone suffering from extreme hunger can effectively exercise either their right to freedom of religion or their right to a fair trial. Equally, the duty to allow people to participate in the political life of their community falls within the right to political participation, not the right to privacy or to health. This is so even if, as a matter of empirical fact, those who have the former right respected are better able to secure the latter rights, as is suggested by the social scientific literature showing that democratic governance is key to the upholding of human rights generally.

Now, the remarkable thing about the standard understanding of the human right to health—reflected in numerous international instruments, such as the General Comments issued by the relevant UN treaty bodies, as well as in the works of leading academic writers on global health justice—is that it is taken to be *extremely* capacious in scope. It encompasses not only duties pertaining to such matters as medical care or public health measures but also entitlements to goods such as the following: food, housing, life, education, privacy, access to information, sex-based equality, work, social inclusion, and freedom from torture and other cruel and inhuman or degrading treatment or punishment (see UN Committee on Economic, Social, and Cultural Rights 2000; Office of the United Nations Commissioner for Human Rights and the World Health Organization 2008; Gostin 2014). The result is that the subject matter of the right to health massively overlaps with other rights listed in the Universal Declaration of Human Rights, including the rights to an adequate standard of living, political participation, freedom from torture, access to work, and so on. The right to health is not the only human right that exemplifies this phenomenon of bloated scope, nor is it a phenomenon restricted to socio-economic rights—the comparative newcomers to human rights discourse. The recent General Comment 36 on the right to life, for example, construes this classic civil right as a 'right to enjoy a life with dignity', and interprets it in a way that massively encroaches on the scope of many other rights, including notably socio-economic rights (see UN Human Rights Committee 2018).

The bloated interpretation of the scope of rights presumably finds its rationale in the assumption that the scope of a right extends as far as the interest under-lying that right (health, life with dignity, etc.), or at least as far as that interest generates, or forms part of the case for generating, duties owed to every human being simply in virtue of their humanity. But this bloated view suffers from numerous defects. First, it vitiates the rationale of having a list of distinct human rights, because, according to such a view, any given right pretty much includes all other rights within itself in a Russian doll-style manner. Second, it makes immensely harder the practical task of assessing to what extent a given human right is respected, given the vast number of duties it subsumes. Third, it obscures the normative focus of each right, in the sense of the distinctive kind of ethical concern that it reflects. All of these unfortunate tendencies are, in turn, exacer-bated by the WHO's wildly capacious definition of health—"a state of complete physical, mental and social well-being and not merely the absence of disease and infirmity" (see World Health Organization 1946)—which equates health with the totality of human well-being, rather than construing it as one element of well-being among others, such as knowledge, friendship, etc.

A better view, I have argued elsewhere, is to construe the scope of the human right to health as encompassing duties pertaining to three subject matters: (a) medical treatment, (b) public health measures, and (c) certain social determin-ants of health. Determining the precise content of these duties is a further matter, and it is entirely possible that this content evolves over time, partly in response to changes in our available resources, including our technological capacities (see Tasioulas and Vayena 2020). But the focus on duties that fall within the subject matter delimited by (a)–(c) means that various health-affecting wrongs—such as torture, exclusion from primary education, deprivation of work, and racial discrimination—can be interpreted as human rights violations, without all of them being treated as violations of the right to health.

How this bloated conception of the scope of the right to health came to be part of human rights orthodoxy is complicated. No doubt one dimension of the problem is strategic, since rights with very wide scope maximize the chances of litigants successfully invoking a given right in defence of their claim—a matter that assumes special significance when the relevant legal instrument, e.g. a national constitution, explicitly lists only some rights (e.g. the right to life) but not others (e.g. the right to health). But in the specific case of the right to health, part of the problem stems from the idea, propagated by the great American public health figure Jonathan Mann, that "health and human rights are complementary approaches to the central problem of defining and advancing human well-being" (see Mann 2010). To this, the correct response is both yes and no. Yes, insofar as one cannot cogently defend human rights without reference to human interests, including the interest in health. But no, insofar as (a) there is more to human well-being than health, and (b) human rights are not the same as the interests that are constitutive of human well-being, but instead consist in certain duties generated by the interests of each individual. These rights-based duties may create important barriers to our ability to advance human well-being, including health, by ruling out such things as laws criminalizing smoking or overeating, or by incentivizing good health by denying medical treatment to those who have neglected to take adequate care of their own health. These individual-directed duties are the distinctive 'added value' that the discourse of rights brings, as compared with the discourse of well-being (see Tasioulas 2012). But, as above, the question then arises of which rights are associated with which duties. Human rights are standardly grounded in a plurality of interests, often including our interest in health, yet this does not render all such rights components of the right to health. Sadly, the opposite conclusion is the orthodoxy enshrined in leading human rights documents.

3.3 Content

The foregoing worry about the scope of the right to health is deepened when we add a further problem flowing from neglecting the importance of the distinction between the right to health and the interest in health—this time regarding *content*. The problem of bloated *content* arises even if we confine the scope of the duties associated with the right to health to the three kinds of subject matter that I have recommended: (a) provision of medical care, (b) public health measures, and (c) certain social determinants of health. In other words, even if the proposed duties fall within the scope of the right to health—understood as its broad subject matter, because they concern putative duties pertaining to (a), (b), and (c)—the specific content of those duties is too extensive to be credible. This differs from duties—such as the duty not to torture people, or the duty to provide people with work opportunities—that do not even fall within the scope of the right to health, as discussed in the previous section.

Orthodox discussion increasingly accepts an account of the content of these duties that expands to encompass any measure falling within (a)–(c) that would benefit our health, irrespective of the cost of securing that measure, including its impact on other rights. This undiscriminating approach is even extended to what, in human rights law, are referred to as the "minimum core obligations" associated with the right to health—i.e. those obligations that must be fulfilled immediately by all states, and which are not subject to progressive realization over time (see Tasioulas 2017b and 2017c). Commenting on General Comment 14's lavish specification of the minimum core obligations associated with the right to health, a leading expert on that right in international law, John Tobin, has aptly written that it is fatally "disassociated from the capacity of states to realize this vision" (Tobin 2014: 240). It is therefore unsurprising that development economists, lawyers, and political philosophers have condemned the right to health as useless in guiding policy since it constitutes a seemingly limitless and unstructured claim on resources (see Easterly 2009; Posner 2014; Weale 2012).

It might be asked: why should we not accept this extremely demanding interpretation of the right to health as an aspirational ideal—an intimation of utopia?[1] Well, perhaps human rights have indeed come to function in this way for many people. But there is a cost to this approach. Human rights, if they are truly rights, cannot primarily be ideals, but must instead generate corresponding duties. The latter are categorical demands on us, the violation of which is morally wrong. Given that it is constitutive of the nature of duties that they are standards it is wrongful to transgress, and that transgressing renders us blameworthy, it must be feasible for duty-bearers to comply with them ('ought implies can'). Elsewhere, I have argued that this entails the threefold requirement that duties associated with rights must be individually possible to comply with, that the cost of doing so must not be excessive, and that as a body duties associated with human rights must be compossible in the general run of cases, leaving aside emergency situations (see Tasioulas 2015).

If we do not constrain the content of the duties associated with human rights in this way, we risk an endless proliferation of wide-ranging human rights entitlements, with the consequent need to trade them off against each other (or other values) in particular cases when, as will habitually be the case, they cannot be jointly satisfied. Such extensive trade-offs seem opposed to the very idea of a duty. This is because the idea of a duty or obligation implies a reason that applies to us

---

[1] See O'Neill (2005) for related thoughts on the aspirational reading of human rights, though I differ from her in seeking to retain socio-economic rights as bona fide human rights.

categorically—i.e. independently of our subjective inclinations, and which is overridden or defeated only in extreme or emergency situations. Nevertheless, the conception of rights as proliferating endlessly, constantly coming into conflict, and regularly being traded off against each other, has been enshrined as orthodoxy by the 'proportionality' approach to human rights law, which is widely accepted in Europe, Latin America, and elsewhere.[2]

A prominent recent defender of this view is the American legal scholar Jamal Greene. Greene advocates importing the proportionality approach into the United States constitutional system, which has up until now resisted the tendency to treat all significant interests as pro tanto rights (Greene 2021). Contrary to my distinction between universal interests and rights, Greene regards the reduction of rights to significant interests as a feature, rather than a bug, of the proportionality doctrine. Hence his clear-sighted emphasis on the ubiquity of rights, given that they encompass pretty much all interests that people find important. According to Greene, '[r]ights are not precious. They are all around us' (Greene 2021: xxv). The point is memorably illustrated by his gloss on a German constitutional rights case relating to a law prohibiting the feeding of pigeons in certain public places: 'If pigeon feeding was an important part of what made this woman's life meaningful, then she had a right to feed pigeons. That's what a right *is*' (Greene 2021: 92). And hence also Greene's embrace of the natural corollary of the ubiquity thesis, which is the systematic need to trade rights off against each other and other values—'[c]onflict is a right's natural state' (Greene 2021: 114).

Engaging with Greene's arguments is a complex matter, partly because it is necessary to disentangle ideas about moral rights from those about legal rights, and then to disentangle legal rights in general from the special problems raised by constitutional rights adjudication in the United States context. On the latter point, one can certainly join Greene in decrying the absence of socio-economic rights from the United States Constitution without invoking the doctrine of proportionality as the appropriate remedy for filling this gap. However, the key difficulty with his analysis is his assumption that the practical alternatives are exhausted by (a) the excessively restrictive, binary, and unnuanced approach to rights adopted within United States constitutional adjudication, and (b) an alternative, free-wheeling democratic approach that identifies rights with significant interests, which are subject to extensive trade-offs in an overall calculus of interests—a calculus that looks suspiciously like the utilitarianism that rights discourse was supposed to replace.

What Greene's set-up discounts is the possibility that there is a principled way of distinguishing between interests—however strong—and legally enshrined moral rights, construed as interests of individuals capable of generating

---

[2] For a discussion of proportionality, see Verdirame (2015).

obligations to respect and protect those interests in various ways. A principled approach of this kind would offer an explication of why an individual's interest in not being tortured generates a duty on others not to torture them, but their interest in romantic love, no matter how powerful, does not put anyone under even a defeasible positive obligation to love that individual romantically. In addition, Greene underplays the extent to which a principled approach that draws a distinction between rights and interests can nonetheless adopt a nuanced conception of the duties associated with rights—one that admits of various exceptions (e.g. hate speech as an exception to the general right to free speech), in contrast to the tendency he decries in United States constitutional adjudication to treat, for example, pretty much all forms of 'speech' as meriting the protection of the right to freedom of speech.

Now, one of the great sources of moral confusion in the public discourse about the liberty-restricting measures adopted by various countries in response to the COVID-19 pandemic—measures such as bans on international travel, mask mandates, and lockdowns—is the facile tendency to conceptualize the situation as one involving rampant rights conflicts. On one familiar rendering, many of these conflicts are between the right to liberty and the right to health. Admittedly, laws making the wearing of masks compulsory do involve a restriction on one's liberty for the sake, in part, of safeguarding the health interests of others. But it is a considerable, and I believe unwarranted, jump to infer that such laws necessarily involve a curtailment—even a justifiable curtailment—of one's *right* to liberty. The latter is not coextensive with one's interest in liberty, which is indeed obviously impaired by such laws, but only with the duty to protect and respect that interest which is generated in the case of each right-holder. To take an extreme and, to my mind, clear-cut example: a convicted murderer's right to liberty is not defeated, even permissibly, when they are justly imprisoned after a fair trial, because the content of the duty associated with that right incorporates such situations as an exception. Similarly, forms of usually innocuous activity, such as the use of public transport without a mask, that are protected by the right to liberty in normal circumstances, fall within an exception to that right in circumstances in which there are good reasons to believe that such activity would pose a significant threat to the health interests of others, including threats that rise to the level of seriously risking a violation of their right to health. Among these circumstances are those in which there is a significant risk that those required to wear masks may be the unwitting carriers of an infectious and potentially lethal virus.

The failure to appreciate that we need to do the often difficult work of specifying the content of the respective rights' associated duties so as to avoid habitual conflict among them, rather than taking as axiomatic a conflict between liberty and health rights in the way the 'proportionality' approach does, has distorted public reasoning about the pandemic. This is not simply because the proportionality approach may lead to the wrong bottom-line conclusion as to whether or not measures such as lockdowns or mask mandates are all-things-considered justified. More fundamentally, it is because it is often mistakenly assumed that, even if such restrictive measures are justified, they necessarily come at the cost of widespread infringements of the right to liberty. This assumption entails that such laws wrong—albeit justifiably—those who are subject to them. But this is to neglect the crucial distinction between a right being (permissibly) defeated or overridden and its incorporating an exception. The normal response to a right being justifiably overridden is to apologize to or compensate the right-holder, in acknowledgment of the wrong that has been done to them. But this seems out of place in the case of justified mandatory masking laws. This 'proportionality' analysis simply skates over the possibility that the right to liberty has not been infringed, even though interests in liberty have been set back, because the pandemic-control measures fall within an exception to the duties associated with that right. And this likely has the side effect of needlessly inflaming negative reactions to liberty-restricting measures in response to the pandemic.

The task of specifying the duties associated with a given right in such a way as to meet the relevant requirements bearing on its content—e.g. of general compossibility of compliance with duties associated with other rights—is hardly a straightforward matter. This is partly because it will often be a difficult matter to specify their precise content, including the exceptions, and partly also because the use of pure reason might not be able to single out one specification as superior to all others. In other words, there may be multiple specifications of the duties associated with a given right, none of which is superior to the others, although they are all as a set superior to certain other specifications. However, in order to ensure effective social coordination in complying with rights—as well as adequate safeguards against the abuse of governmental power, among other reasons—we will often need to set down more determinate guidelines. For reasons such as these, we need processes of social decision to determine authoritatively the content of rights, especially in a pluralistic society. Among these processes, law plays a key role. It is a further question, of course, what the respective roles of the judicial, legislative, and executive arms of government should be in specifying the content of our legally enshrined rights. Here I would endorse Greene's claim that fixing the content of legal rights is a central task for democratic politics, and not largely to be delegated to the judiciary. But I would untether this claim from Greene's assumption that the content of deliberation in such cases is helpfully seen as engaged in a trade-off of multiple interests, all of which accurately present themselves under the aegis of rights. Democratic deliberation can, as Greene says, be about justice capaciously understood—but the core of justice is rights, and they are not simply to be assimilated to the large and open-ended category of interests.[3]

---

[3] On the importance of legislatures in specifying the content of human rights, see Webber et al. (2019).

3.4 Common Goods

If we adopt the more analytically rigorous conception of human rights that I have advocated, then we will discover two things about health policy: (1) that in formulating such policy we cannot appeal exclusively to the right to health, contrary to authors such as Lawrence Gostin, but that instead we must also give an important place to other human rights, including the rights to education and liberty of the person; and (2) that we cannot confine ourselves to human rights in general, but must in addition also appeal to other values. Regarding point (2), the other values in play include imperfect duties with no counterpart right-holder, such as duties of charity (one manifestation of which would be a duty of participation in clinical trials for the development of vitally needed drugs), and duties to one's self (one manifestation of which is the duty to take requisite care of one's health, even though one does not violate one's own right to health in failing to do so). However, the category of 'other values' I wish to focus on here is common goods, since their relationship to human rights is often poorly understood as essentially dichotomous and confrontational.

Health-related common goods include a culture of general health consciousness and physical fitness, and a culture of altruism and solidarity in which customs of helping those in need are widely upheld. Mark Carney, former Governor of the Bank of England, identifies this latter sort of common good as a key factor in effective responses to the COVID-19 pandemic:

> People went beyond compliance with the law and engaged in mass efforts of community altruism. People sewed masks, delivered food to vulnerable populations and publicly cheered the heroism of frontline workers. As private voluntary groups to address community needs burgeoned, governments started formal volunteer campaigns. In the United Kingdom...an appeal for NHS volunteers received over one million applicants. Governments encouraged such altruism by emphasizing the good that social distancing did for others.   (Carney 2021: xii)

What does it mean to say that cultures of health consciousness and physical fitness, of altruism and solidarity, are common goods? I do not have in mind the utilitarian notion, set aside in the introduction to this chapter, that they maximize overall aggregate welfare. Instead, they are common goods in the Aristotelian sense that they serve the interests of everyone in the community, that they serve those interests in the same way, and, most importantly, that they serve them in a non-rivalrous fashion, such that any one person's benefiting from such a culture is not necessarily at the expense of anyone else's ability to benefit in the same way.[4] If we conceive of common goods in this way, we can develop a more integrated or

---

[4] For relevant discussions of the common good, see Finnis (2011) and Raz (1992).

harmonious interpretation of their relationship to human rights. By contrast, utilitarianism tends to generate a picture of rights as being in a dichotomous relationship with the common good, so that rights are seen as external 'trumps' against the common good, in the familiar metaphor of Ronald Dworkin.

On the alternative conception defended here, we can affirm two points. First, that some common goods are essentially concerned with securing human rights: e.g. a system of fair trials, or a vaccination programme to secure herd immunity against COVID-19. Second, that some common goods go beyond anything we can reasonably claim as a matter of individual rights: e.g. a culture that is health-conscious and exhibits high levels of solidarity and citizen participation. But in neither case are we saddled with the ever-present and systematic tendency of rights coming into conflict with common goods that is generated by aggregative conceptions of the latter.[5]

Does this mean that there can never be a conflict between someone's individual right and the common good? No. Although human rights cannot be systematically subject to conflict and defeat, on pain of losing their status as genuine rights, I have suggested that there are emergency cases in which they may be defeated. These are cases that cannot be credibly presented as falling within an exception to the duties associated with the relevant right. Compare, for example, the case of a murderer who is justly sentenced to a term of imprisonment with the case of someone whose property is destroyed by the government to extinguish a bushfire that is threatening the lives of members of a local community, or with the case of someone who is quarantined because they are suffering from a lethal and extremely contagious disease for which there is no available cure. In the latter cases, it seems appropriate to speak of rights as having been overridden— justifiably defeated. And one consequence of this, unlike the case of the murderer, may be the triggering of secondary obligations to apologize to the owner of the destroyed property and to the quarantined individual, and to compensate them for their respective losses. Distinguishing exceptions from overrides in cases of emergency is a very complex matter, and not one I can pursue further here, but I take the distinction to be intuitively compelling even if its principled basis is often obscure and contestable. The distinction is essential to arriving at a conception of human rights according to which, in the words of James Griffin, they are 'resistant to trade-offs, but not completely so' (Griffin 2008: 76).

Since the idea of the common good is, today, making a welcome comeback in contemporary legal and political theory, I should clarify that my view of the relationship between rights and common goods differs from that of the American constitutional lawyer, Adrian Vermeule. In relation to vaccine mandates, Vermeule has written that their imposition in the furtherance of the common good

---

[5] For a fuller discussion, see Tasioulas and Vayena (2020).

does not "override" individual rights because the content of the duties associated with such rights is determined by the common good itself:

> The common good does not "override" individual rights. Rather the common good determines the boundaries of those rights from the beginning since, in the end, the goods of individual and family life can only be enjoyed in a healthy and flourishing polity…Even our physical liberties are rightly ordered to the common good of the community when necessary. Just ask those drafted for military service in a national emergency. Our economic liberties can also be subordinated to the common good: consider those whose property is destroyed by the government to prevent the spread of a fire. Covid-19 is like a spreading wildfire, and the vaccine mandate is analogous in principle to such crisis measures. Our health, our lives and our prosperity, are intertwined in ways that make it entirely legitimate to enforce precautions against lethal disease—even upon objectors.
> (Vermeule 2021; see also Vermeule 2022: 16)

While I concur with Vermeule's conclusion that measures like vaccine mandates can be justified during crises like a pandemic, we differ in the reasoning that leads us to this conclusion. For Vermeule, rights can never conflict with the common good since their content is simply a function of the common good. But this analysis seems to lose the distinctive character of basic moral rights, including their nature as moral standards grounded in the interests and status of each individual considered in themselves (see Tasioulas 2015). On my view, however, measures that protect rights serve the common good, but such measures can—in exceptional circumstances—come into conflict with measures needed to protect other elements of the common good, including other rights. The fact that rights form part of what is secured by the common good, as I understand it, doesn't entirely insulate them from conflict with other values, including other rights, or from being justifiably overridden by these other values. Rights, on my view, generate *pro tanto* reasons in the process of determining what is, all things considered, the right thing to do, and may on exceptional occasions have to be traded off against each other and other values. My suspicion is that Vermeule has a different view partly because he veers towards a conclusory interpretation of the common good, as that which is good, all things considered, in the ordering of a political community, and a corresponding view of the content of rights as a component of this good. This threatens to lose sight of the occasional tragic conflicts that we face even when we do that which is, all things considered, good, some of which may involve the justified violation (infringement) of individual rights.

Now, someone might respond that it has long been recognized that we need both individual rights and public health goods in formulating a defensible health policy, including at the global level. There is an interesting discussion of this issue from a legal historical perspective in John Fabian Witt's book *American*

Contagions: Epidemics and Law from Small Pox to Covid-19 (Witt 2021). Witt refers to the famous American public health official Jonathan Mann, and his pioneering work on HIV/AIDS, both for the United States and for the UN's Global Programme on AIDS. Mann's insight was that rights and public health could be harmonized because 'respect for human rights' leads to 'markedly better prevention and treatment'. Adopting coercive measures that breach human rights undermines the trust required for people to comply with public health measures—it drives the disease underground and facilitates its spread. So it turns out, just as a matter of contingent fact, that human rights and public health goods, like achieving herd immunity, are not starkly opposed.

But this reconciliation, although important so far as it goes, is a precarious one—it is merely contingent, dependent on circumstances that may change drastically over time. And Witt helpfully identifies one major change in circumstances that may make it no longer the case that voluntary compliance is the most efficient way to achieve public health goods. Here the threat to rights is seen as coming from capabilities created by new digital technologies. As Witt puts it,

> [N]ew technologies such as apps for cell phones and cell phone tracing threatened to alter the precarious balance between liberty and health. If states or other powerful institutions were able to develop technologies capable of testing, tracking and tracing individuals in ways that defeated evasion, then the calculus [between individual rights and public health] may change.
>
> (Witt 2021: 106)

What Witt puts forward here as a hypothetical possibility has acquired a kind of concrete reality, as shown by the fact that some authoritarian or less than liberal democratic societies in Asia, such as Singapore, had greater success in stemming the COVID-19 pandemic than liberal democracies like the United Kingdom, France, and the United States. So, implicated here is a broader ideological contest between liberal democracies and emergent authoritarian powers in the world today—one focused on the question of the kind of regime that is best equipped to protect people from public health crises like the COVID-19 pandemic.

I believe that Witt has raised an important question that needs to be engaged with seriously. But we can already see that his formulation of it embodies some highly contestable assumptions, given what has been said in this chapter about human rights and their relation to common goods. The first is the assumption that relations between human rights and public health goods are fundamentally contingent, whereas I have argued that they can also be constitutive—for example, that the common good of a programme for securing herd immunity to COVID-19 is justified primarily by the protection it affords to human rights to life and health. The second is that he has likely been led to his framing of the issue by an aggregative conception of the common good—one that I have argued we should resist.

3.5 Democracy

Still, Witt's discussion underscores the broader question of whether democracies might lose out against authoritarian rivals in the battle to secure the right to health, and the wider public health goods of which it is a component, such as herd immunity from COVID-19. This leads to a consideration of how human rights are related to democracy—another topic on which there is considerable confusion. In my view, some theorists posit an excessively tight connection between human rights and democracy. One way this is done is by building respect for human rights into the very idea of democracy. By contrast, I agree with Josiah Ober that democracy, conceived as limited collective self-government by free and equal citizens, does not entail compliance with the totality of norms that are human rights (Ober 2017). In this sense, an illiberal democracy, or a democracy that fails to respect certain human rights demands, could still be a full-fledged democracy, albeit deficient in other respects. Another way an excessively tight connection is forged is by making the content of human rights the upshot of fair democratic procedures—an idea defended by Norman Daniels (Daniels 2011). But this is in tension with the reality that democracies can get the content of human rights wrong. More fundamentally, democracy is an answer to the question of what the best (or least bad) system of government is—or perhaps more specifically to what the most legitimate system of government is in modern circumstances. It is not an answer to the question of what the criterion is that constitutively determines the truth of human rights claims, even if we were inclined to accord democratic decisions about rights considerable epistemic value.

In contrast to these views, many others propound a deep conflict between human rights and democracy, conceiving of human rights as 'counter-majoritarian norms'. I believe these views are also misguided, and that they are likely influenced by aggregative conceptions of the common good combined with the assumption that democratic processes are institutional mechanisms for giving effect to the common good so understood. However, the most plausible position on the empirical question of the instrumental relation between human rights and democracy is Kathryn Sikkink's hypothesis that the single most important factor that works for the fulfilment of human rights is creating and sustaining a democratic government (Sikkink 2017). Applying this to the pandemic context, Danielle Allen's recent discussion of the challenges posed to democracies by the COVID-19 pandemic underlines the way in which authentically democratic processes can, by generating a sense of common purpose among the citizenry, help foster forms of voluntaristic participation that are vital in controlling a pandemic without the need to transgress individual rights (Allan 2022: 19). And building on this, I want to suggest, in response to Witt's challenge, that although digital technology may have a dark, authoritarian potential, it also has a bright, democratic aspect. Indeed, it may help facilitate more radically participatory forms of democratic governance, as theorists such as Hélène Landemore have argued (see Landemore 2021).

We have a concrete example of the potential of democracies to use digital technology in order to secure public health goals while simultaneously respecting human rights in the case of Taiwan.[6] Under the leadership of the country's first Digital Minister, Audrey Tang, participative, community-built digital tools have been used to create a more democratic, open, and inclusive form of government. Taiwan achieved a 'best in the world' result regarding COVID-19: with only 3 per cent of people vaccinated it had the lowest per capita death rate in the world while avoiding lockdown and despite having mainland China on its doorstep. A digital platform called *polis* gathered and analysed diverse opinions from citizens, synthesizing them into insights that could be channelled into decision-making processes, with 80 per cent of platform discussions leading to government action. Among other Taiwanese examples of digital tools in aid of democracy are those for combatting disinformation campaigns (tools that are especially important during a pandemic) without resorting to censorship, including the tactic of "humour over rumour", in which state agencies are required to correct false claims within two hours by employing humorous debunking methods.

Of course, these successes have only been possible owing to favourable background conditions, such as transparency in governmental decision-making processes, widespread digital education, universal healthcare, and universal broadband access—some of which are arguably required by full respect for human rights. But the hopeful lesson from Taiwan is that democracy seems to be a vital part of the ethos that best secures human rights and public health goals alike. But learning this and other lessons will require established democracies such as the United Kingdom and United States to overcome their ingrained ethnocentric prejudice that when it comes to global health they have much to teach other countries but little to learn (Sridhar 2022: 134).

3.6 Conclusion

The sombre realities of the COVID-19 pandemic should prompt deep reflection by governments, civil society, and ordinary citizens, on how we might better prepare ourselves for the next, probably rather different, pandemic. One element of this preparedness that should not be discounted is a clearer conception of the role of human rights, including the right to health, in global health policy, so that the quality of future democratic deliberation and decision-making in a health crisis can be enhanced. In this chapter, I have argued that this will involve serious

---

[6] I rely in this paragraph on Divya Siddarth (2020).

revisions of our understanding of the scope and content of rights, such as the human right to health, so as to respect the categorical difference between universal interests—however important—and human rights. Failure to respect this difference only strengthens the baleful grip of utilitarian modes of thinking in public health policy, since it reduces rights to ubiquitous interests that have to be constantly traded off against each other in an overall welfarist calculus. When we adopt a more rigorous understanding of the idea of human rights, we are led to see that much of great ethical significance to health policy in a pandemic cannot be exhaustively encompassed within that idea. Among other value concepts, we also need to appeal to common goods, such as practices of citizen solidarity and participation, and also to the value of democracy. But when we do so, we must avoid familiar misconceptions about the relationship between human rights and these other values. In particular, we should resist the oppositional notion that human rights are fundamentally constraints on the pursuit of common goods or the operation of democratic processes. On the contrary, key common goods— such as laws making mask wearing compulsory, or programmes of vaccination aimed at achieving herd immunity—can themselves be justified as protections of human rights. Meanwhile, strong democratic institutions and practices can help to foster vital common goods—such as practices of solidarity and participation— that enable the human right to health, as well other health-related values, to be secured in a way that is maximally consistent with human rights.

Acknowledgements

For helpful comments on previous versions of this chapter, I am grateful to Rebecca Lowe, Owen Schaefer, the editors of this volume, and an anonymous referee.

Bibliography

Allen, D. (2022), *Democracy in the Time of Coronavirus* (Chicago and London: University of Chicago Press).

Carney, M. (2021), *Value(s):Climate, Credit, Covid and How We Focus on What Matters* (London: William Collins).

Daniels, N. (2011), 'Health Justice, Equality and Fairness: Perspectives from Health Policy and Human Rights Law', *The Equal Rights Review* 6 (2011): 127–38.

Easterly, W. (2009), 'Human rights are the wrong basis for healthcare', *Financial Times*, 12 Oct. 2009, http://www.ft.com/cms/s/0/89bbbda2-b763-11de-9812-00144feab49a.html#axzz3ym5AIA9w.

Finnis, J. M. (2011), *Natural Law and Natural* Rights, 2nd ed. (Oxford: Oxford University Press).

Global Health Security Index (2019), *Building Collective Action and Accountability*, https://www.ghsindex.org/wp-content/uploads/2019/10/2019-Global-Health-Security-Index.pdf.

Gostin, L. O. (2014), *Global Health Law* (Cambridge, MA: Harvard University Press).

Greene, J. (2021), *How Rights Went Wrong: Why Our Obsession with Rights is Tearing America Apart* (Boston: Houghton Mifflin Harcourt).

Griffin, J. (2008), *On Human Rights* (Oxford: Oxford University Press).

Landemore, H. (2021), 'Open Democracy and Digital Technologies', in L. Bernholz, H. Landemore, and R. Reich (eds.), *Digital Technology and Democratic Theory* (Chicago: University of Chicago Press).

Mann, J., et al. (2010), 'Health and Human Rights', in L. O. Gostin (ed.), *Public Health Law and Ethics* (Berkeley: University of California Press), 259–63.

Ober, J. (2017), *Demopolis: Democracy before Liberalism in Theory and Practice* (Cambridge: Cambridge University Press).

Office of the United Nations High Commissioner for Human Rights and the World Health Organization (2008), 'The Right to Health: Fact Sheet No. 31', https://www.ohchr.org/en/publications/fact-sheets/fact-sheet-no-31-right-health#:~:text=The%20Fact%20Sheet%20explains%20what,international%20accountability%20and%20monitoring%20mechanisms.

O'Neill, O. (2005), 'The Dark Side of Human Rights', *International Affairs* 81/2: 427–39.

Posner, E. (2014), *The Twilight of Human Rights Law* (Oxford: Oxford University Press).

Raz, J. (1992), 'Rights and Individual Well-Being', *Ratio Juris* 5: 127–42.

Siddarth, D. (2020), *Taiwan: Grassroots Digital Democracy that Works*, RadicalxChange Foundation, https://www.radicalxchange.org/media/papers/Taiwan_Grassroots_Digital_Democracy_That_Works_V1_DIGITAL_.pdf.

Sikkink, K. (2017), *Evidence for Hope: Making Human Rights Work in the 21st Century* (Princeton, NJ: Princeton University Press).

Sridhar, D. (2022), *Preventable: How a Pandemic Changed the World and How to Stop the Next One* (London: Penguin).

Tasioulas, J. (2012), 'On the Nature of Human Rights' in G. Ernst and J-C. Heilinger (eds.), *The Philosophy of Human Rights: Contemporary Controversies* (Berlin: de Gruyter), 17–59.

Tasioulas, J. (2015), 'On the Foundation of Human Rights', in R. Cruft, M. Liao, and M. Renzo (eds.), *Philosophical Foundations of Human Rights* (Oxford: Oxford University Press).

Tasioulas, J. (2017a), 'Exiting the Hall of Mirrors: Morality and Law in Human Rights', in K. Bourne and T. Campbell (eds.), *Political and Legal Approaches to Human Rights* (London: Routledge), 73–89.

Tasioulas, J. (2017b), *Minimum Core Obligations: Human Rights in the Here and Now*, World Bank, https://openknowledge.worldbank.org/handle/10986/29144.

Tasioulas, J. (2017c), *The Minimum Core of the Human Right to Health*, World Bank, https://openknowledge.worldbank.org/handle/10986/29143.

Tasioulas, J., and Vayena, E. (2020), 'Just Global Health: Integrating Human Rights and Common Goods', in T. Brooks (ed.), *The Oxford Handbook of Global Justice* (Oxford: Oxford University Press, 2020), 139–62.

Tobin, J. (2014), *The Right to Health in International Law* (Oxford: Oxford University Press).

UN Committee on Economic, Social, and Cultural Rights (2000), *General Comment No. 14: The Right to the Highest Attainable Standard of Health*, U.N. Doc E/C.12/2000/4.

UN Human Rights Committee (2018), *General Comment No. 36*, art. 6, U.N. Doc. CCPR/C/GC36.

Verdirame, G. (2015), 'Rescuing Human Rights From Proportionality', in R. Cruft, M. Liao, and M. Renzo (eds), *Philosophical Foundations of Human Rights* (Oxford, Oxford University Press).

Vermeule, A. (2021), 'Biden's Vaccine Mandate Serves the Common Good', in https://bariweiss.substack.com/p/vaccine-mandates-the-end-of-covid?s=r.

Vermeule, A. (2022), *Common Good Constitutionalism* (Cambridge, Polity).

Weale, A. (2012), 'The Right to Health versus Good Medical Care?', *Critical Review of International Social and Political Philosophy* 15: 473–93.

Webber, G., et al. (eds) (2019), *Legislated Rights: Securing Human Rights through Legislation* (Cambridge: Cambridge University Press).

Witt, J. F. (2021), *American Contagions: Epidemics and Law from Small Pox to Covid-19* (New Haven, CT: Yale University Press).

World Health Organization (1946), *Constitution of the World Health Organization*, https://apps.who.int/gb/bd/PDF/bd47/EN/constitution-en.pdf.

PART II
LIBERTY

4

Bringing Nuance to Autonomy-Based Considerations in Vaccine Mandate Debates

Jennifer Blumenthal-Barby

The COVID-19 pandemic began in the early spring of 2020. By the late spring of 2021, safe and effective vaccines were widely available for most adults in many countries. In the US, for example, all adults were eligible to receive a vaccine by May 2021. In the early weeks and months of vaccine availability, many citizens clamored to get a vaccine and priority allocation frameworks needed to be established. As time passed, however, policymakers faced (and continue to face) a new reality: those who are vaccine hesitant, skeptical, or refusing. In early October 2021, only 55% of the US population was fully vaccinated, 24% were unwilling, and 6% were uncertain. In the UK, 66% of the population was fully vaccinated, 22% were unwilling, and 4% were uncertain. In Japan, 62% of the population was fully vaccinated.[1] All three of these countries had universal availability of vaccines at the time that these numbers were reported.

Several policy proposals have been made for how to address the problem of the unvaccinated, including public health education, persuasion, nudging, incentives, and mandates. Vaccine mandates became increasingly common in the summer and fall of 2021 as the pandemic raged on and vaccination slowed down. For example, in the US, over 1,000 colleges mandated vaccination for fall 2021 enrollment, several states and school districts required their teachers to be vaccinated or be fired, several healthcare organizations required their employees to be vaccinated or fired, and several large companies deployed vaccination or termination mandates for employees—including United Airlines and Tyson Foods. In September 2021, President Biden issued an executive order mandating vaccines or termination for federal workers and contractors as well as for employees working in institutions that receive Medicare or Medicaid reimbursements (virtually all hospitals). The President also made use of Occupational Safety and Health

---

[1] Data on what percentage was unwilling or uncertain were not available. For those curious about the most highly vaccinated country, the United Arab Emirates led the way with 83% of its population fully vaccinated in October 2021. All data from https://ourworldindata.org/covid-vaccinations.

Jennifer Blumenthal-Barby, *Bringing Nuance to Autonomy-Based Considerations in Vaccine Mandate Debates* In: *Pandemic Ethics: From COVID-19 to Disease X.* Edited by: Dominic Wilkinson and Julian Savulescu, Oxford University Press. © Oxford University Press 2023. DOI: 10.1093/oso/9780192871688.003.0005

Administration regulations to mandate vaccines (or weekly testing) for employees working in businesses with over 100 employees.

The main argument against mandates is that they infringe on or violate individual autonomy. It is for this reason that some ethicists and policymakers eschew mandates altogether or favor them as a "last resort" after other "less restrictive alternatives" such as education, persuasion, and various types of nudges and incentives. In the middle of a raging pandemic, however, concerns about individual autonomy are often set aside in favor of an appeal to consequentialist-based public health arguments along with a Millian harm principle about the freedom to harm oneself but not others. It is this framework that is used to justify vaccine mandates. While I ultimately think that vaccine mandates can be justified, I do believe that the standard approach to justifying them tends to lack important philosophical nuance with respect to autonomy-based considerations and the application of the harm principle. In this chapter, I aim to bring some of that required nuance to bear on the debate.

4.1 The Standard Approach: Appeal to the Harm Principle

Many public health ethics frameworks anchor on John Stuart Mill's "Harm Principle," whereby restrictions to individual liberty are justified in cases where the exercise of that liberty would cause harm (not mere offense) to others.[2] So first, it needs to be true that those who exercise their liberty to not get vaccinated harm others. The coronavirus (particularly the Delta variant) is easily spread and has caused over 4.5 million deaths as of September 2021. Not being vaccinated puts others at risk of harm—especially persons who are not eligible for the vaccine themselves (e.g. young children as of September 2021) or people who are immunocompromised. Failure to get vaccinated contributes to continued spread even to vaccinated persons via "breakthrough cases," which results in ongoing cycles of closings and reopenings of various aspects of the economy. Unvaccinated individuals also contribute to overwhelmed hospitals and providers, limiting access for other patients in need. In short, exercising the liberty to not vaccinate clearly imposes harm on others, so the standard account goes.

An example of the standard account can be found in a November 2021 *New York Times* opinion piece written by Paul Krugman. The article was titled "No, Vaccine Mandates Aren't an Attack on Freedom." Krugman writes, "...personal choice is fine—as long as your personal choices don't hurt other people. I may deplore the quality of your housekeeping, but it's your own business; on the other hand, freedom doesn't include the right to dump garbage in the street. And going unvaccinated during a pandemic does hurt other people—which is why schools,

---

[2] According to Mill, "To constitute a harm, an action must be injurious or set back important interests of particular people, interests in which they have rights" (Brink 2022).

in particular, have required vaccination against many diseases for generations." Krugman adds, "...And the harm done to others by rejecting vaccines goes beyond an increased risk of disease. The unvaccinated are far more likely than the vaccinated to require hospitalization, which means that they place stress on the health care system. They also impose financial costs on the general public, because given the prevalence of insurance both public and private, their hospital bills end up being largely covered by the rest of us."

Another example of an appeal to the harm principle to justify mandates can be found in a *Health Affairs* piece by US ethicists Wynia, Harter, and Eberl titled "Why A Universal COVID-19 Vaccine Mandate Is Ethical Today." They write,

> It is the risk of harm to others—impinging on their liberty to be safe while driving, breathe clean air, or not be shot or trampled—that makes it ethical to place limits on personal choices....In terms of limiting people's choices about vaccination during the COVID-19 pandemic, we must consider whether one person going unvaccinated today is likely to cause harm to other people. Nearly all people interact and come into physical contact with others on a daily basis, and a person with COVID-19 can infect several others even before showing symptoms. The risk of one person harming many others, even inadvertently, provides ethical jus-tification for limiting the choice to go unvaccinated during a pandemic.
>
> (See Wynia et al. 2021)

4.2 Application of the Harm Principle to Vaccine Mandate Debates

While the standard approach of appealing to the harm principle to justify vaccine mandates during a pandemic seems straightforward enough, there are some com-plications. First. the harm principle becomes activated to justify liberty-infringing intervention when one person's behaviors cause harm to another person. But is non-vaccination during COVID-19 sufficient to satisfy the conditions of the harm principle? Some might argue that it is not, because the unvaccinated are not causing harm to others by their failure to vaccinate—they are merely *imposing a risk of* harm, which is not the same as an *actual harm*.

In response, the first point to note is that it is not at all unusual for the harm principle to apply to risk of harm. Take the example of drunk driving: we do not allow individuals to drive drunk because of the risk they pose to others (see Jamrozik et al. 2016: 764). Second, a philosophical argument can be made that risk of harm is itself a harm. Shelly Kagan has taken this position when he argues that harm prohibition and prevention should include consideration of risk of harm. Kagan gives the example of an electronic harpoon that has a fixture that lets the person pulling the trigger set the probability of it firing. According to Kagan, it is not just that pointing the harpoon at someone's heart, setting it to

100% probability, and pulling the trigger (i.e. causing harm) is problematic. So, too, is setting the device at anything beyond zero (i.e. risking harm) (see Kagan 1989: 88). Adriana Placani (2017: 77–100) has argued that what is harmful about putting someone else at nontrivial risk for harm is that it shows a lack of respect for them. John Oberdiek (2009: 376–8) has argued that what is harmful about imposing risk of harm is that it limits autonomy. Oberdiek gives the example of a person who walks through a minefield without stepping on a mine. The risk of harm resulted in a limitation of the person's options, which was harmful (see Oberdiek 2009: 378).[3] Kritika Maheshwari (2021) has argued that risk of harm is contingently harmful insofar as (when) it causes harmful consequences to the risk-bearers, such as psychological distress.

But there is a second complexity in the application of the harm principle to COVID-19 vaccine mandates. It is as follows: What amount of risk and for what type of harm is sufficient to trigger the harm principle and justify vaccine mandates? Those against vaccine mandates will argue that the risk that they impose on others is low. To tie this complexity back to Kagan's harpoon example, there is certainly a difference between someone who sets the harpoon at 5% probability of firing and someone who sets it at 90%. Those against mandates will argue that the risk they pose to others is closer to 5% (and much lower even). They will point to the fact that the case fatality rate from COVID is relatively low depending on country (e.g. 1.1% in Japan, 1.5% in the UK, 1.6% in the US) and that these numbers are even much lower now compared to the start of the pandemic, especially for those who are vaccinated or have immunity (see *Mortality Analyses* 2021). They will argue that the unvaccinated may not even pose increased transmission risks. A cohort study published in *The Lancet Infectious Diseases* conducted in the UK between September 13, 2020, and September 15, 2021, analyzed transmission risk by vaccination status for 231 contacts exposed to 162 epidemiologically linked Delta-variant-infected index cases. They found that "…the secondary attack rate among household contacts exposed to fully vaccinated index cases was similar to household contacts exposed to unvaccinated index cases (25% [95% CI 15–35] for vaccinated *vs* 23% [15–31] for unvaccinated)" (see Singanayagam et al. 2021: 6). This is because "vaccinated individuals with breakthrough infections have peak viral load similar to unvaccinated cases and can efficiently transmit infection…" (see Singanayagam et al. 2021: 1).[4] Additionally, opponents will point to the very low likelihood of vaccinated individuals suffering hospitalization or severe disease even if transmission does occur. Collectively, these data call into question whether unvaccinated people pose sufficient risk of harm to others to justify mandates.

---

[3] I would also imagine that it caused the person quite a bit of psychological distress.

[4] At the same time, there is evidence to support the view that vaccinated individuals do transmit less effectively. See Mostaghimi et al. (2022) and Richterman et al. (2022).

In response, although it could be argued that the risk that the unvaccinated pose to most other individuals (especially if they are vaccinated) is quite low in terms of severe disease or death, it is worth remembering that not everyone is able to get vaccinated for reasons of eligibility, access, or medical reasons, and some people have compromised immunity. The risks to these persons are higher. Vaccines significantly reduce the risk of contracting COVID, and if a person does not have COVID then they cannot pass it on to someone else who may be more vulnerable. Second, there are risks other than death and hospitalization. Little is known about the long-term impacts of COVID; however, a metanalysis found that 80% of individuals infected with COVID-19 developed one or more long-term symptoms. Common long-term symptoms included fatigue (58% of patients), headache (44%), attention disorders (27%), hair loss (25%), and dyspnea (24%) (see Lopez-Leon et al. 2021: 7). Third, it is also worthwhile to note that a large amount of unvaccinated people grouped together in one geographic location could lead to "variant factories." The more that COVID-19 spreads, the more opportunities there are for the virus to mutate. This poses a dual risk to others, regardless of vaccination status: the mutations can lead to viral strains with higher transmission or mortality rates, and the COVID-19 vaccines currently on the market may have variable efficacy rates among variants with higher morbidity and mortality. Fourth, and perhaps most importantly, the harm to others that the unvaccinated pose is not just the harm of transmission. It is the harm of overburdened healthcare workers and systems. From April 4 to July 17, 2021, in the US, 92% of COVID cases, 92% of hospitalizations, and 91% of COVID-related deaths were reported among individuals not fully vaccinated (see Scobie et al. 2021: 1285). The rate of COVID-related hospitalizations was about seventeen times higher in unvaccinated persons (see Havers et al. 2021: 12). From June to August 2021, preventable COVID-19 hospitalizations among unvaccinated adults cost US $5.7 billion, and this number is likely an underestimation, as it does not account for outpatient treatments. The occupation of hospitals with unvaccinated patients continues to result in many hospitals being at capacity with little to no room to care for other patients and forced to turn patients away, even twenty months into the pandemic (see Yan and Elmaroussi 2021 and Paz 2021). Healthcare workers are understandably burnt out and frustrated (see Galanis et al. 2021 and Pappa et al. 2020); 62% of healthcare workers report that worry or stress of COVID-19 has negatively impacted their mental health (see Clement et al. 2021). Some even describe the experience of moral injury, feeling that they are not able to care for their patients as well as they feel they should be able to (see "How Nurses Are Feeling" 2021).[5]

---

[5] Some might object that we should not give much weight to the harms of hospital burden and clinician burnout because hospitals are generally understaffed and overwhelmed due to policies and practices of their own choosing. I thank Jessica Flanigan for this objection. I would, however, point to

In sum, there is empirical and philosophical nuance in the application of the harm principle in defense of COVID vaccine mandates. The application can be justified, but it is far from straightforward.

4.3 Mandates and Freedom of Occupation

Supposing that the conditions for the harm principle have been met, justifying state (or employer) intervention on individual choice, we need to also consider the nature of the mandate itself. In other words, what is the disjunct in "Get your COVID vaccine or…."? In some cases, it is "or get tested daily or weekly." However, in many cases, in the US at least, it is "or lose your job."[6] Indeed, hundreds (5% of unvaccinated workers, 1% of all adults) have left or lost their job due to vaccine mandates, and 25% of adults polled in a Kaiser Family Foundation survey (n = 1,519) say they know someone who has left their job due to mandates (see Hamel et al. 2021). In essence, the vaccine mandate is a burden on freedom of occupation. Is this burden a reasonable and defensible one? There are several points to make here. First, this version of the mandate is more defensible than a mandate that burdened freedom of bodily integrity. Consider a version of the mandate "Get your COVID vaccine or we will jab a needle in your arm against your will." To my knowledge, no one is employing that version of the mandate. But this is merely a lesser-of-two-evils kind of defense. There is also relevant and defensible precedent to draw on here. Consider the following examples: employers often require mandatory drug testing as a condition of employment, truck drivers are required to wear corrective lenses on their face or in their eyes if their vision is impaired, pilots were required to forego certain eye surgeries such as LASIK out of concern that altitude and gravitational force would negatively affect their eyesight. These are all instances where we burden freedom of occupation with conditions that someone do something (or not do something) to their body for workplace safety. COVID-19 vaccination mandates are no different from typical burdens on freedom of occupation. Indeed, certain vaccine mandates (e.g. Hepatitis B) already exist for healthcare and lab personnel for reasons of workplace safety.

Some might argue, however, that COVID-19 vaccine mandates are more coercive than is necessary to ensure workplace or public safety. These objectors might argue that instead of "Get your COVID vaccine or lose your job," the mandate ought to take the shape of "Get daily testing or lose your job," or "Show proof of

---

the harms to the individual overwhelmed workers (who are not hospital administrators and have no say in policy) as well as to the other hospitalized patients who get worse care due to overrun hospitals and clinicians (also through no fault of their own).

[6] It is important to note that, in the US at least, there are legal requirements for medical and religious exemptions.

immunity through recent infection or lose your job." If daily testing or immunity from previous infection would lower the risk of transmission to others to a level close to vaccination, then they ought to be acceptable options. Are they? Let us consider immunity through previous infection first. There is still significant disagreement among experts about viral- versus vaccine-induced immunity for COVID. Some argue that immunity wanes ninety days after infection and that lab studies have shown that previously infected individuals show inconsistent responses against several strains of COVID. A recent study in Kentucky showed that, of 179 residents with a confirmed reinfection, 73% were unvaccinated and 27% were vaccinated (see Cavanaugh et al. 2021: 1081). A nine-state study sponsored by the Centers for Disease Control showed that among patients hospitalized with COVID-like illness, the adjusted odds of a confirmed COVID-19 diagnosis was 5.9 times higher for unvaccinated patients with previous infection compared to fully vaccinated patients (95% confidence interval = 2.75–10.99) (see Bozio et al. 2021: 3).[7] For this reason, as of November 2021, the Centers for Disease Control and The Infectious Diseases Society of America are both recommending vaccination, even for those with previous infections (see Bozio et al. 2021 and Williams 2021). On the other hand, other studies have found a steady presence of helper T-cells and a durable response eight months after infection (see Block 2021: 1). A December 2020–May 2021 study of 52,238 employees of the Cleveland Clinic Health System in Ohio found that not one of 1,359 previously infected employees who remained unvaccinated had a SARS-CoV-2 infection over the duration of the study (five months) (see Shrestha et al. 2021: 10). A multisite study in the UK with over 25,000 participants found that "A previous history of SARS-CoV-2 infection was associated with an 84% lower risk of infection, with median protective effect observed 7 months following primary infection" (see Hall et al. 2021: 1459). And finally, as mentioned earlier in this chapter, a study was conducted in the UK between September 13, 2020, and September 15, 2021 where researchers analyzed transmission risk by vaccination status for 231 contacts exposed to 162 epidemiologically linked Delta-variant-infected index cases. They found that "...the secondary attack rate among household contacts exposed to fully vaccinated index cases was similar to household contacts exposed to unvaccinated index cases (25% [95% CI 15–35] for vaccinated vs 23% [15–31] for unvaccinated)" (see Singanayagam et al. 2021: 1).

Let us next consider whether a mandate option in the form of "Get daily testing or lose your job" would lower the risk of transmission to a level close to vaccination.[8] While possibly effective, this option faces several feasibility challenges. In high-risk settings with ongoing community-based transmission,

---

[7] Vaccination or previous infection occurred three to six months prior.
[8] Whether regular testing requirements involve PCR tests or LFT tests (which may be easier to access and implement, but less accurate) would need to be specified.

twice-weekly asymptomatic viral testing may be required to prevent outbreaks and reduce cases of COVID (see Chin et al. 2020: 6 and Lyng et al. 2021). Less frequent testing may be sufficient in settings with low community-based transmission, especially when it is implemented with additional infection control measures, but delays in returning test results would impact effectiveness of routine testing strategies (see Chin et al. 2020: 6–7). Regular PCR screening for the general population is logistically impossible and inefficient (see Grassley et al. 2020: 1387), and testing for only symptomatic individuals would at best prevent only about 26% of transmission (see Grassley et al. 2020: 1387). There are also the economic and environmental costs of twice weekly or daily testing. On the estimate that a test costs $60 US dollars, for a company with 100 unvaccinated employees testing them twice per week, that would cost $12,000 per week (see Cutler and Summers 2020: 1495). If the federal government were to assume the costs, consider that a policy of, say, 30 million tests weekly would require an additional $75 billion of spending during the next year, and adding the cost of contact tracing would increase the total to approximately $100 billion (see Cutler and Summers 2020: 1496). It would also be unfair to require employers to bear those costs. If an employee is willing to assume the cost and responsibility of daily or twice weekly testing, however, that may be a reasonable alternative to a vaccine mandate.

4.4 Just a Prick? Bodily Autonomy, Trust, and Psychosocial Harm

There is a temptation to take the view that the mandate involves only a small infringement on liberty—after all, we are just talking about a small needle prick. We are not requiring people to undergo something particularly onerous or risky. This view may have been what led President Biden to scoff at or mock those against vaccination during a discussion about mandates in a presidential town hall: "I have the freedom to kill you with my COVID—come on, freedom?" (see Villarreal 2021).

It is true, the procedure is relatively painless, and the risks associated with the vaccine are minimal. A study on the safety and efficacy of the mRNA Covid-19 Vaccine published in *The New England Journal of Medicine* reported that reactions included mild-to-moderate pain at the injection site within seven days of receiving vaccination, with less than 1% of individuals reporting severe pain (see Polack et al. 2020: 2606). Severe systemic events after the first dose had a frequency of 0.9% or less (see Polack et al. 2020: 2606), and severe systemic events were reported in less than 2% of vaccine recipients after either dose (see Polack et al. 2020: 2606). Fatigue and headache were the commonly reported side effects.

Few participants in either group (vaccine or placebo) had severe adverse events, serious adverse events, or adverse events leading to withdrawal from the trial (see Polack et al. 2020: 2608). The vaccine had a 95% efficacy rate, with a 95% confidence interval of 90–98% (see Polack et al. 2020: 2608). A follow-up study found that the vaccine is safer and has lower incidence of side effects (especially serious side effects) than COVID (see Barda et al. 2021: 1079).

While it is true that a needle prick is painless and the vaccine has been deemed safe and low-risk, it is too quick to dismiss the resulting autonomy infringement as insignificant. There are two reasons for this. First, a coerced vaccine is, categorically, a violation of bodily autonomy. Any violation of bodily autonomy is recognized by most liberals as a significant autonomy infringement.[9] John Stuart Mill famously argued that an individual should be sovereign over her own body and mind. Mill also drew distinctions between liberty interests that should be immune from interference, ones that deserve a presumption in favor of liberty, and ones that deserve no such presumption. Liberty interests that are particularly weighty and deserve immunity or a presumption in favor of them, according to Mill, are ones that relate to "...choices that are consequential for an individual's overall life prospects and focally related to control over the shape of a self-determining life as a whole" (see Powers et al. 2012: 10). This leads to a second point about the view that "it's just a pin prick." Coerced vaccines do not just involve complaints about unwanted bodily intrusion as a physical violation, but also complaints about violations of core beliefs and expression—e.g. expressions of autonomy as "my body, my choice." For some people, this represents a deep and significant infringement and psychosocial harm. This may particularly be the case in situations of complex power dynamics and trust issues between those doing the mandating and those receiving the mandates. For instance, Black Americans may be more hesitant than white Americans due not only to historical events such as the Tuskegee experiments but also to everyday racism encountered in the healthcare system (see Bajaj and Stanford 2021: 1).[10] Mandates may be experienced as a deeper autonomy infringement for some populations compared to others.[11]

---

[9] This is compatible with the view that some violations of bodily autonomy might be more significant than others (e.g. compare coerced seatbelts pushing into my body, a coerced pinprick on my finger, a coerced vaccination, a coerced caesarean section).

[10] In the United States, as of November 1, 2021, across 43 states, 55% of white people had received at least one COVID vaccine dose, 53% of Hispanic people had received at least one dose, and 48% of Black people received the first dose; 71% of Asian people received at least one dose of the vaccine. "Latest Data on COVID-19 Vaccinations by Race/Ethnicity" in KFF on November 3, 2021. By Nambi Ndugga et al. See also: Covid Data Tracker, CDC.

[11] This does not necessarily lead to a totally subjective view of autonomy infringement—it is just to say that subjective perceptions of autonomy infringement do matter to some extent, morally—and it is also to recognize that some groups might experience perceived or actual autonomy infringements more negatively than others.

4.5 Reasons for Refusal and Implications for Autonomy

One tempting way to view the situation is that the choice to decline a vaccine is not likely very autonomous to begin with due to a host of factors including cognitive and affective biases and distortions in belief. If this is the case, mandates would not clearly and automatically violate autonomy in the way that their opponents claim. One could even make a soft-paternalist argument that mandates could protect and promote individual autonomy by preventing people from making harmful, misinformed, and/or non-voluntary choices and are thus defensible.

Are COVID vaccine refusals driven by misinformation, false beliefs, and cognitive biases? There is reason to think that many of them are (see Azarpanah et al. 2021, Berenbaum 2021, Ling 2020, and Stolle et al. 2020).[12] And I have argued elsewhere that these factors compromise the exercise of autonomous decision-making (see Blumenthal-Barby 2016 and 2021). However, the reasons that unvaccinated adults with access to the vaccine give for not vaccinating are many and varied. A June 2021 Kaiser Family Foundation (KFF) survey of 1,888 US adults found that half of those unvaccinated believe that current cases are so low that there is no need for more people to get vaccinated (see Lopes et al. 2021). For the other half, 53% cited worries about side effects and the newness of the vaccine, 43% just did not want to get it, 38% cited lack of trust in the government, 38% believed they do not need the vaccine, 37% did not believe that COVID-19 vaccines are safe, and 26% did not trust vaccines in general (see Lopes et al. 2021). A US-based consortium issued a September 2021 report titled "A 50-State COVID-19 Survey Report: The Decision to Not Get Vaccinated, From the Perspective of the Unvaccinated." This survey provided additional insight regarding perception of risks of side effects, including concerns about allergic reactions, blood clots and inflammation, and contracting COVID from the vaccine (see Uslu et al. 2021: 6). Uncertainty regarding the risks the vaccine poses were driven by concerns over long-term effects or how quickly the vaccine was developed. Finally, lack of trust in institutions was often directed at the federal government and organizations like the CDC (see Uslu et al. 2021: 8). Some persons of color voiced skepticism at whether health institutions or the government were truly beneficently disposed towards them, given personal or historical grievances. For example, one woman said, "I do not trust the government as a black woman, they are pushing a little too hard for people to take this when other infectious diseases are treated as cash cows. This is highly suspicious to me" (see Uslu et al. 2021: 8).

---

[12] It is important to also consider the cause of anti-COVID vaccine stances that are due to false beliefs or cognitive biases. Social media, the internet, and various news outlets often propagated misinformation. And, arguably, ill-considered public messaging campaigns may have negatively impacted public decision-making (perhaps by triggering various cognitive biases).

While we might be tempted to draw a distinction between (a) vaccine refusals based on an informed, thoughtful, principled basis and (b) vaccine refusals based on anti-science rhetoric, distorted beliefs, or misinformation, and believe that type (a) refusals are autonomous and epistemically justified and type (b) are not, this is a distinction with fuzzy boundaries. It is problematic to say that a person is not autonomous or reasons-responsive because they picked "the wrong side" to trust, given that there are complicated and conflicting issues relating to epistemic trust that cannot all be boiled down to people being misinformed, biased, or ignorant. The experts are not always perfect decision-makers or communicators, which might lead to legitimate skepticism or mistrust. Indeed, many refusals likely fall into a middle category between type (a) and type (b)—we might refer to these as semi-principled refusals, characterized by an attitude of intelligent skepticism about the new vaccines, which is different from being simply scared, being stubborn to evidence, or having some sort of anti-newness bias.

One might wonder why we should even care about figuring out if an individual's choice to not vaccinate is reasons-responsive or autonomous or not.[13] In my view, given that there are some potential weak spots in the application of the harm principle to justify vaccine mandates, there would be a potential justificatory boost from weakening claims about autonomy infringement. Yet, as I have shown in this section, matters here are also far from straightforward.

4.6 A Word about the Least Restrictive Alternative—Mandates vs. Nudges and Incentives

Some argue that for vaccine mandates to be an ethically defensible public harm mitigation strategy, they must be the "least restrictive alternative"; meaning that there does not exist a harm mitigation strategy that would be just as effective but less burdensome (see Kass 2001: 1780). It is for this reason that some argue in favor of other options such as nudges and incentives. Nudging refers to using insights from behavioral economics and decision psychology to predictably shape people's decisions in ways that do not forbid or overly burden choice options. Examples of nudges to vaccinate include messenger effects (picking a messenger who people will identify with or want to be like), the use of social norms (letting people know that most other people, especially people in a group they identify with, are getting vaccinated), defaults (showing up with ready-to-administer vaccines), salience (making the harms of not vaccinating and benefits of vaccinating salient), affect (sharing emotional stories of people who died of COVID), and appeals to ego (appealing to the desire to help do good, especially for vulnerable

---

[13] Most Western philosophical accounts of autonomy rely on some notion of reasons-responsiveness.

groups). Unfortunately, nudge strategies have not been effective quickly enough in the US. The devil is in the details in terms of how much or for how long we need to try these alternative approaches; but suffice it to say that, in a situation of a rapidly spreading virus, every moment lost to continuing to try new methods of education or persuasion costs lives and public welfare. Incentives have also been experimented with, but they are not cost-effective or effective on the truly vaccine-hesitant or skeptical (see Fischels 2021, Gneezy et al. 2011, Kreps et al. 2021, Loewenstein and Cryder 2020, Robertson et al. 2021, Taylor et al. 2020, and Walkey et al. 2021).

4.7 Conclusion

In conclusion, this chapter points to some of the nuances and complexities around autonomy-based considerations and vaccine mandates in a pandemic. Many believe that they can set aside considerations related to individual autonomy by appealing to the harm principle to justify vaccine mandates, arguing that individual liberty interests can be overridden when they cause harm to others. I have argued that this move requires a philosophical account of risk as harm, clarification regarding a threshold for when risk and harm to others is significant enough to trigger the harm principle, and consideration of whether there are alternative forms of mandates that would protect others the same amount as vaccine mandates while imposing less of a strain on individual autonomy (e.g. mandated daily testing or mandated proof of previous infection). In the case of COVID-19, I have argued that the harm principle may reasonably be applied, especially considering the harm posed to hospital workers and systems in addition to the transmission harm to individual others. I have also argued that, based on current data, mandated proof of previous infection should be considered as an alternative to mandated vaccination, but that daily testing mandates are for the most part not feasible or cost-effective alternatives. Finally, I have argued that even if vaccine mandates can be justified under the harm principle, they ought not to be dismissed as a minor autonomy infringement as some are keen to do.

While my focus here has been on the case of the COVID-19 pandemic, there are lessons that we can draw for future pandemics. The main take-home is that vaccine mandates (or any mandates, for that matter) are only justified if the unvaccinated pose a substantial risk of harm to others (beyond a threshold), and this depends on the details of the unvaccinated population. Policymakers ought to be careful to calculate and analyze this carefully in future pandemics rather than making loose and broad appeals to the "harm principle" to justify mandates. Ethicists ought to be involved in these analyses because there is quite a bit of normative nuance to be worked out (e.g. regarding risk thresholds and risk to whom). Second, even in cases where the scientific evidence supports the effectiveness of some pandemic intervention such as a vaccine, there will be some people whose refusals are thoughtful and autonomous, and it may be hard to differentiate between those who have "good reasons" to refuse and those who do not. Third, mandates that infringe on individual autonomy may ultimately be justified under certain conditions, but these autonomy infringements ought not to be dismissed or minimized. Autonomy infringements that might appear minor to many may not actually be minor for certain groups—e.g. those who have been historically mistreated through autonomy violations or other harms.

Bibliography

Amin, K., and Cynthia Cox (2021), 'Unvaccinated COVID-19 hospitalizations cost billions of dollars', *Peterson-KFF Health System Tracker* (1 August 2021), https://www.healthsystemtracker.org/brief/unvaccinated-covid-patients-cost-the-u-s-health-system-billions-of-dollars/ (accessed 3 Nov. 2021).

Azarpanah, H., et al. (2021), 'Vaccine hesitancy: evidence from an adverse events following immunization database, and the role of cognitive biases', *BMC Public Health*, 21(1): 1686, doi:10.1186/s12889-021-11,745-1.

Bajaj, S. S., and Stanford, F. C. (2021), 'Beyond Tuskegee—Vaccine Distrust and Everyday Racism', *New England Journal of Medicine*, 384(5): e12, doi:10.1056/NEJMpv2035827.

Barda, N. et al. (2021), 'Safety of the BNT162b2 MRNA Covid-19 Vaccine in a Nationwide Setting', *The New England Journal of Medicine*, 385 (12): 1078–90. doi.org/10.1056/NEJMoa2110475.

Berenbaum, M. R. (2021), 'On COVID-19, cognitive bias, and open access', *Proceedings of the National Academy of Sciences*, 118(2), p. e2026319118. doi:10.1073/pnas.2026319118.

Block, J. (2021), 'Vaccinating people who have had covid-19: why doesn't natural immunity count in the US?', *BMJ*, 374:n2101, doi:10.1136/bmj.n2101.

Blumenthal-Barby, J. S. (2016), 'Biases and Heuristics in Decision Making and Their Impact on Autonomy', *American Journal of Bioethics*, 16(5): 5–1, doi:10.108 0/15265161.2016.1159750.

Blumenthal-Barby J. S. (2021), *Good Ethics and Bad Choices* (Cambridge, MA: MIT Press).

Bozio, C. H. et al. (2021), 'Laboratory-Confirmed COVID-19 Among Adults Hospitalized with COVID-19–Like Illness with Infection-Induced or mRNA Vaccine-Induced SARS-CoV-2 Immunity — Nine States, January–September 2021', *Morbidity and Mortality Weekly Report*, 70, doi:10.15585/mmwr.mm7044e1.

Brink, D. (2022), 'Mill's Moral and Political Philosophy', *Stanford Encyclopedia of Philosophy*, edited by Edward N. Zalta and Uri Nodelman. https://plato.stanford.edu/archives/fall2022/entries/mill-moral-political/.

Cavanaugh, A. M., et al. (2021), 'Reduced Risk of Reinfection with SARS-CoV-2 After COVID-19 Vaccination — Kentucky, May–June 2021', *Morbidity and Mortality Weekly Report*, 70(32): 1081–3, doi:10.15585/mmwr.mm7032e1.

Chin, E. T., et al. (2020), 'Frequency of routine testing for COVID-19 in high-risk healthcare environments to reduce outbreaks', *medRxiv*: 2020.04.30.20087015, doi:10.1101/2020.04.30.20087015.

Clement, Scott, Cece Pascual, and Monica Ulmanu (2021), 'Stress on the front lines of covid-19', *Washington Post* (6 April 2021), https://www.washingtonpost.com/health/2021/04/06/stress-front-lines-health-care-workers-share-hardest-parts-working-during-pandemic/ (accessed: 3 Nov. 2021).

Cutler, D. M., and Summers, L. H. (2020), 'The COVID-19 Pandemic and the $16 Trillion Virus', *JAMA*, 324(15): 1495–6, doi:10.1001/jama.2020.19759.

Fischels, J. (2021), 'Get $100 For A Vaccine? Cash Incentives Work for Some, Others Not So Much', *NPR*, 30 July 2021, https://www.npr.org/2021/07/30/1022567245/vaccine-cash-incentives-100-dollars-lotteries-effectiveness (accessed 15 Oct. 2021).

Galanis, P., et al. (2021), 'Nurses' burnout and associated risk factors during the COVID-19 pandemic: A systematic review and meta-analysis', *Journal of Advanced Nursing*, 77(8): 3286–302, doi:10.1111/jan.14839.

Gneezy, U., Meier, S., and Rey-Biel, P. (2011), 'When and Why Incentives (Don't) Work to Modify Behavior', *Journal of Economic Perspectives*, 25(4): 191–210, doi:10.1257/jep.25.4.191.

Grassly, N. C., et al. (2020), 'Comparison of molecular testing strategies for COVID-19 control: a mathematical modelling study', *The Lancet Infectious Diseases*, 20(12): 1381–9, doi:10.1016/S1473-3099(20)30630-7.

Hall, V. J., et al. (2021), 'SARS-CoV-2 infection rates of antibody-positive compared with antibody-negative health-care workers in England: a large, multicentre, prospective cohort study (SIREN)', *The Lancet*, 397(10283): 1459–69, doi:10.1016/S0140-6736(21)00675-9.

Hamel, Liz, et al. (2021), *KFF COVID-19 Vaccine Monitor: KFF*. (28 October 2021), https://www.kff.org/coronavirus-covid-19/poll-finding/kff-covid-19-vaccine-monitor-october-2021/ (accessed 4 Nov. 2021).

Havers, F. P., et al. (2021), *COVID-19-associated hospitalizations among vaccinated and unvaccinated adults ≥18 years—COVID-NET, 13 states, January 1 – July 24, 2021*. preprint, doi:10.1101/2021.08.27.21262356.

Jamrozik, E., Handfield, T., and Selgelid, M. J. (2016), 'Victims, vectors and villains: are those who opt out of vaccination morally responsible for the deaths of others?', *Journal of Medical Ethics*, 42(12): 762–8, doi:10.1136/medethics-2015-103327.

Kagan, S. (1989), *The Limits of Morality* (Oxford: Clarendon Press).

Kass, N. E. (2001), 'An Ethics Framework for Public Health', *American Journal of Public Health*, 91(11):1776–82.

Kreps, S., et al. (2021), 'Public attitudes toward COVID-19 vaccination: The role of vaccine attributes, incentives, and misinformation', *npj Vaccines*, 6(1): 1–7, doi:10.1038/s41541-021-00335-2.

Ling, R. (2020), 'Confirmation Bias in the Era of Mobile News Consumption: The Social and Psychological Dimensions', *Digital Journalism*, 8(5): 596–604, doi:10.108 0/21670811.2020.1766987.

Loewenstein, George, and Cynthia Cryder (2020), 'Why Paying People to Be Vaccinated Could Backfire', *New York Times* (15 December 2020), https://www.nytimes. com/2020/12/14/upshot/covid-vaccine-payment.html (accessed 17 Oct. 2021).

Lopes, L., et al. (2021), 'KFF COVID-19 Vaccine Monitor: June 2021 - Findings', *KFF*, 30 June 2021, https://www.kff.org/report-section/kff-covid-19-vaccine-monitor-june-2021-findings/ (accessed 4 Nov. 2021).

Lopez-Leon, S., et al. (2021), 'More than 50 long-term effects of COVID-19: a systematic review and meta-analysis', *Scientific Reports*, 11(1):16144, doi:10.1038/s41598-021-95565-8.

Lyng, G. D., et al. (2021), 'Identifying optimal COVID-19 testing strategies for schools and businesses: Balancing testing frequency, individual test technology, and cost', *PLOS ONE*, 16(3):e0248783, doi:10.1371/journal.pone.0248783.

Maheshwari, K. (2021), 'On the Harm of Imposing Risk of Harm', *Ethical Theory and Moral Practice*, 24(4): 965–80, doi: https://doi.org/10.1007/s10677-021-10227-y.

Mortality Analyses (2021), Johns Hopkins Coronavirus Resource Center, https://coronavirus.jhu.edu/data/mortality (accessed 4 Nov. 2021).

Mostaghimi, D., Valdez, C. N., Larson, H. T., Kalinich, C. C., and Iwasaki, A. (2022), 'Prevention of host-to-host transmission by SARS-CoV-2 vaccines', *The Lancet Infectious Diseases*, 22(2): 52–8, doi: https://doi.org/10.1016/S1473-3099(21)00472-2.

New York Times. (2021), 'How Nurses Are Feeling: Tired, Angry and Hopeless', (25 August 2021), https://www.nytimes.com/2021/08/25/opinion/letters/nurses-covid.html. (accessed 28 Nov. 2022).

Oberdiek, J. (2009), 'Towards a Right against Risking', *Law and Philosophy*, 28(4), doi: https://doi.org/10.1007/s10982-008-9039-5.

Pappa, S., et al. (2020), 'Prevalence of depression, anxiety, and insomnia among healthcare workers during the COVID-19 pandemic: A systematic review and meta-analysis', *Brain, Behavior, and Immunity*, 88: 901–7., doi:10.1016/j.bbi.2020. 05.026.

Paz, I. G. (2021), 'Colorado hospitals are nearly full as the state battles a growing caseload', *New York Times* (3 November 2021), https://www.nytimes.com/2021/11/03/us/colorado-hospitals.html (accessed 4 Nov. 2021).

Placani, A. (2017), 'When the Risk of Harm Harms', *Law and Philosophy*, 36(1): 77–100, doi: https://doi.org/10.1007/s10982-016-9277-x.

Polack, F. P. et al. (2020), 'Safety and Efficacy of the BNT162b2 mRNA Covid-19 Vaccine', *New England Journal of Medicine*, 383(27): 2603–15, doi:10.1056/NEJMoa2034577.

Powers, M., Faden, R., and Saghai, Y. (2012), 'Liberty, Mill and the Framework of Public Health Ethics', *Public Health Ethics*, 5(1): 6–15, doi:10.1093/phe/phs002.

Richterman, A., Meyerowitz, E. A., and Cevik, M. (2022), 'Indirect Protection by Reducing Transmission: Ending the Pandemic With Severe Acute Respiratory

Syndrome Coronavirus 2 Vaccination', *Open Forum Infectious Diseases*, 9(2), ofab259, doi: https://doi.org/10.1093/ofid/ofab259.

Robertson, C., et al. (2021), 'Paying Americans to take the vaccine—would it help or backfire?' *Journal of Law and the Biosciences*, 8(2): lsab027, doi:10.1093/jlb/lsab027.

Scobie, H. M., et al. (2021), 'Monitoring Incidence of COVID-19 Cases, Hospitalizations, and Deaths, by Vaccination Status — 13 US Jurisdictions, April 4–July 17, 2021', *MMWR. Morbidity and Mortality Weekly Report*, 70(37): 1284–90, doi:10.15585/mmwr.mm7037e1.

Shrestha, N. K. et al. (2021), 'Necessity of COVID-19 vaccination in previously infected individuals' (5 June 2021), doi:10.1101/2021.06.01.21258176.

Singanayagam, A., et al. (2021), 'Community transmission and viral load kinetics of the SARS-CoV-2 delta (B.1.617.2) variant in vaccinated and unvaccinated individuals in the UK: a prospective, longitudinal, cohort study', *The Lancet Infectious Diseases*, 0(0), doi:10.1016/S1473-3099(21)00648-4.

Stolle, L. B. et al. (2020), 'Fact vs Fallacy: The Anti-Vaccine Discussion Reloaded', *Advances in Therapy*, 37(11): 4481–90, doi:10.1007/s12325-020-01502-y.

Taylor, S., et al. (2020), 'A Proactive Approach for Managing COVID-19: The Importance of Understanding the Motivational Roots of Vaccination Hesitancy for SARS-CoV2', *Frontiers in Psychology*, 11: 2890, doi:10.3389/fpsyg.2020.575950.

Uslu, A. A., et al. (2021), 'The Decision to Not Get Vaccinated from the Perspective of the Unvaccinated', The COVID States Project #63: 16, https://osf.io/fazup/.

Villarreal, Daniel (2021), 'Biden mocks vaccine skeptics: "I have the freedom to kill you with my COVID"', *Newsweek*, https://www.newsweek.com/biden-mocks-vaccine-skeptics-i-have-freedom-kill-you-my-covid-1641485 (accessed 4 Nov. 2021).

Walkey, A. J., Law, A., and Bosch, N. A. (2021), 'Lottery-Based Incentive in Ohio and COVID-19 Vaccination Rates', *JAMA*, 326(8): 766–7, doi:10.1001/jama.2021.11048.

Williams, Tyler (2021), 'IDSA Response to CDC's Recommendation for People Previously Infected with COVID-19 to get Vaccinated', IDSA (31 October 2021), https://www.idsociety.org/news--publications-new/articles/2021/idsa-response-to-cdcs-recommendation-for-people-previously-infected-with-covid-19-to-get-vaccinated/ (accessed 4 Nov. 2021).

Wynia, Matthew K., Thomas D. Harter, and Jason T. Eberl (2021), 'Why A Universal COVID-19 Vaccine Mandate Is Ethical Today', *Health Affairs Blog*, https://www.healthaffairs.org/do/10.1377/hblog20211029.682797/full/ (accessed 4 Nov. 2021).

Yan, Holly, and Aya Elamroussi (2021), 'Unvaccinated Covid-19 patients are filling up hospitals, putting the care of others at risk, doctors say', *CNN* (3 November 2021), https://www.cnn.com/2021/08/01/health/us-coronavirus-sunday/index.html (accessed 3 Nov. 2021).

5

The Risks of Prohibition during Pandemics

Jessica Flanigan

During a pandemic, public officials may pass laws that penalize risky behaviour or they may pass laws that penalize transmission that results from risky behaviour. For example, public officials may enforce lockdown policies, mask mandates, vaccine mandates, or social distancing requirements that aim to prevent people from transmitting a contagious illness. Or they may directly penalize people who knowingly or recklessly harm others via contagious transmission.

In this chapter I argue against the penalization of risky behaviour and transmission. For most of this chapter, I focus on the policies that officials enforced to prevent the spread of COVID-19. But I also describe how these considerations could inform public health policies that relate to the transmission of other contagious diseases.

Proponents of a prohibitive approach to the prevention of contagious transmission may justify these policies either on the grounds that people who transmit or risk transmitting viruses are liable to be interfered with or on the grounds that a prohibitive approach is good for public health in general. Neither of these justifications succeeds, however, and there are serious risks to empowering public health officials to enforce prohibitive policies on these grounds.

In Section 5.1, I argue that the kinds of interference entailed by a prohibitive approach to public health cannot be justified by appeal to claims about liability. For one thing, many of the people who are subject to prohibitive public health policies are not liable to be interfered with. For another, public health policies are often excessively burdensome, even to those who are in principle liable to be interfered with for the sake of public health.

In Section 5.2, I make the case that prohibitive public health policies also cannot be justified on the grounds that they promote public health in general. There are many reasons to doubt officials' claims that prohibitive approaches effectively promote public health. First, some of the prohibitive policies that were enforced during the COVID pandemic, for example, were not supported by evidence. Second, even where there is evidence that some behavioural modification can effectively promote public health, there is not generally evidence that requiring

Jessica Flanigan, *The Risks of Prohibition during Pandemics* In: *Pandemic Ethics: From COVID-19 to Disease X.*
Edited by: Dominic Wilkinson and Julian Savulescu, Oxford University Press. © Oxford University Press 2023.
DOI: 10.1093/oso/9780192871688.003.0006

that modification would promote public health. Third, even if prohibitive public health policies do effectively promote public health, if there are non-prohibitive ways of achieving the same outcome, then officials should favour those means instead.

In Section 5.3, I then argue that officials may also lack the standing to enforce prohibitive public health requirements to the extent that they are also enforcing prohibitive policies that undermine public health in other ways. For example, if officials are actively impeding people's access to testing or vaccination, they lack the standing to impose burdensome pandemic mitigation requirements on people. Even where there is evidence that a prohibitive policy would promote public health, officials often overlook the possibility of backlash or the risks of stigmatizing and penalizing members of disadvantaged populations.

In Section 5.4, I consider how this argument applies beyond the example of COVID. My argument establishes a presumption against prohibitive public health policies, but it is not decisive. To the extent that an illness is more contagious or deadlier than COVID, the case for prohibitive policies is stronger. The case for more prohibitive policies is also stronger to the extent that an illness is more harmful to children. And it is even harder to justify prohibitive policies and mandates that aim to prevent the transmission of illnesses that are more easily avoided.

Section 5.5 concludes by reflecting on the broader implications of this argument for public health. I suggest that public health officials should hold themselves to the same standards as other public officials when it comes to the regulation of risky conduct, which would effectively mean that public health officials should not prohibit or regulate risky behaviour most of the time.

5.1 Policing Pandemic Risks

During a pandemic, public officials may enforce prohibitive policies that limit people's freedom for the sake of reducing rates of contagious transmission. These policies include mask mandates, testing requirements, enforced lockdowns, social distancing requirements, and vaccine mandates. In this section, let's assume for the sake of argument that these policies are effective. These policies may then be justified on the grounds that they protect people's rights against being infected with a deadly illness.

To illustrate this justification for prohibitive policies, consider an analogy that I develop further elsewhere (Flanigan 2014):

Gunfire Analogy: On Independence Day you are sitting outside watching fireworks when your patriotic neighbours begin shooting guns in the air to celebrate. Seeing that you are at risk, you make you way inside to avoid injury. Before you make it to your door, a bullet lodges in your arm. Later, you attend a

Memorial Day party with your children. Some of your neighbours bring their unvaccinated children, one of whom is coughing and gasping. Seeing that you are at risk, you gather your children and leave the party. But it's too late. Ten days later your child is diagnosed with pertussis. Your child is very ill for two months, he requires antibiotic treatment, and he misses several weeks of school.

I initially proposed this analogy to illustrate the point that people who recklessly transmit contagious illnesses violate other people's rights, just as people who recklessly fire guns in the air violate people's rights. In principle then, this analogy justifies prohibitive policies that protect people's rights against contagious transmission just as public officials are justified in enforcing policies that protect people's rights against being shot.

In other words, if people have rights against being put at risk or injured by others' reckless behaviour, then potential transmitters of contagious illnesses are liable to be interfered with. People who recklessly expose their neighbours to the risks of contagious transmission forfeit their rights against governmental interference in proportion to the risk they impose on others.

In principle, this argument can justify officials' enforcement of coercive policies in the context of a pandemic. Throughout the COVID pandemic, commentators have cited the gunfire analogy in arguments for vaccine mandates. The argument is that citizens who are potentially vectors of COVID transmission forfeit their rights against governmental interference to a degree that justifies a vaccine mandate. Before vaccines, one could have made similar case for lockdowns or mask mandates.

But in practice the applicability of the gunfire analogy to coercive COVID policy is less clear. During a pandemic, not everyone is liable to be interfered with on the grounds that they are likely to transmit a contagious illness. People who choose not to interact with the public and people who are immune to an illness do not put others at risk, and hence they are not liable to be interfered with on these grounds. So, at minimum, it would be difficult to justify a legal vaccine mandate for people who live in remote areas or for people who already had COVID.[1]

Another reason to doubt the applicability of the gunfire analogy to the case of prohibitive COVID policy is that the analogy assumes that people in public places cannot reduce their risk of being seriously injured by gunfire or contagious transmission. This analogy is apt for harmful diseases where vaccines are not very effective at preventing severe illness or where those most at risk are ineligible for vaccination. But once the COVID vaccine was available, those who were most at risk could generally avoid severe illness by getting vaccinated.

---

[1] This is to the extent that natural immunity produces a similar immunological response to vaccination, which is unclear (Castro Dopico et al. 2021; Waldman 2021).

Moreover, even if people were liable to be interfered with on the grounds that they could transmit COVID, liability on its own is not a sufficient justification for prohibitive policy. Even if someone forfeits their rights against interference when they expose others to a risk of COVID, it doesn't follow that public officials should interfere with them. It could be the case that any feasible way of enforcing a coercive vaccine mandate would be disproportionately burdensome to those who are liable, even if they have forfeited their rights against interference to some extent.[2]

And even if a person is liable to be interfered with and interference would not be disproportionate to their liability, this claim only establishes that a prohibitive policy would not violate people's rights against interference. It does not establish that public officials should, all things considered, enforce a prohibitive policy. Prohibitive policies can be costly even if they target people who are liable to be interfered with because any policy that relies on law enforcement puts people at risk of being treated unjustly by law enforcement. Also, a policy that primarily targets people who are liable to be interfered with can still be unjustified if it is enforced in a discriminatory or unequal way.

5.2 Prohibition and Public Health Outcomes

Considerations of liability cannot justify prohibitive responses to COVID, but perhaps that is unsurprising because many public health policies cannot be justified on the basis of liability. For example, people are not liable to be interfered with when they ride unbelted in cars, yet most public health authorities nevertheless think that seatbelt mandates are justified on the grounds that seatbelt mandates promote health or wellbeing to an extent that the moral cost of interfering with non-liable people is worth it. On this view, welfarist considerations can justify a coercive policy if the welfarist benefits are substantial and the harm of coercion is minor enough. Or, maybe I'm wrong about the moral significance of people's rights against interference, and public officials should aim instead to simply maximize population health or aggregate wellbeing.

Yet even if coercive public health policies can in principle be justified by an appeal to the good outcomes they promote, this justification for a prohibitive approach cannot justify the prohibitive policies that were enforced during the COVID pandemic, because officials often did not have solid evidence that proposed behavioural changes would be effective at promoting public health. And even when officials did have evidence that a behavioural change would effectively promote public health, they didn't have good evidence that coercive interventions requiring those behaviours would. And even if officials did have good evidence

---

[2] I defend this conception of liability further in *Duty and Enforcement* (Flanigan 2018).

that enforcing a prohibitive policy would effectively promote public health, they would also need to show that the coercive approach had better results than a non-coercive policy, which they generally did not do.

Consider first the claim that officials often did not have solid evidence that their proposed behavioural changes would effectively prevent COVID transmission. This isn't true for all behavioural interventions. The evidence that vaccination reduces rates of infection and transmission is very clear. But officials do not have such solid evidence for their masking guidance, lockdown policies, social distancing guidance, or school closures.

In the case of masking, officials in the United States first stated, without evidence, that masks were unnecessary for protecting people from COVID. Then officials said that masks were needed to protect people from COVID. The truth is probably somewhere in between these two claims. There is some observational evidence that community mask wearing reduces COVID transmission by preventing contagious people from infecting others and by protecting uninfected people (Brooks and Butler 2021; Leech et al. 2021). On the other hand, randomized controlled trials (RCTs) of masking are generally inconclusive, and few find a statistically significant correlation between mask wearing and protection from infection (Anderson 2021; Brosseau and Sietsema 2020).

One might reply to this line of argument that the evidence for the effectiveness of masking was evolving throughout the pandemic, and that officials did not know whether masking could be an effective intervention. On this view, officials might have thought it best to play it safe and mandate masking rather than permitting people to go maskless and potentially transmit COVID.

In response to this line of argument, I'm suggesting that there was not sufficient evidence for public health authorities or officials to confidently conclude not only that masking was effective at reducing COVID transmission but also that widespread mask wearing was so effective that public officials should mandate it. My point here is not to suggest that masking or mask mandates are ineffective. Several international studies suggest that mask mandates can reduce the rate of COVID infection (Karaivanov et al. 2021; Lim et al. 2020; Mitze et al. 2020). International comparisons are generally favourable to mask mandates for COVID (Adjodah et al. 2021). One influential study of the United States finds that mask mandates for employees are effective at reducing transmission rates, measured as weekly growth in cases and deaths by more than 10 per cent (Chernozhukov, Kasahara, and Schrimpf 2021a).[3] However, the evidence is difficult to interpret because even these studies establish only that mask mandates are correlated with better health outcomes; they do not establish that mask mandates would have been effective in the places that did not adopt them because it could be that mask mandates were

---

[3] See Chernozhukov, Kasahara, and Schrimpf (2021b) for a discussion of the validity of this study.

implemented by local officials in places where the population was also more cautious, supportive of masking, and compliant with public health guidelines.

Some researchers have attempted to find causal evidence for the effectiveness of widespread masking, which could provide evidence in favour of a mandate. Specifically, in 2021 researchers conducted a large-scale RCT of masking in Bangladesh as evidence of masks' effectiveness (Peeples 2021). But the Bangladesh study was not well designed to determine the efficacy of masking, and, in any case, the protective effect of masking was small (Recht 2021). If this is the strongest evidence that public officials can muster to justify a blanket requirement that citizens wear masks in public, they have not provided enough evidence to override maskless people's presumptive rights against interference.

What about the effectiveness of staying at home? Surely when people stay home, they are less likely to transmit COVID and they are less likely to be infected with COVID. But it's less clear that staying at home will protect someone in the long run, if it merely delays their exposure to COVID. The evidence for government-mandated lockdowns is fairly weak. Unless a community can entirely close its borders, short-term lockdowns are not a feasible solution to disease transmission because they only delay increases in the incidence of infection until the lockdown ends and disease transmission begins again (Scherbina 2020).

Granted, it could be good for officials to encourage people to stay home for short terms in limited cases. For example, if hospital systems are temporarily overwhelmed, undersupplied, and understaffed, then people may have moral reasons to stay home in an effort to avoid further contributing to an overburdened health system. However, policymakers that consistently underfund their health systems cannot generally rely on the public's goodwill as a means of keeping medical costs down, nor should they during a pandemic. Just as it would be wrong for policymakers to prohibit people from riding motorcycles, jumping on trampolines, or smoking, as a means of keeping down publicly subsidized healthcare costs, so too it is wrong for officials to mandate lockdowns for the sake of reducing stresses to the health systems they failed to adequately fund.

The claim that lockdown policies effectively reduced excess mortality is not clearly supported by the available evidence (Agrawal et al. 2021). And lockdowns were potentially harmful, on balance, in low-income countries (Ma et al. 2021). To the extent that lockdowns are effective during an outbreak, it is not clear that the lockdown is necessary because people stay home during outbreaks anyhow (Goolsbee and Syverson 2020). For this reason, proponents of lockdowns overestimate the benefits of lockdowns (Allen 2021). As the Swedish example suggests, voluntary behavioural changes have a similar effect to lockdowns, but this approach is less coercive and less costly (Lemoine 2021).

In both cases, the added benefits of enforcement do not seem justified, given that people can also voluntarily engage in masking behaviour or they may choose to stay home. The evidence for other policies is similarly shaky. For example, the 'two metre rule' or the 'six feet of social distancing' guidance was not based on accurate assumptions about how COVID is transmitted (Jones et al. 2020). Similarly, school closure guidelines also were not clearly supported by the evidence, which finds that reopening schools did not substantially increase community case rates (Ertem et al. 2021; Oster 2020).

For all these policies, I am not suggesting that the evidence clearly shows that public officials are doing more harm than good when they enforce lockdowns, mask mandates, distancing requirements, or school closures. Rather, I'm suggesting that public officials don't have sufficient evidence to justify coercive interventions, either because there is weak evidence in favour of the intervention, evidence that the intervention would be ineffective, or evidence that the intervention could be harmful on balance.

In contrast to these policies, the evidence in favour of vaccination as a way of preventing COVID-related infection, hospitalization, and death, is much clearer. RCTs and many observational studies find that vaccination dramatically reduces the prevalence and the severity of COVID. If public officials were *only* considering the health and welfarist benefits of a coercive response to the COVID pandemic, the best case for a coercive policy is in favour of a vaccine mandate.

But there are also risks to mandating vaccination that officials ought to consider. First, if a community could achieve mass immunization through private businesses' mandates and public incentive programs, such as prizes or payments for vaccination, then these non-coercive interventions would be preferable, insofar as there is some moral cost to exposing people to punishment or coercive penalties.

And counterintuitively, the case for a COVID vaccine mandate is weaker to the extent that the COVID vaccine is highly effective and widely available. As I argued in the previous section, the best case for any vaccine mandate appeals to the idea that it is wrong to transmit a harmful illness to people who cannot avoid infection. But if effective COVID vaccines are freely available to everyone, then people can generally avoid infection and avoid the harms of infection by becoming vaccinated. The case for a vaccine mandate is stronger for a disease like pertussis, because the pertussis vaccine is not as effective as the COVID vaccine and pertussis is most harmful to children who cannot be vaccinated. In the case of COVID, though, the disease is most harmful to older people who have access to a highly effective vaccine, so the justification for a COVID vaccine mandate (unlike other vaccine mandates) would be paternalistic, rather than based on the value of preventing harm to others.

More generally, prohibitive approaches to public health can be counterproductive to the extent that they contribute to the stigmatization of illness. For example, people who knowingly transmit a contagious illness may in principle be liable to punishment or required to pay compensation (Caplan et al. 2012). But enforcing such a policy could discourage people from getting tested, as happened previously when some US states criminalized the transmission of HIV

(Centers for Disease Control and Prevention 2021). Prohibitive approaches to public health policy can also contribute to broader socioeconomic disparities to the extent that people with lower socioeconomic status are more subject to state surveillance and law enforcement.

5.3 Public Health Hypocrisy

In response to the foregoing argument, a proponent of coercive pandemic policies may reply that I am holding public officials to an unfairly high standard. After all, many laws coerce non-liable people for the sake of the greater good. Many laws are paternalistic. And public officials often enforce coercive policies even if an equally effective non-coercive alternative is available. But officials' decision to use coercive policies to address the COVID pandemic is distinctively objectionable in part because officials were simultaneously enforcing prohibitive policies that violated people's rights and made the pandemic worse. Here I am referring to the enforcement of policies that prevented people from accessing testing and premarket approval policies that impeded the development and distribution of vaccines. Not all public officials were responsible for upholding these counterproductive policies, but those who were lacked the standing to enforce or even recommend coercive laws aimed at slowing the spread of COVID.

In addition to the aforementioned lockdowns, mask mandates, vaccine mandates, and school closures, public officials also enforced prohibitive public health regulations that made the COVID pandemic worse. In the United States, for example, these include restrictions on private provision of testing during the early weeks of the pandemic (Boburg et al. 2020) and officials' delayed approval of rapid antigen tests (Przybyla 2021; Rubin 2020). Officials delayed approval of vaccines (McGinley and Johnson 2020), failed to invest in manufacturing capacity (Athey et al. 2020), and failed to approve all effective vaccines (Irfan 2021)—policies that contributed to the pandemic's death toll by delaying access to vaccines. Officials also continue to prohibit people from participating in challenge trials, which slowed vaccine development and continues to impede researchers' ability to understand COVID (Flanigan 2021). Regulators' delayed approval of vaccination for children alongside the prohibition of off-label prescribing for children potentially increased rates of transmission during the wave of Delta-variant infections (Jenco 2021; Savo Beers 2021).

Many of these public health regulations are justified as a way of preventing researchers and manufacturers from harming patients. But these prohibitive policies do not protect patients, they prevent people from voluntarily accessing the means to treat or prevent illness in the case of vaccine development, or from knowing their medical status in the case of testing. Elsewhere, I have argued that preventing people from accessing tests, participating in trials, or purchasing and using vaccines violates people's bodily rights. And since we now know that

COVID vaccines are highly effective, we can see that delaying vaccination cost lives. Regulators' cautionary approach was especially harmful because rates of infection grow exponentially, so addressing outbreaks early saves many more lives.

In defence of a cautionary approach, some have argued that regulators sought to avoid a public health event, such as an unsafe vaccine, which would erode the public's trust in the health system (e.g. Gupta et al. 2021). But to the extent that public officials are genuinely concerned with preserving public trust, they should first look inward at the misleading and false messaging they engaged in at the beginning of the pandemic (Powell and Prasad 2021).

Public health officials who were concerned with public trust would also aim to avoid excessively partisan messaging in order to ensure that negative political polarization would not undermine vaccination efforts (Nahum, Drekonja, and Alpern 2021). And trust-sensitive officials would also aim to avoid accusations of double standards in their public health guidance, which officials encountered when they advocated for a ban on religious gatherings and anti-lockdown protests, but not other political protests (Powell 2020). Additionally, public officials should research the determinants of public health compliance more rigorously and assess whether the risks to public trust in the event of a drug disaster warrant the deadly delays associated with a cautious regulatory approach. Officials should also consider whether their communications about the risks of transmission may be counterproductive in populations that engage in risky socializing when presented with a potential threat (Forsyth 2021).

In response to this line of argument, one may argue that even if public health officials lack the standing to impose coercive restrictions on citizens, if those restrictions are in fact effective, then public officials should nevertheless enforce them.[4] After all, in many cases a bad messenger is better than no messenger at all. However, a bad messenger is not better in cases where their message backfires and further undermines compliance with public health guidance. In light of the foregoing considerations, it is reasonable for citizens to view coercive public health policies with suspicion because public officials made the pandemic worse than it needed to be in many ways, and in some cases they misled the public. In cases like this, when officials lack standing to credibly claim that their proposed coercive and prohibitive pandemic responses are necessary or justified, public health interventions carry the risk of backfiring in this way.

5.4 General Principles for Prohibition and Pandemics

To this point, my argument has proceeded as follows. I first argued that public officials do not have the right to enforce prohibitive public health policies that

---

[4] I am thankful to Govind Persad for encouraging me to consider this objection.

coerce non-liable citizens who are not engaged in wrongdoing. I then argued that even policies that coerce liable people are often enforced in ways that are disproportionate to people's liability. Next, I considered the view that officials may have a right to coerce non-liable people if doing so would promote better public health outcomes. In response to this view, I suggested that coercive policies often fail to meet this standard and there are significant risks to adopting a prohibitive approach if alternatives are available.

These arguments apply more generally, beyond the COVID pandemic. Public health officials should generally adopt a presumption against enforcing prohibitive policies because they have historically been overly quick to violate people's rights while advancing policies that were not effective. For example, officials plausibly violate tobacco manufacturers' rights against compelled speech when they required them to include graphic warning labels about the dangers of smoking (Haynes, Andrews, and Jacob 2013), though there is not sufficient evidence that these kinds of labels are effective at reducing smoking behaviour (Strong et al. 2021). Similarly, in the case of the COVID pandemic, most public health officials heartily endorsed coercive policies in the absence of sufficient evidence that these policies would effectively reduce the severity of the pandemic.

This is not to say that a coercive approach can never be justified. In some cases, a mandate or prohibition may be necessary as a last resort. Several factors should inform officials' decision to enforce coercive policies. These include the rate of contagious transmission, the severity of illness, the extent that infection is avoidable, and the extent that a disease is harmful to children.

A non-coercive, non-prohibitive approach to pandemics begins by removing burdensome regulations that impede people from effectively preventing or treating illness. For example, during the COVID pandemic many states relaxed or removed scope of practice regulations for healthcare providers and regulations that previously made it difficult for people to access telemedicine. In addition to these regulations, officials should also consider relaxing or removing regulations that restrict people's access to testing, rapid tests, and opportunities to participate in medical research through challenge trials. Rather than framing questions of pandemic policy in terms of trade-offs between freedom and public health, officials should look for deviations from the status quo that effectively promote both values.

Where officials do resort to coercion, they should be mindful of several things. First, officials who implement a coercive policy for the sake of public health should have solid evidence that the policy is mandating an effective behavioural change and that the mandate itself would effectively promote that behavioural change *before* they implement the coercive policy. One may reply that this requirement is unrealistic in the context of a quickly evolving pandemic because it is infeasible for officials to gather high-quality evidence about how to effectively change behaviour. Yet this reply assumes that coercion is presumptively justified, and should only be abandoned when a public policy is evidently ineffective. Whereas, on my view, public officials should be mindful of the moral risks of coercion. One of the risks of using coercion is that a public health intervention can backfire if it becomes politicized or if it stigmatizes sickness in a way that prevents people from seeking treatment or refraining from risky conduct. But more generally, coercion is always presumptively morally risky, so if a non-coercive policy is available, officials should consider bearing significant costs to avoid the risk of unjustifiably violating people's rights (Guerrero 2007; Moller 2011).

Public officials should also be able to show that the effects of their proposed coercive policy are good *on balance,* not just good in terms of narrow pandemic-related outcomes. This is difficult to achieve when people who work for public health agencies, which are primarily responsible for reducing negative health outcomes from the pandemic, are also responsible for making public health policy. This arrangement provides insufficient incentives for officials to consider whether the overall burdens of complying with a prohibitive policy are proportionate to the good that is achieved through the policy and that the burdens of the policy are equitably distributed.[5]

So while in principle some prohibitive policies can be justified as a way of protecting people's rights, in practice these policies are costly and morally risky. For these reasons, public officials should err on the side of a permissive approach, rather than a prohibitive approach. One critic of a permissive approach to vaccine development has argued that it's better to enforce coercive mandates that require things like masking and social distancing because the burdens of pandemic management should be shared among citizens in a democratic society (Bramble 2021). But even if a more permissive approach lets some people off the hook, and even if it's valuable for citizens to share the costs of prevention, these benefits of enforcing coercive pandemic policies are not worth the moral risks of enforcement and the costs of prohibition. In most cases, the best way for officials to respond to pandemic risks is to first get out of the way of researchers and to provide honest and accurate information to the public while avoiding coercion.

5.5 Conclusion

Public officials are often faced with trade-offs related to risk. They must decide how much risk to tolerate, and when to protect people from risk. Judgments about acceptable risk are normative judgments. For example, when a mayor decides that there is too much lead in the public water supply or when a regulator

---

[5] This is similar to Klosko's claim that policies which require people to contribute to public goods should distribute the burdens of providing a benefit in a way that is fair and that the burdens are proportionate to the value of the benefit (Klosko 1987).

decides that a factory produces too much air pollution, they are judging that the risks of injury from lead or pollution are not morally acceptable. When a judge decides that a prisoner should not be paroled, they are judging that the prisoner poses an unacceptable risk to public safety. Likewise, whenever a public official enforces a coercive policy for the sake of public health, they are imposing their judgment about whether the risk of an activity is acceptable on an entire population of people who may have different levels of risk tolerance.

I have claimed that public officials should generally take a permissive approach to pandemic-related risks. Because people have different levels of risk tolerance, a permissive approach amounts to letting people manage risks in their own lives as much as is possible. This principle favours a broadly non-paternalistic approach to public policy, where citizens are free to put their health at risk. But this principle also supports a fairly non-prohibitive approach to choices that expose others to risks that they cannot consent to. In these cases, officials must decide whether the benefits of prohibiting a risky choice exceed the moral risks of enforcing a prohibitive policy, but they should seriously weigh the practical costs of enforcement even if coercion can be justified in principle.

There isn't a formula to determine whether and when officials should intervene to minimize risks to innocent bystanders. However, to the extent that officials tolerate activities such as driving and alcohol consumption, both of which expose non-consenting bystanders to some level of risk of death, then they should also tolerate other activities that expose non-consenting bystanders to a lower level of risk or which risk less severe harms. This principle provides further guidance for officials who are considering enforcing prohibitive policies during a pandemic. If the risks of contagious transmission are less than the risks associated with driving or consuming alcohol, then officials should refrain from enforcing coercive policies to address a pandemic.

A less prohibitive approach to public health during a pandemic could also enable officials to concentrate resources where they will do the most good. Instead of trying to control everyone's behaviour, public health would be better served if officials focused on preparing for and avoiding the worst outcomes while re-establishing the legitimacy they lost during the COVID pandemic.

Bibliography

Adjodah, Dhaval, Karthik Dinakar, Matteo Chinazzi, Samuel P. Fraiberger, Alex Pentland, Samantha Bates, Kyle Staller, Alessandro Vespignani, and Deepak L. Bhatt (2021), 'Association between COVID-19 Outcomes and Mask Mandates, Adherence, and Attitudes', *PLOS ONE* 16(6): e0252315, https://doi.org/10.1371/journal.pone.0252315.

Agrawal, Virat, Jonathan H. Cantor, Neeraj Sood, and Christopher M. Whaley (2021), 'The Impact of the COVID-19 Pandemic and Policy Responses on Excess Mortality',

Working Paper 28930. Working Paper Series. National Bureau of Economic Research, https://doi.org/10.3386/w28930.

Allen, Douglas W. (2021), 'COVID-19 Lockdown Cost/Benefits: A Critical Assessment of the Literature.' *International Journal of the Economics of Business* 0(0): 1–32, https://doi.org/10.1080/13571516.2021.1976051.

Anderson, Jeffrey (2021), 'Do Masks Work? A Review of the Evidence.' *City Journal*, August 10, 2021, https://www.city-journal.org/do-masks-work-a-review-of-the-evidence.

Athey, Susan, Michael Kremer, Christopher Snyder, and Alex Tabarrok (2020), 'Opinion: In the Race for a Coronavirus Vaccine, We Must Go Big. Really, Really Big.' *New York Times*, May 4, 2020, sec. Opinion, https://www.nytimes.com/2020/05/04/opinion/coronavirus-vaccine.html.

Boburg, Shawn, Robert O'Harrow Jr, Neena Satija, and Amy Goldstein (2020), 'Inside the Coronavirus Testing Failure: Alarm and Dismay among the Scientists Who Sought to Help.' *Washington Post*, Apr. 2, 2020.

Bramble, Ben (2021), 'The Ethics of Human Challenge Trials: COVID-19 and Beyond.' *Cato Unbound*, March 9, 2021, https://www.cato-unbound.org/issues/march-2021/ethics-human-challenge-trials-covid-19-beyond.

Brooks, John T., and Jay C. Butler (2021), 'Effectiveness of Mask Wearing to Control Community Spread of SARS-CoV-2.' *JAMA* 325(10): 998–9, https://doi.org/10.1001/jama.2021.1505.

Brosseau, Lisa M., and Margaret Sietsema (2020), 'Masks-for-All for COVID-19 Not Based on Sound Data.' *Center for Infectious Disease Research and Policy*, April 2020, https://www.cidrap.umn.edu/news-perspective/2020/04/commentary-masks-all-covid-19-not-based-sound-data.

Caplan, Arthur L., David Hoke, Nicholas J. Diamond, and Viktoriya Karshenboyem (2012), 'Free to Choose but Liable for the Consequences: Should Non-Vaccinators Be Penalized for the Harm They Do?' *Journal of Law, Medicine & Ethics: A Journal of the American Society of Law, Medicine & Ethics* 40(3): 606–11, https://doi.org/10.1111/j.1748-720X.2012.00693.x.

Castro Dopico, Xaquin, Sebastian Ols, Karin Loré, and Gunilla B. Karlsson Hedestam (2021), 'Immunity to SARS-CoV-2 Induced by Infection or Vaccination.' *Journal of Internal Medicine* 291(1), https://doi.org/10.1111/joim.13372.

Centers for Disease Control and Prevention (2021), 'HIV and STD Criminalization Laws', CDC, October 25, 2021, https://www.cdc.gov/hiv/policies/law/states/exposure.html.

Chernozhukov, Victor, Hiroyuki Kasahara, and Paul Schrimpf (2021a), 'Causal Impact of Masks, Policies, Behavior on Early COVID-19 Pandemic in the U.S', *Journal of Econometrics*, 220(1): 23–62, https://doi.org/10.1016/j.jeconom.2020.09.003.

Chernozhukov, Victor, Hiroyuki Kasahara, and Paul Schrimpf (2021b), 'A Response to Philippe Lemoine's Critique on Our Paper 'Causal Impact of Masks, Policies, Behavior on Early COVID-19 Pandemic in the U.S." *ArXiv:2110.06136*, https://arxiv.org/abs/2110.06136.

Ertem, Zeynep, Elissa M. Schechter-Perkins, Emily Oster, Polly van den Berg, Isabella Epshtein, Nathorn Chaiyakunapruk, Fernando A. Wilson, et al. (2021), 'The Impact of School Opening Model on SARS-CoV-2 Community Incidence and Mortality.' *Nature Medicine*, October, 1–7, https://doi.org/10.1038/s41591-021-01563-8.

Flanigan, Jessica (2014), 'A Defense of Compulsory Vaccination', *HEC Forum*, 26:5–25, http://link.springer.com/article/10.1007/s10730-013-9221-5.

Flanigan, Jessica (2018), 'Duty and Enforcement', *Journal of Political Philosophy* 27(3): 341–62. https://doi.org/10.1111/jopp.12173.

Flanigan, Jessica (2021), 'The Case for Challenge Trials.' *Cato Unbound*, March 9, 2021, https://www.cato-unbound.org/2021/03/09/jessica-flanigan/case-challenge-trials.

Forsyth, Rachel B. (2021), 'When Motivated Responses to Threat Backfire: Risky Socializing During the COVID-19 Health Crisis.' *Social Psychological and Personality Science* 13(5), https://doi.org/10.1177/19485506211045885.

Goolsbee, Austan, and Chad Syverson (2020), 'Fear, Lockdown, and Diversion: Comparing Drivers of Pandemic Economic Decline 2020.' Working Paper 27432. National Bureau of Economic Research, https://doi.org/10.3386/w27432.

Guerrero, Alexander A. (2007), 'Don't Know, Don't Kill: Moral Ignorance, Culpability, and Caution.' *Philosophical Studies* 136(1): 59–97.

Gupta, Ravi, Jason Schwartz, Joseph Ross, and Genevieve Kanter (2021), 'During COVID-19, FDA's Vaccine Advisory Committee Has Worked To Boost Public Trust – It Can Still Do More' Health Affairs Blog, February 26, 2021, https://www.healthaffairs.org/do/10.1377/hblog20210225.712221/full/.

Haynes, Bryan M., Anne Hampton Andrews, and C. Reade Jacob (2013), 'Compelled Commercial Speech: The Food and Drug Administration's Effort to Smoke Out the Tobacco Industry through Graphic Warning Labels.' *Food and Drug Law Journal* 68(4): 329–56.

Irfan, Umair (2021), 'AstraZeneca's Absurd and Unprecedented Dispute with Regulators, Explained.' *Vox*, March 25, 2021, https://www.vox.com/22346789/astrazeneca-covid-19-vaccine-oxford-efficacy-results-nih-fda.

Jenco, Melissa (2021), 'AAP: Don't Use COVID-19 Vaccine off-Label for Children.' *AAP News*, October, https://www.aappublications.org/news/2021/08/23/fda-covid-vaccine-licensure-082321,/news/2021/08/23/fda-covid-vaccine-licensure-082321.

Jones, Nicholas R., Zeshan U. Qureshi, Robert J. Temple, Jessica P. J. Larwood, Trisha Greenhalgh, and Lydia Bourouiba (2020), 'Two Metres or One: What Is the Evidence for Physical Distancing in COVID-19?' *BMJ* 370 (August): m3223, https://doi.org/10.1136/bmj.m3223.

Karaivanov, Alexander, Shih En Lu, Hitoshi Shigeoka, Cong Chen, and Stephanie Pamplona (2021), 'Face Masks, Public Policies and Slowing the Spread of COVID-19: Evidence from Canada', https://doi.org/10.1101/2020.09.24.20201178.

Klosko, George (1987), 'Presumptive Benefit, Fairness, and Political Obligation', *Philosophy & Public Affairs* 16(3): 241–59.

Leech, Gavin, Charlie Rogers-Smith, Jonas B. Sandbrink, Benedict Snodin, Robert Zinkov, Benjamin Rader, John S. Brownstein, et al. (2021), 'Mass Mask-Wearing

Notably Reduces COVID-19 Transmission', https://doi.org/10.1101/2021.06.16.21258817.

Lemoine, Philippe (2021), 'The Case against Lockdowns.' *CSPI Center* (blog). March 4, 2021, https://cspicenter.org/blog/waronscience/the-case-against-lockdowns/.

Lim, S., H. I. Yoon, K.-H. Song, E. S. Kim, and H. B. Kim (2020), 'Face Masks and Containment of COVID-19: Experience from South Korea', *Journal of Hospital Infection* 106(1): 206–7, https://doi.org/10.1016/j.jhin.2020.06.017.

Ma, Lin, Gil Shapira, Damien de Walque, Quy-Toan Do, Jed Friedman, and Andrei A. Levchenko (2021), 'The Intergenerational Mortality Tradeoff of COVID-19 Lockdown Policies.' Working Paper 28925, National Bureau of Economic Research, https://doi.org/10.3386/w28925.

McGinley, Laurie, and Carolyn Johnson (2020), 'FDA Poised to Announce Tougher Standards for a COVID-19 Vaccine That Make It Unlikely One Will Be Cleared by Election Day.' *Washington Post*, September 22, 2020, https://www.washingtonpost.com/health/2020/09/22/fda-covid-vaccine-approval-standard/.

Mitze, Timo, Reinhold Kosfeld, Johannes Rode, and Klaus Wälde (2020), 'Face Masks Considerably Reduce COVID-19 Cases in Germany', *Proceedings of the National Academy of Sciences* 117(51): 32293–301, https://doi.org/10.1073/pnas.2015954117.

Moller, Dan (2011), 'Abortion and Moral Risk.' *Philosophy* 86(3): 425–43.

Nahum, Ari, Dimitri M Drekonja, and Jonathan D Alpern (2021), 'The Erosion of Public Trust and SARS-CoV-2 Vaccines— More Action Is Needed', *Open Forum Infectious Diseases* 8(2), https://doi.org/10.1093/ofid/ofaa657.

Oster, Emily (2020), 'Opinion: Schools Are Not Spreading COVID-19. This New Data Makes the Case', *Washington Post*, November 20, 2020, sec. Opinions, https://www.washingtonpost.com/opinions/2020/11/20/covid-19-schools-data-reopening-safety/.

Peeples, Lynne (2021), 'Face Masks for COVID Pass Their Largest Test Yet', *Nature*, September, https://doi.org/10.1038/d41586-021-02457-y.

Powell, Kerrington, and Vinay Prasad (2021), 'The Noble Lies of COVID-19', *Slate*, July 28, 2021, https://slate.com/technology/2021/07/noble-lies-covid-fauci-cdc-masks.html.

Powell, Michael (2020), 'Are Protests Dangerous? What Experts Say May Depend on Who's Protesting What', *New York Times*, July 6, 2020, sec. U.S, https://www.nytimes.com/2020/07/06/us/Epidemiologists-coronavirus-protests-quarantine.html.

Przybyla, Heidi (2021), 'Critics Say Regulatory Holdup Is Delaying Key Weapon in Coronavirus Fight', NBC News, March 18, 2021, https://www.nbcnews.com/politics/congress/critics-say-regulatory-holdup-delaying-key-weapon-coronavirus-fight-n1261337.

Recht, Benjamin (2021), 'Effect Size Is Significantly More Important than Statistical Significance', Arg Min Blog, September 13, 2021, http://benjamin-recht.github.io/2021/09/13/effect-size/.

Rubin, Rita (2020), 'The Challenges of Expanding Rapid Tests to Curb COVID-19', *JAMA* 324(18): 1813–15, https://doi.org/10.1001/jama.2020.21106.

Savo Beers, Lee (2021), 'Letter to Janet Woodcock, Acting Commissioner, Food and Drug Administration', American Academy of Pediatrics, https://downloads.aap.org/DOFA/AAP%20Letter%20to%20FDA%20on%20Timeline%20for%20Authorization%20of%20COVID-19%20Vaccine%20for%20Children_08_05_21.pdf.

Scherbina, Anna (2020), *Determining the Optimal Duration of the COVID-19 Suppression Policy: A Cost-Benefit Analysis*, AEI Economic Policy Working Paper, American Enterprise Institute, May 1, 2020.

Strong, David R., John P. Pierce, Kim Pulvers, Matthew D. Stone, Adriana Villaseñor, Minya Pu, Claudiu V. Dimofte, et a (2021), 'Effect of Graphic Warning Labels on Cigarette Packs on US Smokers' Cognitions and Smoking Behavior After 3 Months: A Randomized Clinical Trial.' *JAMA Network Open* 4(8): e2121387, https://doi.org/10.1001/jamanetworkopen.2021.21387.

Waldman, Meredith (2021), 'Having SARS-CoV-2 Once Confers Much Greater Immunity than a Vaccine—but Vaccination Remains Vital', *Science*, August 26, 2021, https://www.science.org/content/article/having-sars-cov-2-once-confers-much-greater-immunity-vaccine-vaccination-remains-vital.

6

Handling Future Pandemics

Harming, Not Aiding, and Liberty

F. M. Kamm

6.1 Introduction

All over the world there have been protests over restrictions legally imposed to deal with the COVID-19 pandemic (such as mask wearing, lockdowns, and required vaccination for participation in many activities). In addition, there has been libertarian-like resistance to the idea that there are moral grounds for such restrictions even when they are not legally enforced. (It is because some deny (or do not act on) moral grounds that legal mandates arise.) I will be concerned with the moral issue in this chapter.[1]

Can we decrease the probability of similar opposition in future pandemics? This is in part an empirical question about causal mechanisms. But it is also a question about what mechanisms are morally justifiable. Assuming that it would be wrong to make people more docile and regimented or to manipulate them, one justifiable approach is communicating to the general public essential moral distinctions related to liberty, responsibility, and distribution of burdens.

Future pandemics and the means to combat or mitigate them may be very different from what is true about COVID-19. This is so even when the "future" is near-term rather than so distant that it involves only future generations. When I refer to measures for dealing with COVID-19 (e.g. masks or vaccines), they should be taken as mere stand-ins for different possible measures needed in the future that require similar costs or burdens. The types of issues related to liberty-focused views that I discuss are sufficiently general that versions of them can be expected to arise in future pandemics. My suggestions for dealing with these issues from a moral (rather than a legal) point of view take seriously libertarian-like views that emphasize rights not to be interfered with and only minimal (if any) duties to provide aid. Hence, my suggestions could be useful both (a) in addressing those who hold such views and (b) in helping others who address

---

[1] Some libertarian-like views are limited to government action. I shall not be speaking to those views.

F. M. Kamm, *Handling Future Pandemics: Harming, Not Aiding, and Liberty* In: *Pandemic Ethics: From COVID-19 to Disease X*. Edited by: Dominic Wilkinson and Julian Savulescu, Oxford University Press.
© Oxford University Press 2023. DOI: 10.1093/oso/9780192871688.003.0007

them to appreciate that certain measures are justifiable in principle to those with libertarian-like views even if the latter do not grasp this. There are many positions about when a justification to another person is in principle sufficient and appropriate. I will rely on being able to derive implications from that other person's views.[2]

The chapter is divided into two sections. The first section offers twelve proposals for elucidating the right not to be harmed and duties not to harm others, distinguishing these from the right to be aided and duties to provide aid. The second section delves into aspects of the twelfth proposal, investigating how to weigh costs to some against "benefits" to others. It draws implications from this discussion for whether elective procedures should be postponed and lockdowns imposed on some to prevent imminent deaths of others.

6.2   Distinguishing Not Harming from Aiding

Emphasizing the distinction between not harming and aiding should be important to those with libertarian-like views, since libertarians typically emphasize negative moral rights not to be harmed (at least in certain ways and without one's consent) even if they do not emphasize positive moral rights to be aided and duties to aid.[3] The distinction is based, roughly, on rights over oneself as a separate person which implies that others have weak or no right to one's efforts except to prevent one's interfering with others' rights over themselves. Hence, universalizing a right not to be harmfully interfered with by others (in certain ways) implies a correlative duty not to harmfully interfere with others who have the same rights.[4]

Each of the twelve proposals could be included in public health messaging to increase understanding of what moral rights are at stake, and why libertarian-like views need not conflict with many best community practices during a pandemic.

(i) There are different types of illnesses. As simple as it sounds, it is important to appreciate and communicate the difference between contagious versus non-contagious illnesses. Many of those who protest restrictions repeat the mantra that what happens in and to their own bodies is up to them. (They here rely on widespread agreement that paternalistic interference and duties not to harm

---

[2] That a position is justifiable "to" someone need not mean it is justifiable. This can happen if the position is implied only by that person's mistaken views. Nevertheless, in a democracy it could sometimes be justifiable to justify positions to people who hold unjustifiable views on the basis of their views.

[3] Not all ways of harming others, such as competition that harms someone's business, are ruled out by libertarian-like views. In competition, one business offers a consumer a benefit which they are free to accept if they have no duty to help another business. This indirectly leads to making that other business worse off in a permissible way.

[4] Even those who recognize strong moral duties to aid could distinguish morally between harming and not aiding, as shown by (other things equal) lower costs required to aid than not to harm and the priority of not harming some rather than aiding others in a forced choice. On this see Kamm (1996) and (2007).

oneself have limits in liberal societies.) They might not emphasize this if they appreciated that when they have a contagious illness, its effects do not remain in their own bodies (like a cancer) but can affect others outside their bodies in a harmful way. This can occur by way of transmission of the illness. Furthermore, it is important to communicate that someone who is asymptomatic could transmit an illness that makes others seriously ill.

Having a contagious illness is different from possibly having it; in both cases, but especially in the latter, there is only a risk that one can transmit illness. However, if there are many people and each has a low risk of carrying a virus, by the so-called law of large numbers it is certain that someone will have the virus and infect some other people. On an ex post view, the focus is on the number who will be infected and seriously harmed. (This is typically the public health approach.) There may be a tendency to impose large costs on individuals to pre-vent much serious ex post harm, but imposing large costs on each individual in a large population who has only a small chance ex ante of harming others and also of being someone who will be harmed seems unreasonable regardless of the ex post numbers.[5] However, when the costs of preventing serious effects of infection (e.g. death) are low (e.g. wearing a mask), a moral duty to prevent oneself from causing or risking serious harm to others seems justified, at least if this is the only means available for stopping the large amount of serious ex post harm.

If the harm that either will or may occur becomes less serious, this is a reason for reducing the cost that may permissibly be imposed on a threatener. But how should we calculate the seriousness of a harm? It is an aspect of being infected with some diseases that surviving them gives the benefit of increased immunity to future illness of the same type. Suppose the worst effect of an illness is less than death or else the risk of death is very low. Should the possible benefit of increased immunity be taken into account when deciding whether to permit the initial harm? Seana Shiffrin has argued that one should refrain from imposing an initial harm on someone even if one knows they will benefit overall. For example, she claims that one may not (without consent) break someone's arm to produce more than compensating wealth for him though one might break his arm to prevent a worse outcome such as his death.[6] The issue then becomes how much of a risk of death or other significant harm one may present to others when this provides them subsequent immunity to death or other significant harm. (Even taking a vaccine imposes a very small risk of death in order to greatly decrease overall chance of death.) If data show that allowing natural infection and immunity lead

---

[5] Similarly, when each person has a small chance of winning a lottery, depriving each of that chance can result in someone not winning big. However, the loss to each in being deprived of a small chance of winning is small and so there might justifiably be less concern that one of these people who has a small chance of winning will be negatively affected in a big way ex post. By contrast, taking away the winning lottery ticket from one person is a big loss to him.

[6] See Shiffrin (1999). For some criticism of her argument see Kamm (2013a).

to many more deaths than preventing transmission, doing the latter at low cost imposed on each person seems justified.[7]

(ii) There may be various ways to harm others. It is important to appreciate and communicate that besides transmission of a virus there may be additional ways to harm others. Allowing one's body to be a location in which a virus can mutate so that it can evade currently effective vaccines may be another way to harm others.[8] This might be so even if one doesn't transmit the mutated virus directly to others but an intervening entity (e.g. an insect) carries it to others. Analogously, suppose that dust that accumulates on one's property attracts insects who multiply on it and fly off on their own to infect people. Since insects are not intervening moral agents, one could be said to harm others if one does not get rid of the dust. It is even clearer that one harms others if only something one does (e.g. move around) causes these insects to fly off to others.

Another way to harm others could be by overburdening healthcare systems. Suppose victims of a viral pandemic seek medical care so that others in need go untreated. Then the latter are at least made worse off by those who spread a virus and/or do not prevent their own illness. (Note that some of those who cannot access treatment may also not have taken care to avoid their illnesses. Their seeking care would worsen victims of a pandemic who then cannot get care.)[9]

(iii) It is possible to harm someone without intending to do so. It is important to appreciate and communicate that harmful interference with others by those who transmit disease can occur without anyone intending harm; one can run over another person with a car though one does not intend this. Indeed, philosophers have discussed what they call "morally innocent threat" cases in which someone becomes a threat to others even though he performs no action. For example, a third party or the wind hurls a person at someone else or causes him to emit death rays.[10] Those with libertarian-like views should contrast not aiding with both harming (if this requires doing something)[11] and inactively presenting a threat. Those who breathe out virus are doing something (breathing) that benefits them,[12] but they can be considered morally innocent harmers if they non-negligently lack awareness of doing something harmful and the costs of refraining would be great (e.g. not breathing). Further, those who transmit a disease usually interact with other people through their own acts, so they are at least minimally responsible agents (though not necessarily at fault for the harm they cause).

---

[7] On this see Mishra (2021).

[8] However, if mutations tend to result in less harmful versions of a virus, being a locus for mutation might be seen as providing an overall benefit even if it is against one's self-interest.

[9] Even if there is no impact on others receiving healthcare, someone's becoming ill and using socially provided healthcare can financially harm others. I shall not discuss financial harm in this chapter.

[10] Robert Nozick discussed one type of innocent threat in Nozick (1974).

[11] As suggested by John Deigh.

[12] Connie Rosati suggests they are like polluters whose behavior and its effects libertarians can agree to limit or mitigate.

Assuming knowledge of the threat one presents, even completely inactive innocent threats may have a moral duty to interfere with their being a threat at some reasonable cost to them (e.g. by redirecting themselves). Those who become threats by actively engaging with others may have a duty not to actively engage (e.g. isolate) or protect themselves from transmitting disease (e.g. by wearing a mask). If they do not do so, they would no longer be morally innocent but at fault for the harm they do.

Are distinctive issues raised by taking a vaccine to prevent one's harming others (if it prevents transmission) because it introduces something foreign into one's body? Although taking pills also does this, pills generally have short-term effects whereas the best vaccines' effects can be long-lasting or permanent. One may worry about something whose effects last long or are permanent if those effects are bad (as one might be concerned about wearing a mask that could not be removed for a year).

However, someone's using such a vaccine to reduce harboring and transmitting a virus might not involve any cost to him if it reduces his own chance of being harmed by the virus. By then choosing not to take this no-cost action to prevent being a threat to others, he could unjustifiably cause or risk causing harm. It is important to see that in this argument the fact that a vaccine or highly self-protective mask would prevent harm to the vaccinated person is not used to justify paternalism but only to show that no cost is required to prevent harm to others. Though this nonpaternalistic argument is weakened if the vaccine does not significantly reduce transmission, it would still reduce harm to others that comes from one's use of medical facilities and being a locus for virus mutation.

However, suppose alternatives such as working from home alone would interfere with being a threat to others. If one's employer required in-office presence that put one in a position to transmit or acquire disease merely as a pretext to promote vaccination, this would not be consistent with a libertarian-like moral view.

(iv) There is a difference between "saving" others and preventing oneself from harming them. It is important to appreciate and communicate that preventing oneself from harming others is not equivalent to "saving" or otherwise benefiting others. When I save a person who is in harm's way due to an accident or a third party, I improve the condition of that person from what it would have been without my involvement (when living is good for him). This means that I benefit the person by raising him up relative to his lower expected baseline and keep him in the condition he was in before being threatened with decline. If I don't save the person, I do not make him worse off either than he was before falling into harm's way or than he would otherwise have been without my involvement.[13] By contrast, when I harm another I make him worse off than he was (or would otherwise

---

[13] This is a rough approximation to a more complicated truth.

have been); I lower him relative to his baseline.[14] When I prevent myself from harming another person (e.g. by wearing a mask to stop transmitting a virus), I do not make him better off than he was or would have been without my involvement; I merely counteract a threat I would have presented to him. I have not "saved" him if I had no right to harm him when I merely avoid making him worse off than he was or would have been without my involvement.

Public messages that portray measures that prevent one's harming others as instead ways to "save the lives" of others are misleading and can also raise objections by those with libertarian-like views. This is because a libertarian objecting to being interfered with merely to aid others is objecting to being interfered with merely to make others overall better off relative to their baseline. Similarly, messages that emphasize "protecting" others by wearing a mask or taking a vaccine do not make clear that what one would be protecting them from is a threat of harm one would present that would drive them below their baseline.[15]

(v) **Preventing a person from causing harm to others may supersede that person's moral right not to be interfered with.** It is important to appreciate and communicate that another party's interference with one's body can be morally permissible when doing so is necessary to prevent one causing harm to others, even if one's right to liberty may morally prohibit such interference when only one's own well-being or the provision of benefits to others is at stake. Each person's moral right to noninterference gives rise to a correlative moral duty on the part of each not to interfere with others. If one fails to carry out the duty (e.g. by spreading disease when doing so is easily preventable), it can be morally permissible for others to interfere in self- or other-defense when interference is necessary and proportionate (e.g. imposing use of a mask if only that prevents transmission).

(vi) **Understanding how methods of prevention work increases their effectiveness.** It is important to appreciate and communicate how some methods of interfering with a threat work. The need for clarity is shown, for example, by the mantra of "choice" repeated by those in the COVID pandemic who did not oppose others choosing to wear masks in schools but did not see a moral duty to wear one in that context. The sorts of masks recommended for use by the general public during the first two years of the COVID-19 pandemic primarily interfere

---

[14] I am simplifying and not considering cases where one preemptively causes someone the same harm someone else would have caused him. The distinction between an agent harming and his not aiding is different from the distinction between an agent behaving in a way that results in a person falling or not being raised from his baseline. For whether (a) you don't prevent someone's falling from his baseline due to a threat you didn't present or (b) you don't lift him from his baseline, you would fail to aid rather than harm him.

[15] This is consistent with public health officials themselves saving others by encouraging those who would harm others to not do so. Public health messages might portray people as saving others by wearing masks because it is attractive to think of oneself as a hero (doing something beyond minimal duty). But even at low cost, going beyond what is strictly required may not be appealing from a libertarian-like perspective.

with transmission *from* a person. They do not to a high degree protect the wearer against virus coming *to* them. If many people choose not to wear such a mask, those who do are still subject to a higher risk of illness if they have to interact with unmasked people, some of whom are likely to transmit the virus. Moreover, unmasked people may be unharmed due to those who *do* wear a mask lowering others risk of infection.

Hence, it might seem that an argument for everyone wearing such masks is that it is unfair that mask-wearers prevent transmission to others who do not prevent transmission to them. The non-maskers seem like free-riders in a system that should be reciprocal. John Rawls claimed (following H. L. A. Hart) that there is a duty of fair play and when one benefits due to others' restraint, one has a duty to do likewise. However, Robert Nozick argued against such a duty of fair play when one does not (a) seek to benefit or (b) encourage others to restrain their behavior so that one is benefited.[16] I argued earlier that wearing a mask is not best understood as a case of benefiting others in the way that saving a life is. But Nozick's point can still apply to nonreciprocal prevention of harm to others: If nonmaskers do not expect others to wear masks and do attribute to them an equal moral right not to, then there may be no unfairness even if there is unequal interference with transmission. The crucial moral issue is not unfairness but that some people may harm others who do not consent to be harmed.

(vii) **Someone may truly aid others (as opposed to merely not harm them) in many cases.** Appreciating and communicating this may prevent other sorts of moral duties being required of and inciting resistance by those concerned about their liberty. Suppose that when most people wear a mask that interferes with transmission, something akin to herd immunity occurs. Here people who prevent transmission by wearing the device not only do not cause harm—they can *aid* those who cannot protect themselves against a virus. They do this if they increase the likelihood that the vulnerable will interact with nontransmitters instead of with those who do not wear devices that impede transmission.

That choosing to circulate in public while wearing a mask is in this way to aid the vulnerable is shown by what happens if many of these device-wearers stay at home. Here, the vulnerable will more likely interface with transmitters and become worse off than they would have been had maskers been present. Nevertheless, the people who stay home do not thereby cause harm. They only fail to aid. The same would be true where true herd immunity is to be achieved by reaching a critical mass of vaccinated people but the vaccinated choose to stay home rather than circulate in the community. Here the vaccinated fail to provide a beneficial service (interfacing with the vulnerable), but this does not mean that they are harming others.

---

[16] See Rawls (1971) and Nozick (1974).

In these cases, there could be a genuine libertarian-like moral objection based on personal liberty not to aid in creating herd immunity by serving as "cocoons" for others. When public health pronouncements call for people to be vaccinated in order to protect those who cannot yet be vaccinated (e.g. the very young), those who have libertarian-like moral views may object to this argument for vaccination that is based on aiding (rather than not harming) others.

(viii) **There is a distinction between harming and wronging.** In some pandemics, everyone can present a threat to everyone else and everyone can take measures to avoid threatening others. It is important to appreciate and communicate that in this situation, individuals might weigh the burden to them of not threatening others against the harm they avoid by others bearing a like burden not to threaten them. It is possible that each decides it is in his interest to risk disease rather than bear the burden of not threatening others. Then individuals who are harmed by others would at least have no complaint against them since everyone would, in essence, have waived his right not to be harmed at least by those who would not deliberately harm him. Taking liberty seriously may involve morally recognizing such waivers.

This possibility shows that harming someone does not always involve wronging someone, as wronging involves at least unconsented-to infringement of a moral right. Of course, even if these people who transmit disease or remain loci of viral mutations do not wrong each other, they may still wrong others who have not similarly waived their moral rights against harm, and transmitters may need to use protective devices in those others' presence. Those who agree to risk disease but do not waive their right to medical care (assuming there are such rights in the society) may also wrong those who must care for them or who lose the opportunity for treatment in an overburdened medical system.

(ix) **Encourage self-reliant self-defense.** It is important to appreciate and encourage the general public to use self-defense measures that they control (and that do not harm others even as an unintended side effect or by redirecting a threat back to a threatener). Examples of such self-defense in a viral pandemic include wearing a mask that primarily protects the wearer (e.g. an N95) or getting a vaccine that reduces the vaccinated person's risk of contracting or experiencing serious effects of the virus.

There are various moral reasons for encouraging such self-defense. In some pandemics a particular group, like the elderly, is particularly susceptible to serious disease. Those who can infect them, except for fellow elderly, are not as susceptible to infection. In this situation, some who might bear a burden to prevent their infecting others (e.g. by masking, vaccination, or being in lockdowns) are not the ones who thereby avoid illness. Some have suggested that it would be better if those who "benefit" from not being harmed (using the term "benefit" even for cases in which someone is not raised above their baseline) would also bear the burden of preventing harm to themselves.[17] This could be a moral argument for defensive measures being the responsibility of those who would otherwise be harmed. But this argument ignores the fact that the burden on those who do not benefit is meant to interfere with the harm that they would otherwise do to others. There need be no unfairness in a burden being imposed on a potential harmer to prevent the harm he would otherwise do to his potential victim. This is another instance where using "benefiting" when someone prevents a harm he would do leads to the wrong conclusion.

Those who hold libertarian-like views typically support forms of self-defense that place the biggest burden of harm prevention on a wrongful threatener (e.g. shooting an attacker to defend oneself). Others may think that in situations where those who harm would be morally innocent or minimally responsible, it is morally appropriate to share the costs of preventing harm between potential victims and threateners. For example, imagine a case where an innocent threat would have to swerve into a wall and be severely injured to avoid hitting someone. If the potential victim can instead move out of the way at the cost to himself of only minor injury, he should bear the burden. In this case one self-defends by bearing a lesser cost in order to prevent a much greater cost to the morally innocent threatener. By contrast, if a guilty aggressor would succeed in deliberately harming someone, the burden of preventing the harm should (arguably) solely fall on the aggressor.

How should the burden of avoiding harm be allocated if someone would transmit a virus that causes serious harm only because the potential victim has not easily self-defended (e.g. with a vaccine)? Even when there is no deliberate harming, it does not seem correct to entirely eliminate the burden on the transmitter to prevent transmission. Analogously, suppose someone carries a gun that could go off, seriously harming others who could easily have worn a bullet-proof vest. Should the gun carrier be relieved of using easy means to make the gun safe because others do not easily self-defend? It would clearly be wrong to relieve the gun carrier as a means of increasing pressure on others to wear the protective vests (or analogously, to get vaccinated).

In a pandemic, a reason to engage in self-reliant self-defense besides reducing the burden on potential harmers is concern about the unreliability of depending on others to prevent harm to oneself. (For example, when only the elderly are at risk, they might defend themselves rather than relying on the young to minimize the threat they present to the elderly.) In the COVID-19 pandemic the most effective self-protective equipment before the vaccine, N95 masks, were originally reserved for healthcare workers. It is possible that much disease

[17]   For example, Profs. O. Yakusheva and J. Bhattacharya in each one's Princeton Center for Human Values presentation, December 20, 2021.

might have been prevented by massively increasing the production of good self-protective equipment for the general public. Although this would have been more expensive than producing cloth masks intended primarily to prevent transmission, self-interest might have been a stronger motivator (even if it does not generate a moral duty) to wear masks than respect for the rights of others (even as part of a scheme for mutual protection). If fewer people would then have become seriously ill, lower healthcare costs could have resulted in overall savings despite the increased cost of masks. In future pandemics, more should be done to make self-defense possible by one's own efforts, especially if the burden of this (e.g. wearing an N95) is no greater than or the same as the burden of each not threatening others (e.g. wearing masks that prevent only transmission).

The possibility of excellent self-reliant self-defense could diminish public conflict such as occured over requirements for universal mask wearing in schools. In arguing for universal mask wearing among children returning to in-person learning, some have emphasized that unless all wear masks, there is little good coming to the one child who wears a mask.[18] But this depends on the sort of mask that child wears; if it is an N95, it will do her a lot of good even if others do not wear masks.

(x) **The safety of some need not depend on the safety of all.** The possibility of good self-reliant self-defense implies that one's safety need not depend on everyone's being safe, contrary to the COVID-19 public health mantra that "no one is safe until everyone is safe." The mantra makes an empirical claim and may increase the number of those who are safe if individuals think that taking measures to promote the safety of others (including those in foreign countries) is the best means to their own safety. Hence, the mantra may be designed to appeal to those who do not recognize strong moral duties not based on self interest to aid others like those with libertarian-like moral views.

Nevertheless the mantra may not be true. Taken literally, it implies that one unsafe person makes everyone else in the world unsafe too, which hardly seems true. (It would certainly reduce one's self-interested motivation to promote the safety of others if one believed both that [i] it is futile to try to make literally everyone safe, especially given many people's resistance to preventive measures, and [ii] making everyone safe would be the only way to make oneself safe.)

The mantra would also be untrue if certain types of self-defense measures (e.g. vaccines) did provide protection from a virus for some even when others were not similarly safe. Of course, the degree of safety for the vaccinated decreases if the unvaccinated harbor virus that mutates to a new vaccine-resistant form. But the more successful vaccines are in protecting individuals against even mutated virus, the more they give lie to the mantra that no one is safe until everyone is.

---

[18] For example, Dr. Danny Benjamin on PBS Newshour, August 10, 2021; https://www.pbs.org/newshour/show/as-millions-of-students-return-to-the-classroom-parents-remain-divided-on-mask-mandates.

Since such "supervaccines" would reduce the self-interested incentive to protect everyone, some might oppose their development. This would change the empirical claim ("no one is safe until everyone is safe") into a moral claim ("no one *should* be safe until everyone is safe"). Such a moral claim might be supported on the ground that equality is valuable either as an end or as a means. That is, if the valuable end were increasing the number of those who are safe, it might be suggested that the best way to accomplish this is arranging for no one to be safe until everyone is, even if it is empirically true that some could be safe when others are not.

Opposition to creation of supervaccines that resist mutant viruses is independent of concern about the proper distribution of scarce vaccines. In the case of COVID-19 there was opposition to rich countries providing each of their citizens with multiple vaccinations for superior defense since this reduced the vaccine available to poorer countries. But suppose a single shot of a supervaccine sufficed for complete protection against any variant. Opposition could still arise if those who were protected in one country then had no interest in funding more production and wider distribution of the vaccine even though they were not using multiple doses when others had none. Rather, the opposition would be to their not helping make the vaccines less scarce by producing more.

Arranging for no one to be safe until everyone is (e.g. by hindering the production of supervaccines that could resist any new variant) would interfere with the liberty of some people to maximally self-defend. It might be suggested that it would maximize liberty overall were more people at liberty to self-defend with non-supervaccines when that would reduce the possibility of mutations arising. But libertarian-like views need not conceive of liberty as a value that should be maximized even by interfering with the liberty of some for the sake of liberty for others. Rather, they may conceive of the liberty of an individual as what Robert Nozick referred to as a side-constraint that should not be violated even in order to increase liberty overall.

Nevertheless, suppose the same degree of protection for some people could be achieved by either (a) their using supervaccines or (b) all people using non-supervaccines. Voluntarily choosing route (b) in order to maximize the number protected, including those who would be protected in route (a), seems morally right and also consistent with a concern not to violate a side-constraint of individual liberty. Suppose route (a) were chosen. This could be because it is scientifically easier or because route (b) would require imposing protective measures on the unwilling. Then some would lack a self-interested reason to make everyone safe but a moral reason to try could still exist. Those with libertarian-like views may just deny that this reason gives rise to a moral duty.

(xi) **Not avoiding illness by easy means may diminish rights to assistance.** It is important to appreciate and communicate that people who could have avoided illness by easy means may have forfeited (or diminished the strength of) their right to healthcare, at least when scarcity of resources means not everyone can be helped.[19] (Those with libertarian-like views may deny that there is a right to healthcare stemming from need, but they may not be opposed to rights based on voluntary insurance.) At a certain point, COVID-19 was described as a "pandemic of the unvaccinated" and in the US many of those to whom this phrase referred chose not to use low-risk vaccines when information about and access to them was widely available. Their having a diminished right to healthcare could prevent them from reducing others' chances of being treated. Being liable to such diminishment is not the same as deserving it, which would imply that it is positively good that these people not be treated. Liability only implies that, because of their risky behavior, they should go without care when someone must.

This claim about forfeiture or diminished strength of a right to healthcare has far-reaching and perhaps unacceptable implications. Should heart attack victims who chose not to take low-cost preventive measures have a diminished right to healthcare relative to heart attack victims who did take such measures? It might be argued that in this case there are enough medical resources to take care of both types of people. But perhaps there is no scarcity only because more money is allocated than should be to care for even those with relatively weakened rights to care thus creating scarcity of other goods and services.

Healthcare providers may have duties stemming from a professional code, not from any rights of the ill. If so, the strength of a patient's right to care might not affect the kind of care they should receive from individual providers. Nevertheless, it could affect the amount of funding society should provide for resources to be used by professionals.

Whether there is a reduced claim to healthcare among those who could have easily avoided illness is a complicated issue that I shall not settle here. However, if one focuses on liberty and is resistant to claims about uncontracted-for aid, one is more likely to think it permissible to hold those who could have easily avoided needing such aid accountable for the consequences of their decisions.

(xii) **Which people should be helped and which burdened depends on whether and why losses to different people may be interpersonally aggregated.** It's important to appreciate and communicate that the permissibility of relieving less serious problems of many people rather than relieving more serious problems of fewer people can depend on whether it is morally permissible to aggregate lesser losses to each of many people so that they outweigh greater losses to each of fewer people. Also, the permissibility of imposing burdens on many people (thus harming them) to prevent losses to fewer people can depend on whether the burdens are imposed on those who would otherwise cause the losses. The first issue

---

[19] Forfeiting, unlike waiving, a right is not voluntary. Note that if there is a choice between treating (i) someone who omitted both to easily protect himself and easily prevent himself from harming someone else or (ii) his victim (who didn't easily self-defend), it is the former who may have forfeited care.

arises in deciding whether to delay certain medical treatments during a pandemic surge; the second issue arises in deciding whether to have lockdowns. I will deal with these issues further in Section 6.2.

6.3 How to Weigh Costs to Some against "Benefits" to Others

Now consider how lesser and greater losses in individuals should be compared in order to decide (1) whether an impartial agent should postpone many medical procedures on some in order to prevent imminent deaths in others, and (2) whether an impartial agent may impose lesser losses on some through lockdowns in order to prevent imminent deaths in others.

A. The following discussion will assume that no one has forfeited, diminished, or waived their right to healthcare. It will also assume (for the sake of argument) that when elective procedures are postponed the cost is small because the problems will be taken care of eventually. Other procedures will not be referred to as "elective" because delaying them results in loss which is significant even if not life-threatening (or life-threatening but not imminently so, for example missed cancer diagnoses). These are both types of cases in which not providing medical aid to some is at issue. By contrast, in a lockdown people have a burden imposed on them (i.e. they must refrain from ordinary movement and business activity). The question then is whether and when there is a moral (aside from legal) case for these policies of not aiding and of harming.

B (i). It has been suggested that the experience of being shut in and suffering economic trauma in a lockdown for a considerable time results in the loss of a year of life for a person. The aim of this calculation is to translate experiential and economic losses due to a lockdown into the language of life lost. Suppose that by adding up all the life-years lost across many people (i.e. interpersonally aggregating), we get 40 million. Some might conclude that this total of life-years lost could outweigh the deaths of individuals that would occur if lockdowns were not imposed and use that as an argument against lockdowns.[20]

But in translating experiential and economic loss into life-years lost we must recognize that if 40 million people each lose one year of life, no one of those people will suffer a loss as great as someone who, for example, loses an additional twenty years of life by dying at 50 instead of at 70 as he otherwise would have. It is a mistake to always aggregate small losses to each of many people and morally equate the total to a large loss to a single person. How a total is distributed across separate persons is morally important. However, if it is only on average that one year of life is lost due to lockdown, some of the 40 million people may lose many

---

[20] I here use data that economist Nick Bloom presented on PBS Newshour Broadcast June 18, 2020.

more years and even as much as (or more than) those who die of a disease at 50 rather than 70. Hence, arguing against lockdowns by relying on the average figure actually weakens the case against lockdowns.

B (ii). There is an alternative to always aggregating smaller losses interpersonally or relying on average losses in a population. This involves separating out types of losses and comparing each type of smaller loss individuals would suffer against each type of larger loss other individuals would suffer. This leads to a form of what is known as "pairwise comparison" though it need not involve comparing each individual person pairwise with every other person since we compare types of losses.

To illustrate this procedure, instead of considering lockdowns that impose losses on some, first consider a healthcare provider or other impartial agent deciding whom to help amongst people whose illness they have not caused when not everyone can be helped. In the COVID pandemic whom to try to save was sometimes decided on the basis of who was most likely to survive or the patient's age. (This was not because older people were not considered the moral equals of younger people. Rather, it might be thought either that the aged would not live many more years in any case or that those who have lived longer already have had a benefit that those who are younger would lack if they died.[21]) However, the issue of rationing aid can also arise in the cases we are now considering in which the issue is not whose life to save but whether to treat those who face imminent death or those who each face lesser losses.

For example, suppose the impartial agent must decide whether to save one person for a significant period of life or to save a great many people from each suffering only a sore throat. In this case, the sore throats, even if constituting a large body of illness when aggregated, should all be irrelevant and the life should be saved. This is because the sore throats will each occur in separate persons and the type of loss due to a sore throat is small when compared with the type of loss to each of those who would die. I have described the sore throat in one person as an "irrelevant good" by comparison to death of another person. Using this reasoning as a model, we should also not aggregate the mere delay in successful treatment to each of many people and weigh the sum against the much greater loss of death to each of fewer people.

Indeed, I have argued that a person has a moral duty to suffer a sore throat to save someone else's life. One form of this duty is not seeking help for a sore throat if that would interfere with another person's life being saved. I would also argue that someone has a duty to accept a delay in elective treatment in order that help may instead be given to save someone's life. If each person had such moral duties, this is an additional reason why from an impartial agent's point of view no

---

[21] For more on this issue (and others dealt with in this chapter) see Kamm (2022).

number of sore throats or elective delays should count against saving one life.[22] (It is no objection that some untreated sore throats will be deadly. This would not support interpersonally aggregating small benefits but only balancing some deaths against others.)

Notice that (a) a duty not to seek help for one's sore throat so that impartial agents may save someone else's life is conceptually and possibly morally different from: (b) a duty not to cure one's sore throat by one's own means that could otherwise be used to save someone else' life; (c) a duty not to cure one's sore throat or have it cured because having a sore throat was itself what would save another's life (e.g. person A would donate money to save B only if C did not cure his own throat); (d) a duty to acquire or allow others to give one a new sore throat because that would save another's life. Some might agree that we have all the duties in (a)–(d), but those especially concerned with liberty might be more resistant to (b)–(d) than to (a).

But what if the choice was between saving someone's life or saving many people from each losing three fingers or a leg?[23] In a pairwise comparison of types of losses, someone's losing three fingers or a leg is not anywhere as bad as losing life, and in that sense they are not "relevant to" another's losing his life. Hence, one view is that an impartial agent should save even one person's life rather than save any number of individuals from losing three fingers or a single leg. This is so even if no one has a moral duty to sacrifice his three fingers or leg to save someone else's life at (least in ways described in [b]–[d]). This view implies that an impartial agent cannot decide what types of lesser losses to each of many people may be aggregated and weighed against more serious losses in others merely by seeing what loss someone has no moral duty to suffer in ways involved in (b)–(d) to save a life. Indeed, even someone's having no duty to refrain from seeking assistance (as in [a]) need not determine what assistance an impartial agent should provide to different groups of people.[24]

However, suppose one person will die and another person would be totally paralyzed. Other things being equal, in a pairwise choice between these two individuals we should help the first person when we cannot help both. (This assumes that death is worse for someone than total paralysis.) Nevertheless, it might be morally right to save one hundred people from total paralysis rather than one person from death when we cannot do both. If so, it is because the lesser loss is "relevant to" the greater loss in another person. It would be morally appropriate

---

[22] See Kamm (1993), among other places, where I make this point. Note that in this case the decision that someone has a duty to suffer the sore throat must be true even when many other people will also be doing this.

[23] These are examples I presented in Kamm (1993).

[24] I presented this view (and considered alternatives to it) in, among other places, Kamm (1993). However, here I am distinguishing further among ways (i.e. [a]–[d]) in which one has or does not have a duty to make a sacrifice.

to count the number of people who would be spared the lesser relevant loss, weighing the total against the total number of lives at stake to decide which group to save.[25]

In sum, on this view it is only after comparison of types of losses to determine the relevance of a lesser loss to the worst loss (and what good would occur if each loss were avoided) that we should consider how many people would suffer that relevant lesser loss by comparison to how many would suffer the greater loss. Then the impartial allocator of assistance could determine if helping the first set of people supersedes saving the lives of others.[26]

A partially contrasting view is offered by Alex Voorhoeve. He agrees that losses each would have a duty to suffer to save someone's life should not be aggregated even if many would suffer the loss. However, he also claims that if an individual who is not helped would suffer a type of loss he would not have a duty to suffer to save a life, then (i) each of those losses is "relevant to" the loss of a life and gives someone a claim to be considered, and (ii) an impartial agent should interpersonally aggregate those individual lesser losses to decide whom to help. (Included in the aggregation is the strength of the individual claim for aid as well as the number of people having the claim. Voorhoeve's (and others') notion of "relevant to" also applies when losses other than of life are at stake.) If there are a sufficient number with weaker claims to aid, it could be morally right to help them rather than save a person's life.[27]

Voorhoeve's sense of "relevant to" differs from the one described earlier. That view denied that any loss one had no duty to suffer in any ways (a)–(d) to prevent someone else's loss is relevant to it and may be interpersonally aggregated by an impartial agent to choose whom to aid. Voorhoeve does not specifically distinguish the various ways in which one might suffer a lesser loss, but he argues that we can reach unanimity on not pressing a claim to have a sore throat treated when another's life is at stake. By contrast, there need be no unanimity on not pressing a claim to avoid some larger lesser loss so that another can benefit. On this ground it should be counted in a decision whether to prevent multiple lesser losses or instead save one life.

One of my concerns about Voorhoeve's view is that it might be that one person who would lose a limb has a duty not to press a claim for treatment against someone who would die even if it is clear that he need not volunteer his limb to save another's life. So perhaps Voorhoeve only means that if someone has no duty to give up his limb (in ways [b]–[d]), interpersonal aggregation of those losses is appropriate in deciding what to do. But why should what each person has no duty to give up in order to save another's life determine what an impartial agent should

---

[25] As discussed in Kamm (1993).
[26] I discuss these issues in greater detail in, among others places, Kamm (1993, 2013b).
[27] See Voorhoeve (2014) and Kamm (2015) for my earlier response to Vooorhoeve.

do with his life-saving resource? After all, no one is being required to decide to give up anything when an impartial agent decides whom he will assist using his (or public) resources.[28] Either way, each of the many may suffer the lesser loss, but it can be morally important how the loss comes about.

For those with libertarian-like moral views who (in the extreme case) think we have no moral duties to aid (including to refrain from seeking to be aided), Voorhoeve's view that any loss one has no duty to suffer for others should be aggregated implies that impartial agents should aggregate curing sore throats in deciding whether to save someone's life. It could also be morally wrong to put off elective procedures in many for the sake of saving fewer lives. Such conclusions could be avoided by denying either that there are no moral duties to aid or that losses beyond what one has a duty to bear should always be aggregated by impartial aiders.

C. Now consider a case in which an impartial allocator of aid must decide whether to help 40 million people to each avoid economic loss and/or loss of a year of life or help fewer people to each avoid death (losing many more years of life). (The allocator does not cause the economic/life year loss.) Also, consider a case in which an impartial allocator of aid must decide whether to help many people each avoid significant permanent physical loss or help fewer people each avoid death. On the first view about aggregation that we considered, in each of these cases the allocator should first pairwise compare these types of losses (and how much each person would benefit from help) to determine whether an individual's lesser loss is relevant to death. If it is relevant, the allocator should then consider how many people would suffer that relevant loss by comparison to how many would suffer the greater loss. Then the impartial agent could determine if helping the first group supersedes saving the lives of others. If the economic loss, lost life-years, or permanent physical loss is much less significant than loss of life, then even if individuals have no duty to give up a year of their life, close their business, or suffer permanent physical loss to save another's life, the impartial allocator need not aggregate the lesser losses. The total could not outweigh loss of life.

On the other hand, suppose preventing the permanent physical loss to each was relevant to preventing death because survival was unlikely even with treatment or the gain from survival was minimal.[29] Then it could be morally correct for the impartial allocator to help prevent the permanent losses in each of many people rather than trying to save lives. If those who would die were taken care of nevertheless, those who suffered the permanent loss could complain that care was incorrectly allocated.

---

[28] At this point we are not considering imposing the lesser loss which is a case of harming.

[29] Determining how bad a death is for someone could factor into the morality of deciding how to allocate care between those who would die without treatment and those who would not die but suffer permanent loss. I discuss this further in Kamm (2022).

D (i). Suppose (for the sake of argument) that an impartial allocator should use pairwise comparison in either of the ways I have considered (or some other way that is a compromise between these two) when deciding whom to help. How should we view interpersonal aggregation of lesser losses when an impartial agent is deciding whether to impose them on, thus *harming,* some people for the sake of helping others? For example, suppose a noncommunicable disease causes death at an early age in some and it could be cured by other people doing what costs each of them one year of life (e.g. participate in research on the disease and so die at 70 rather than 71). Suppose also that a person does not have a moral duty to give up a year of his life to save others from dying at a young age and helping them live many more years. Then on a libertarian-like view, requiring that each of those who can help do so would be a violation of each one's negative moral right not to be imposed on to aid others. Further, the more people who would be required to do this, the greater the number of rights violated. Violation of one right would be serious but violating many would be more serious. In this case, aggregating the smaller losses to each of many people to weigh against the lives lost would be justified because imposing each of the smaller losses would, by hypothesis, involve violation of a moral right.

Hence, suppose one views an imposed lockdown as involving such violation of the moral rights of many not to be harmed for the sake of saving some others' lives. (Or alternatively, one thinks that individuals have no moral duty to remain in lockdown simply to aid others.) Then pairwise comparison of types of losses would *not* be a better way of deciding what should be done than aggregating the smaller losses to many people.

D (ii). Crucially, however, whether such moral rights violations occur could depend on whether those who would be in lockdown would otherwise harm or be at significant risk of harming others (who did not voluntarily accept the risk). (The harms could be any of those discussed in Section 6.2 [ii].) Whether there are moral rights not to be in lockdown could also depend on whether potential victims of harm are morally obligated to bear the cost of self-defense and on whether costs due to lockdown are a burden proportional to the harm (and risk of it) that one might otherwise cause. Suppose it was right to impose the cost on each potential harmer to prevent his harming. Then it would be wrong to interpersonally aggregate the losses to all those who should be prevented from harming others in order to determine the permissibility of lockdowns. If proportionality is violated, it could be appropriate to interpersonally aggregate the out-of-proportion costs when objecting to the costs being required. (For example, suppose each person staying at home for one day a week were a proportional loss to bear rather than harm others but not two days. Then it would be morally permissible to interpersonally aggregate the excess loss to each person in objecting to a two-day requirement.)

In sum: (1) Pairwise comparison of types of losses rather than simple interpersonal aggregation may be the correct method to use when an impartial agent is deciding among people whom to aid. Numbers of people and the losses they would suffer could count only once losses are relevant to those of people who would be worse off if not helped (assuming they would benefit significantly from help). (2) Suppose there are moral rights violations in imposing lesser losses on some for the sake of aiding others or inconsistency between their rights and a moral duty that they suffer the lesser losses to aid others. Then aggregation of these losses may be appropriate in objecting to the imposition of, and the recognition of a duty to suffer, the losses. (3) Suppose losses would be imposed on, or morally required of, those who would otherwise harm others. Then simple aggregation of proportional losses imposed on or required of each person could be inappropriate. Hence, whether interpersonal aggregation of smaller losses is morally wrong could depend on whether the loss is or is not correctly imposed on someone to prevent his harming others.

Conclusion: We have considered moral distinctions between not harming and aiding and between saving others and preventing oneself from harming them. We used these distinctions to help justify some moral requirements in a pandemic even to those most concerned about liberty. We have also examined the limits some moral philosophers recommend on interpersonally aggregating losses and benefits and how this affects the morality of putting off elective medical procedures and having lockdowns to prevent deaths. The conclusion was that foregoing elective procedures and imposing relatively small harms on each of many people could sometimes be justified to those with libertarian-like views even if it resulted in greater overall (aggregated) losses.[30]

Bibliography

Kamm, F. M. (1993), *Morality, Mortality, vol. 1: Death and Whom to Save From It* (New York: Oxford University Press, 1993).

Kamm, F. M. (2007), *Intricate Ethics* (New York: Oxford University Press, 2007).

Kamm, F. M. (2013a), 'Genes, Justice, and Obligations in Creating People: Reflections on *From Chance to Choice* and on Views of Nagel, Shiffrin, and Singer', in F. M. Kamm, *Bioethical Prescriptions* (New York: Oxford University Press, 2013).

Kamm, F. M. (2013b), 'Health and equity', in F. M. Kamm, *Bioethical Prescriptions* (New York: Oxford University Press, 2013).

Kamm, F. M. (2015), '*Bioethical Prescriptions:* Response to Critics', *Journal of Medical Ethics,* 41: 493–95.

---

[30] For comments on earlier versions of this article, I am grateful to the editors of this volume as well as to R. Crisp, J. Deigh, E. Emanuel, J. Fix, G. Persad, T. Pummer, C. Rosati, L. Sager. I also benefited from questions by seminar members at University of Texas Law School and attendees at the Knox Lecture at the University of St. Andrews and at a philosophy colloquium at Oxford University.

Kamm, F. M. (2022), 'Rights and Aggregation in a Pandemic', in F. M. Kamm, *Rights and Their Limits: In Theory, Cases, and Pandemics* (New York: Oxford University Press, 2022).

Mishra, S., et al. (2021), 'Comparing the Responses of the UK, Sweden, and Denmark to COVID-19 Using Counterfactual Modelling', *Scientific Reports* 11, article no. 16,342.

Nozick, R. (1974), *Anarchy, State, and Utopia* (New York: Basic Books, 1974).

Rawls, J. (1971), *A Theory of Justice* (Cambridge, MA: Harvard University Press, 1971).

Shriffin, S. (1999), 'Wrongful Life, Procreative Responsibility, and the Significance of Harm', *Legal Theory* 5/2: 117–48.

Voorhoeve, A. (2014), 'How Should We Aggregate Competing Claims', *Ethics* 125/1: 64–87.

7

Against Procrustean Public Health

Two Vignettes

Govind Persad and Ezekiel Emanuel

7.1 Introduction

Throughout the COVID-19 pandemic, public health responses have frequently been criticized for treating people differently from one another. Differential treatment has been described as biased, castigated as socially divisive, rejected as imperfectly accurate, and even analogized to grave social evils like apartheid and the Holocaust.

Objections to differential treatment have been raised in almost every facet of pandemic response. Commentators have complained about prioritizing some people over others for critical care treatments like ventilators based on differences in their prospect of benefit or their degree of disadvantage. They have complained about treating people working in or patronizing essential businesses like grocery stores differently from those patronizing bars or concert venues, or treating people who wear masks differently from those who do not. Governments have resisted sending more vaccines to places facing more severe COVID-19 surges on the basis that it would treat people differently.

Procrusteanism is insisting that everyone be treated the same regardless of their differences. (In Greek mythology, Procrustes stretched or trimmed his guests to fit into the same bed, regardless of their different heights.) It has been a consistent theme in pushback against COVID-19 responses. And this pushback has come from all sides of the political spectrum. Some on the political left have complained that differential treatment exacerbates preexisting disparities, discriminates, or creates social divisions. Those on the political right have charged that allowing governments to treat people differently amounts to overreach and 'picking winners and losers.'

The appeal of Procrusteanism reflects a common mistake about what justice in general entails, and what a just public health response to a pandemic involves. It claims to prioritize equality over maximizing benefits and helping the disadvantaged. The Procrustean approach appeals to the value of equal treatment, and judges the justice of a policy, including a public health policy, by how similarly

Govind Persad and Ezekiel Emanuel, *Against Procrustean Public Health: Two Vignettes* In: *Pandemic Ethics: From COVID-19 to Disease X*. Edited by: Dominic Wilkinson and Julian Savulescu, Oxford University Press.
© Oxford University Press 2023. DOI: 10.1093/oso/9780192871688.003.0008

those directly affected by the policy are treated. In its pursuit of equality, Procrusteanism often ignores differential needs and vulnerabilities as well as the policy's indirect effects. The Procrustean approach wrongly treats policies' fundamental task as being symbolic recognition of human equality or expression of solidarity. The correct measure of a just public health response should be the outcomes it achieves. A just response should strive to prevent more harm, and in particular to prevent harm to those already disadvantaged, while infringing on individuals' rights no more than needed to achieve those goals.

In this chapter, we identify two ways in which Procrustean reasoning has infected and hampered pandemic response, and explain why in each case it is mistaken. The first is *Procrusteanism about public health restrictions*, which wrongly holds that fairness requires imposing the same public health restrictions on everyone, and in particular imposing the same restrictions on vaccinated people as on those who are unvaccinated. The second is *Procrusteanism about medical interventions*, which wrongly holds that fairness requires providing everyone with the same treatment regardless of their individual risk. In our Conclusion, we identify a problem unifying the two: *lack of research trials*. Because Procrusteanism has often pushed policy too quickly toward identical treatment, we have missed opportunities to conduct rigorous trials that compare different approaches, often stopping when safety is established without taking the next step to optimize efficacy. These could have helped us learn which public health restrictions are most effective at mitigating the harms of the pandemic while producing the least burden, and which medical interventions and mechanisms for delivering them—for instance, which vaccine combinations and dosing schedules—would similarly have averted more harm at lower cost. Instead, policies and protocols that initially were justified by precautionary reasoning rather than comprehensive trials have become entrenched without a continuing examination of how they could be improved. When they have been changed, the changes have often similarly reflected a lack of rigorous scientific underpinning. Our observations focus on the COVID-19 pandemic, but apply to future public health responses as well, where similar issues are likely to recur.

A further problem that Procrusteanism has encouraged is the rise of two unfortunate, though diametrically opposed, policy objectives. One is to simply stack public health policies atop one another as new technologies become available, chasing the unachievable goal of eliminating COVID-19's harmful impact altogether. On this approach, exemplified by current events in China, universal public health restrictions are maintained even when vaccines are widely available and antivirals increasingly available as well (Dyer 2022). This approach may superficially seem to treat everyone the same, and to promise a future where everyone will be equally free from the harms of COVID-19—but, in practice, these restrictions produce inequitable harm that is not justified by the harms they prevent. The other, exemplified by some American courts, is to order the elimination of public health policies designed to mitigate the harms of COVID-19. On this approach, beyond perhaps making vaccines and antivirals available, government can and should do nothing more to mitigate harm: it cannot require vaccination or impose public health measures even in targeted, high-risk settings. Again, this approach may seem to treat everyone identically by applying no public health requirements to anyone, but it also produces needless and inequitable harm by undermining the potential for well-targeted policies. Time may heal grief and sorrow, but the mere passage of time does not diminish the value of a public health response.

In discussing these problems, we focus on the context of vaccination. We select vaccination because for the foreseeable future it is the most impactful and widespread intervention in response to the COVID-19 pandemic. Many of the arguments we make, however, are also applicable to other interventions. For instance, many of the arguments made by people on the political right and left against requiring vaccination to participate in some activities were previously made, prior to the advent of vaccines, against requiring masks for participation (Gatter and Mohapatra 2020). The insistence on standardizing vaccine types and modes of delivery was also adopted with unfortunate effect for other public health interventions, such as testing (Mina and Andersen 2021). And the lack of continuing research to optimize vaccine dosing has been a consistent problem for assessing and optimizing the efficacy of masking and ventilation, and appears likely to recur with antiviral medications as well.

7.2 The Ethics of Considering Vaccination Status to Design Public Health Restrictions

We argue that, after vaccination, public health responses *should* treat people who are vaccinated differently from others, and that this differential treatment is neither discriminatory nor socially divisive but ethically desirable. Throughout the pandemic, and even after the advent of the Omicron variant, people who are vaccinated have faced different risks of contracting, transmitting, and (most importantly) getting very ill from COVID-19, compared to those who are unvaccinated. If COVID-19 had only ever presented risks at the level it presents to vaccinated people, much of the public health response to COVID-19, including closing businesses and borders, would not have been justifiable. It is not reasonable to subject people to public health restrictions that are not justified by the risks that they face or pose to others.

Initially, efforts to combat the COVID-19 pandemic understandably often took a broad-brush form. Public health restrictions, such as limits on indoor activities and on travel, were applied universally to the population despite the different risks that individuals face based on age, sex, comorbidity, living situations, and other factors. Compared to abandoning restrictions in the hopes of achieving herd immunity through infection, these broad restrictions were justified, especially when we knew little about the different risks that different groups faced from the virus. Furthermore, many people were not aware of the risk factors and many people at high risk were in proximity to those at lower risk, making broader restrictions easier to justify.

The arrival of vaccines within less than a year has changed the situation, enabling people to largely protect themselves against the severe impacts that justified initial, broad public health restrictions. Such impacts include death as well as hospitalization, which produced severe pressure on health systems and adoption of crisis standards of care in areas with substantial COVID-19 spread, worsening outcomes for patients both with and without COVID-19. (Even for groups at lower risk of death, such as children, spikes in COVID-19 hospitalization following the Omicron variant put pediatric hospitals under substantial pressure [Cloete et al. 2022].) Vaccination also reduces the duration of infection and the spread of disease, though it does not eliminate infection or spread. Both in this pandemic and others, the vast difference in risk between people who are vaccinated and those who are not supports policies that treat the two groups differently. Certain public health restrictions may be justified with respect to those who are not vaccinated while no longer being justified with respect to those who are vaccinated.

7.2.1 Why Considering Vaccination Status Is Consistent with Freedom and Equality

Understanding the proper baseline to which policies should be compared suggests the flaw in bioethical arguments that considering vaccination status unjustly impinges on individual freedom. The problem is determining the correct baseline for comparisons. Compared to a baseline without any public health restrictions, considering vaccination status in determining what restrictions a person should have to adhere to does directly decrease the formal freedom of unvaccinated people, though it may increase their substantive freedom by reducing exposure to infections that can be deadly. But "no health restrictions" is the wrong baseline. The right baseline is comparing freedoms based on a baseline of the public health restrictions necessary to control the pandemic. Compared to the broad application of public health restrictions, considering vaccination status in determining to whom these restrictions apply actually increases overall freedom, by increasing the freedom of the vaccinated while not worsening the restricted freedom of the unvaccinated.

Others object to policies that consider vaccination status on the basis that they unacceptably differentiate people. But what is ethically unacceptable is differentiating people based on characteristics, such as skin color or religious beliefs, that are irrelevant to legitimate policy goals in a pandemic. Conversely, differentiating people based on relevant differences does not constitute discrimination. And in the case of public health measures during a pandemic, the different level of medical risk due to the virus is a relevant characteristic.

Requiring governments, businesses, or other settings to ignore vaccination status unethically levels people down. Maintaining public health restrictions without differentiating by vaccination status deprives vaccinated people of the freedom to engage in important activities for little public health benefit. This clearly violates the long advocated public health principle that public health restrictions should be the *least restrictive* necessary to achieve the important, legitimate health goal, whatever it is (Childress et al. 2002). Abandoning these restrictions without differentiating by vaccination status, meanwhile, would allow unvaccinated people to freely become infected, placing unacceptable strain on the health system and likely leading to harm not only to them but also to many non-COVID-19 patients who require medical assistance.

The case for considering vaccination status is further bolstered by the fact that the world is now awash in COVID vaccines. Just twelve to fifteen months after their creation, the supply of vaccines is not the limiting factor in vaccination rates. Willingness to be vaccinated is. Supply of vaccines is now and for the foreseeable future not the limiting factor (Guarascio and Rigby 2022). Considering vaccination status differentiates people based not only on a relevant medical difference but on a characteristic that people in wealthy and middle-income countries—and increasingly in lower-income countries as well—are now easily able to choose and thus change at little burden. This differentiates policies based on vaccination status from policies based on unchosen risk factors, such as age, subjection to racism, geography, or medical conditions (Savulescu and Cameron 2020).

7.2.2 Implementation, Ineligible Groups, and Vaccine Scarcity

While the arguments that considering vaccination status violates freedom or equality fail, considering vaccination status is not always justified. But when it is unjustified, the reasons why are invariably dependent on empirical assessments. For instance, considering vaccination status will be unjustified in cases where it does not prevent substantial harm that justifies the expense of maintaining a vaccine verification system. But even in these cases, it is not fundamentally unfair, in the way that it can be unfair to differentiate people based on unchangeable characteristics or fundamental identities. Instead, scaling back, or scaling up, consideration of vaccination status in view of its contribution to harm prevention is akin to other forms of enforcement that might be "switched on" or "switched off" according to pandemic severity, such as mask or testing requirements.

There are some groups for whom considering vaccination status poses special issues. This includes children and people who are medically ineligible for vaccination. In the case of children who are eligible for vaccination, it seems justifiable to permit children whose families opt for vaccination to be excused from public health restrictions that are burdensome to them, such as requirements to quarantine if exposed at school, because their risk is so low and the burden of these requirements to them compared to their risk is substantial. The question of whether these public health restrictions are still appropriate for children at all is important, but distinct from the question of whether to permit vaccination status as an exception to these restrictions. For instance, countries differ on whether mask requirements for children attending school are appropriate or not (Krishnaratne et al. 2022). But regardless of whether such requirements are appropriate, it could be acceptable to exempt children who are vaccinated from them. This can be true even if vaccinated children still present some degree of risk to one another. The goal of public health policy is not to eliminate all risk from infectious disease, or to minimize risk, but to reduce risk to the background level of everyday life using the least burdensome interventions first (Childress et al. 2002). In the process of doing this, some acceptable level of risk will be reached. Countries may reasonably differ on what risk level is appropriate, but any reasonable answer must take into consideration the widespread burdens (even if individually small) of universal restrictions, and will certainly fall above zero risk.

What about children who are still ineligible for vaccination, and other people who are medically ineligible for vaccination? The issue of children's ineligibility depends on whether the goal of considering vaccination status is to reduce the spread of infection to others, or to limit the burden on hospitals. Children are less likely to be hospitalized if infected, meaning that even if a public health restriction may be justified for unvaccinated adults, it is less likely to be justifiable for unvaccinated children, except in an extreme surge. The issue of spread is more complex. Vaccination reduces spread but does not eliminate it. Furthermore, now that vaccines are available, people who wish to avoid severe consequences from infection can largely prevent those consequences by themselves being vaccinated. Therefore, it may be justifiable to exempt ineligible children from most public health restrictions. The main counterargument to this is that some people may not be fully protected by vaccination, or may not be eligible for vaccines. The imposition of public health restrictions on ineligible children to protect these individuals will depend on how often children and high-risk individuals are participating in the same spaces and whether there are other ways of mitigating risks, as well as on the value of the activity at issue for children. For instance, it may be appropriate to allow ineligible children to travel by plane even when vaccination is otherwise required, given the high value of travel for families and children, but not appropriate to allow unvaccinated children into high-risk settings such as infusion centers for medical patients, even where vaccinated companions are permitted.

Medically ineligible adults are similar to children with the added complication that medically ineligible adults tend to be at a higher personal risk of hospitalization and death if infected. Accordingly, it may be justifiable to exclude them from high-risk settings that are accessible to vaccinated adults, even if unvaccinated children who are at lower personal risk are allowed to enter the settings. It may also be appropriate to exclude them from settings that are not essential to them, even if there would be value in their being able to participate. For instance, it is appropriate to exclude a medically ineligible companion even if an infusion patient wanted to have them. While effort should be made to reasonably accommodate those who are medically ineligible, reasonable accommodation can be limited when it imposes risks on others.

Last, people who are ineligible for vaccination due to their own personal beliefs and practices should not be treated analogously to people who are medically ineligible. Part of adopting personal or religious beliefs involves accepting the consequences associated with those beliefs, which may include not being able to participate in certain types of activities. For instance, someone's religious beliefs may preclude them from working in certain occupations or playing professional sports on a Sabbath or holiday. Similarly, if someone adopts a religious belief that prevents them from being vaccinated, they may not be able to work in an occupation that requires vaccination.

Another set of objections to policies that consider vaccination status has to do with settings where vaccines are not widely available, and with differences in efficacy between different vaccine types and vaccination schedules. What these differences suggest is a spectrum of different vaccination-based approvals for different risk settings, analogous to the difference between a general driver's license and a commercial license. For most settings, a wide variety of vaccines may be acceptable, especially if the aim is to reduce serious disease or hospitalization. But if the goal is specifically to reduce transmission, as may be appropriate in high-risk medical settings, then treating recipients of boosters differently, or people who have received lower efficacy vaccinations differently, may be appropriate.

What about settings where vaccines are not widely available? Even in these settings, it still can be acceptable to make some activities conditional on vaccination status, particularly if many important activities are closed to everyone. Most countries attempted to distribute vaccines in short supply in a reasonably fair way. It would have been fair to permit people who are prioritized for vaccination, often on the basis of medical or other risks, to engage in activities they were previously prevented or restricted from engaging in. For instance, it would be fair to allow nursing home patients to visit with others who have been vaccinated. If a country is distributing vaccines in a way that is grossly unfair, for instance favoring elites over others, it would be unfair to then base access to public spaces on these sorts of distributions. It is the fairness of the vaccination prioritization that determines the justification of treating vaccinated people differently, not the underlying fairness of the principle that it is just to impose different restrictions on the unvaccinated compared to the vaccinated. Yet, when a country adopts unfair prioritization of vaccines, it is unlikely that any ethical argument would do much to persuade elites in the country to not fairly enforce a vaccine verification program.

What about the use of vaccination status as a criterion for traveling across national borders? It is again important to compare such a policy against the ethically correct baseline arrangement. There is no right to travel freely across international borders under typical circumstances. Rather, being able to travel internationally often depends on the ability to obtain other costly items, such as passports, visas, airline or train tickets, and accommodation. The use of vaccination status is much more clearly connected to risk and benefit to the residents of the receiving country than the consideration of many factors that are in widespread use.

Permitting people who have been vaccinated to cross international borders might be seen as exacerbating disparities between those who have been vaccinated and those who have not. But the existence of vaccination itself exacerbates disparities: those who are vaccinated have the immensely important protection of being more shielded against COVID-19 than others are. We should not pretend that this difference is irrelevant or level people down who genuinely are more protected than others for the sake of formal equality.

Irrespective of disparity, it is not reasonable to impose restrictions on a fundamental interest, like being able to travel, that are not justified by the risks that people face or present to others. Values like solidarity are not a sufficient reason to impose public health restrictions that would not be justified by risks posed to people. The purpose of public health restrictions is to prevent serious harm—a fundamental ethical value. The purpose of such restrictions is not to realize other values, such as solidarity. The compelling case for closing borders was based on slowing the spread of COVID-19 and thereby reducing the risk that substantial COVID-19 spread might overwhelm hospitals and cause large-scale death. A secondary justification was the large financial costs of someone coming into a country, contracting COVID-19, and then being expensively hospitalized for a period of time when hospitals are already at risk of being overwhelmed. If the risk of overwhelming the health system is substantially diminished, the case for closing borders becomes weaker. If the argument is that closing borders to unvaccinated people does not reduce spread and risk—an empirical question—that is a different point. It is about the actual risk, not about the threat to solidarity or invasion of liberty by limiting the activities of the unvaccinated.

People may also complain about differentiation between recipients of different types of vaccines because they perceive it as unfair. Here it is important to distinguish the use of vaccination type as a pretext for nationality-based exclusions, which is unacceptable, and the use of vaccination type as a reasonable proxy for the COVID-19 risks that people may face or present to others. Again, whether different vaccinations all provide a sufficient level of protection to permit access, or whether some do not, may depend on the type of setting at issue.

7.2.3 Evaluating Discrimination and Related Objections

Objections to policies that consider vaccination status have come in three categories. One set of objections, most often offered from the political right, argues that the use of vaccination status as a criterion for access to public spaces or travel is a form of governmental overreach. But whatever we make of this critique, it is not a specific critique of using vaccination status. Presumably, simply closing those spaces would be an even greater form of governmental overreach. So, the question is whether, compared to closures, using vaccination status is a form of governmental overreach rather than in fact being liberty-enhancing. The charge of governmental overreach is too simple.

The second complaint is that using vaccination status constitutes discrimination. This complaint has been raised by people from multiple political positions. Those from the right (and some from the left) have tended to argue that considering vaccination status is unacceptable because it is a type of "direct" or "disparate treatment" discrimination (Klas 2021). The problem with this argument is that all policies will treat people differently, and, on this viewpoint, can be described as discrimination. For instance, only permitting people on a plane who have purchased a ticket, or only permitting people who have an appropriate passport or visa to cross borders, could also be described as discrimination against those who lack tickets or passports. The question is *which ways* of treating people differently constitute invidious or unacceptable discrimination. There is a rich and robust literature in law and ethics on this question, but one plausible answer is that treating people differently is unacceptable when based on either animus towards the source of difference or factually inaccurate beliefs about that difference. For instance, excluding people from a business based on their race, sexual orientation, or religion is unacceptable because it usually reflects either animus toward those groups or factually inaccurate beliefs about their participation. In contrast, excluding people who pose a health threat to others, or who are more likely to be injured if they participate in an activity, does not reflect animus or factual inaccuracy. It reflects a factually present difference between people, just as not permitting unticketed people on a plane reflects the fact that people who have not purchased a ticket have not paid for the cost of fuel, the pilot's salary, and so on.

What commentators demanding that unvaccinated people be treated the same as vaccinated ones are really requesting is not simply formal anti-discrimination but an accommodation or subsidy for the unvaccinated at some cost to the public.

In some settings, we do afford accommodations even at a cost to the public. For instance, we accommodate some religious or medical needs even when these needs can impose costs on others—for instance, conducting "bloodless" surgery for Jehovah's Witnesses. But being unvaccinated by choice is different from having a costly religious belief or a medical need. Medical needs are almost always far less chosen than being unvaccinated is. And costly religious beliefs are regarded as much more fundamental to a person's identity than being unvaccinated typically is. Furthermore, even when a religious belief or medical need is fundamental, accommodation is not unlimited. If an accommodation would present an undue burden on others, it is not required. For instance, in the United States, someone with an unchosen medical condition can be excluded from some forms of employment on the basis that they either present an undue risk to others or face an undue risk to themselves (Chevron USA Inc. v. Echazabal, 536 U.S. 73 2002). If this argument suffices in the case of serious medical conditions, it certainly seems to suffice in the case of a chosen vulnerability like remaining unvaccinated.

A different argument which might also be understood as an interpretation of the idea of discrimination is the complaint that differentiation based on vaccination status will have a disparate impact on people who are disadvantaged in other ways, such as racial minority groups or poorer people (Osama et al. 2021). To evaluate this argument, however, we would need to understand both the extent to which vaccination status actually tracks disparities and whether it exacerbates disparities more than extant policies such as requiring people who want to travel on a plane to pay for the privilege. With the widespread availability at zero cost of vaccination in many countries, disparities in uptake have reduced substantially, particularly along racial lines. In the United States, Hispanic Americans and Asian Americans are more vaccinated then white Americans, and Black Americans may now be as well. In the United States, the strongest driver of disparities appears to be political commitments rather than differential access (Hamel 2022).

Second, even if there are residual disparities in access to vaccines, it is not obvious that disparities produced by considering vaccination status are more objectionable than disparities produced by policies like requiring payment to fly by plane. Yet we do not regard the fact that requiring tickets entrenches pre-existing economic disparities as something that makes it unacceptable to require that people traveling by plane pay for their ticket, have a government-issued ID, or have a passport. This point is particularly relevant in countries where access to vaccines may remain disparate. It is immensely important to expand access and reduce disparities in access. However, just like requiring payment to fly, it is not obvious that there is anything uniquely or specially unjust about requiring vaccination to fly. Indeed, since vaccination itself is free in most places, vaccine-based differentiation is unlikely to increase disparities more than payment-based differentiation.

The last argument, which seems to primarily be offered by people from the left, objects to policies that consider vaccination status because they portend a return to normalcy. These commentators object that the ability to require vaccination allows a return to activities like working in jobs and attending school as people did prior to the pandemic. This undermines their hope that the pandemic would lead to a dramatic remaking of society (Gonsalves 2020). These critics are typically not arguing that vaccination status consideration is ethically objectionable because we should instead open everything up. Instead, they are arguing that society should remain universally subject to major public health restrictions in service of some type of solidaristic goal. They seem to be arguing that it is wrong to engage in certain activities, such as attending concerts or going to school without masks, unless and until everybody not only has had the *option* to be vaccinated but has *actually been* vaccinated, and perhaps also until those who cannot be vaccinated or fully protected through vaccination are protected in other ways. Arguments casting a "return to normal" as unethical have increasingly been advanced (Gonsalves 2022), though with little success, in the United States as mask requirements have been dropped and other public health restrictions relaxed.

The problem with this objection is that public health policies should be based on values that are widely shared and that people can reasonably be expected to accept. There are interesting philosophical arguments over whether it would be better to reorganize society, especially the workplace, in drastic ways. But it is not acceptable to use a pandemic to achieve those outcomes when its worst effects can be mitigated in less disruptive fashion. Policymakers have a responsibility to assist the least advantaged, although not everyone who objects to COVID-19 restrictions falls into this category. But they have an obligation to pursue this goal in a way that is least restrictive to others, which is unlikely to be reconcilable with maintaining population-wide restrictions. For instance, before concluding that long-term mask requirements in workplaces or schools are appropriate, or that large gatherings are never appropriate without everyone being tested beforehand, policymakers should start by investigating the least burdensome alternatives, such as improving ventilation and making access to therapies more equitable. The research efforts discussed in Section 7.4 will be an important adjunct to these goals.

7.3 The Ethics of Using "Second-Best" Vaccines

Another issue has involved the availability of different types of vaccines in different places, with mRNA vaccines initially being more widely used in high-income countries while inactivated-virus or viral-vector vaccines were used in lower-income countries. Likewise, boosters initially were widespread in some countries and not others. Vaccine types, scheduling, and doses have varied in different countries and for different patients.

We argue that providing different vaccine types or schedules in different places is ethically permissible and sometimes required. Even in an ideal world, different patients may benefit from different vaccines. And in our actual world, while the first available vaccine may not be the best, the far greater protection of vaccination with any vaccine makes vaccinating people more quickly, even with a vaccine that would be "second best" in a world of plenitude, the ethical choice.

Much attention has been focused on the limited availability of mRNA vaccines outside of the developed world, with many commentators criticizing mRNA vaccine manufacturers for not distributing their vaccines to a wider range of countries. Other vaccine technologies, such as inactivated virus or viral-vector vaccines, have sometimes been criticized as second-class (Peel et al. 2021) due to findings of lower initial efficacy against certain outcomes. More recently, viral-vector vaccines have been viewed as not as good due to rare side effects, such as blood clotting, not present for mRNA vaccines.

These objections go wrong in two ways. First, we are still learning about the long-term durability of vaccine protection for individual recipients and about the optimal vaccine schedule. mRNA vaccines may not be the most durably protective vaccine technologies. Newer studies suggest that the most durable protection might be achieved by heterologous ("mix and match") vaccination, where different types of vaccines are administered as part of a dosing schedule (Mahase 2022). Rather than assuming that the vaccine types and dosing schedules used in wealthier countries are optimal even for individual recipients and without regard to resource constraints, policymakers should update their recommendations in light of evolving data and, more importantly, should collectively invest in research on optimal dosing schedules and combinations.

Additionally, the same dosing schedule and approach may not be optimal for all groups. In the United States, manufacturers have stuck to a tight spacing between doses in current pediatric trials, even though newer studies suggest that a longer spacing may have both safety and efficacy advantages. Similarly, despite highly distinct levels of side effects by sex of complications from the Johnson & Johnson vaccine (Brady et al. 2021), the CDC resisted making a sex-based recommendation because it would be "difficult to implement" (Oliver 2021), notwithstanding the frequent use of sex-based recommendations in other settings (e.g. breast cancer and osteoporosis screening).

Second, optimal direct protection for individual recipients may not be optimal ethically or for the community under scarcity. When vaccines were initially scarce, some countries were willing to vary their vaccination schedules in order to increase the population-wide benefit of vaccines, yet others were hesitant to do so in part because they feel that doing so would unfairly treat recipients differently from one another. And while countries like the UK and Canada have varied their vaccination schedules from manufacturer recommendations, sometimes providing shorter intervals for higher-risk populations, no countries have yet pursued the strategy of fractional dosing, offering less than a full dose for specific populations (Du et al. 2022). This is particularly relevant given that lower doses have been used for pediatric populations, and that a large portion of the population in some developing countries falls within or just above the pediatric range, making it realistic that fractional dosing would be effective. Countries should avoid arrangements that emphasize equalizing the protection enjoyed *by vaccinated people* as opposed to increasing the protection enjoyed *by the population as a whole* (most importantly, by protecting more people), even if doing so involves making medically supported distinctions among vaccinated people. Some commentators have argued that it is ethically required to provide recipients a choice between vaccines (Hughes et al. 2021), but this choice only becomes plausible when vaccines are truly plentiful in a country—and, arguably, globally. And even then, just as many health systems choose to offer limited formularies in order to control costs and improve access (Feldman et al. 2020), it can be reasonable for a health system to offer fewer vaccine options in order to control costs and expand access to available options.

The case for varying vaccine schedules is further strengthened by the fact of limited resources. Rather than purely emphasizing making mRNA vaccines available to the world, it is also important to improve the availability of vaccine types that do not require cold storage or can be produced more cheaply. These vaccines can provide substantial protection, especially against severe illness and death, even if the protection is not theoretically equal to the protection offered by mRNA vaccines. It can be particularly relevant when the population being protected is one that faces lower age-based risk, as is often true in developing countries, but is not able to access high-quality intensive care.

In other contexts, the World Health Organization has been willing to recognize that resource limitations in specific settings can support the use of certain medical interventions, even if these approaches are not commonly used in the developed world (Persad and Emanuel 2016). An example is the use of fractional dosing for yellow fever vaccines (Vannice et al. 2018). A similar approach is warranted for COVID-19 vaccines. In order to effectively vaccinate the world, we should not require that everybody be vaccinated with the same vaccines, on the same schedule, or in the same way. Nor should we pretend that all vaccines are equally effective or protective. Rather, we should aim to improve global protection against COVID-19 even if protection is not equal globally. What matters is protecting the population overall, not whether all vaccinated people are equally well protected. Maximizing or equalizing the protection of each vaccinated person should not be pursued at the expense of vaccinating more people more quickly.

Accordingly, it would be ethically desirable and perhaps even required to continue conducting research on vaccine technologies even on vaccines that might not seem to be as initially effective as mRNA vaccines, if it might be easier to deploy these vaccines in specific settings or for certain populations. This is true not only in low-income countries but for some populations in high-income countries as well. For instance, in groups like children who face comparatively little risk of serious disease from COVID-19, it may be preferable to select vaccines that have fewer side effects, such as inactivated virus or protein-based vaccines (Wu et al. 2021), even if these vaccines are less protective against infection. The risk–benefit balance may, for instance, ultimately favor using inactivated virus or protein-based vaccines in children rather than mRNA vaccines. Even if the main risk averted is fever or another mild side effect, the reduction in side effects could both improve the risk–benefit balance and increase interest in vaccination.

Rather than shying away from acknowledging these risks, public health agencies should make their vaccine recommendations with a view to trying to provide vaccines that provide a favorable risk–benefit balance both for individuals and populations. Successfully vaccinating the whole world—which appears to be stalling not for lack of vaccine supply but due to lack of demand and logistical barriers (Guarascio and Rigby 2022)—will likely require continuing to invest in a variety of vaccine technologies, including nasal vaccines, vaccines with minimal side effects (even if mild), and vaccines that do not require an extensive cold chain.

7.4 Coda: Why Research Remains Imperative

We have argued that a Procrustean approach is a mistake both for public health policies and for the provision of medical interventions like vaccines. Both for public health responses and for vaccine schedules, a further failure of the Procrustean approach has been a lack of ongoing research and optimization of the public health response. At times, countries have too quickly decided that a given approach is "optimal" without conducting research trials to rigorously compare different alternatives. As an example, at the start of the vaccine rollout in the United States, it was claimed that a three-week interval between mRNA vaccine doses (the only interval tested in trials) was "optimal" (Press Briefing 2021). Many countries selected other intervals (Quach and Deeks 2021); clinical research trials comparing alternative schedules were not conducted. Over a year after the initial rollout, the CDC changed its recommendation to suggest a longer interval for some patient groups (Wallace et al. 2022). Similarly, because the antibody levels induced by mRNA vaccines rose rapidly and seemed to offer better protection from severe illness in the first weeks after vaccination, they were presumed to be "better" vaccines. But more recent studies have suggested that other vaccines may provide more durable immunity (Bartlett, 2021). This is all evolving, making it unclear whether there is a "best vaccine" and, if so which one it might be.

While we have saved millions of lives through vaccination, we have failed to conduct the right studies of mixing and matching and altering vaccination schedules to determine the optimal vaccination protocol. Booster vaccination recommendations, such as the dose quantity, interval, and eligibility criteria, have been made based on observational data rather than on clinical trials. And despite the ubiquity of prior COVID-19 infection following the Omicron variant (Clarke,

2022), policymakers have been slow to offer clear recommendations for people who were previously infected other than either waiting to be vaccinated or receiving the exact same vaccine dose and schedule as those without prior infection—a dubious recommendation given preliminary data (Frieman et al. 2021).

Similarly, rigorous real-world trials that, for instance, randomized different settings to different types of masks, or to different ventilation or gathering arrangements, could have helped us learn which policies prevent more harm, allowing policymakers to select a package of interventions that better balances mitigating the direct harms of the pandemic and reducing the indirect harms of public health restrictions. Arguments that such trials are unethical (Clapham and Cook 2021) are baseless: when some locations or jurisdictions are selecting one policy without trials while others, also without trials, are selecting a different policy, it cannot credibly be claimed that it is unethical to rigorously compare the two policies rather than allowing different policies to become entrenched in different places due to initial political variation and path dependence. While initial responses had to be developed without sufficient information, the lack of continuing research efforts to optimize pandemic response has been a failure of the biomedical research community and vaccine regulatory bodies.

7.5 Conclusion

In any pandemic, public health responses need to be measured by how well they reduce the harms from the pandemic and by how well they mitigate disadvantage. In pursuit of these aims, public health policies need to use the least restrictive measures. That is, they need to limit any restrictions or impositions to the fewest people and activities needed to reduce harms to an acceptable level while adequately mitigating disadvantage. Much of the criticism of the ethics of public health policies, both within countries and between high-income and low-income countries, has been based on three types of faulty reasoning.

One type of faulty reasoning involves assessing public health restrictions such as limiting travel or use of facilities. Determining the appropriate degree of restrictions for a specific activity or group should not involve comparison with "normal" life but with the public health restrictions that would need to be universally imposed to achieve the same outcomes. In this comparison, imposing fewer restrictions or imposing restrictions on fewer people to achieve the same public health outcomes is more ethical. Consequently, restricting actions of the unvaccinated but not the vaccinated can be ethical because it achieves the same goals while fewer people have their freedom limited.

A second element of faulty reasoning is charging discrimination whenever policies treat individuals differently or have differential impact. All policies have differential impact. Minimizing harms and mitigating disadvantage and using the least restrictive policies to achieve these aims mean that implementing policies with differential impacts on certain populations is both inevitable and just. Differential impacts do not inherently constitute discrimination or other unjust treatments. It depends on the justification for the differential impacts. They are just when the differential treatment is not linked to animus, unalterable characteristics such as race, or characteristics deeply linked to personal identify, such as religion, and when it serves the justifiable goals of preventing harm and mitigating disadvantage. If differential treatment is based on protecting the public, and is based on factors relevant to that protection, it is just and not discriminatory.

The third element of faulty reasoning is arguing that low-income countries were treated unjustly because they received different, "second best" viral-vector vaccines from AstraZeneca and Johnson & Johnson when high-income countries had "the best" mRNA vaccines. Which COVID vaccines are "best" or "second best" is an empirical question, currently unclear, and seems to depend upon whether they are being compared on immediate protection or durability of protection. More importantly, the key variable is not the abstract measure of which vaccine is best. Compared to no vaccine, even a "second-best" but protective vaccine is better in limiting the population impact from COVID. Furthermore, as we are learning, it is important to consider not just vaccine types and numbers but actual administration. Sending "best" vaccines that expire or never get to people because of problems with countries' ability to ensure a cold chain or distribute vaccine, or because of local hesitancy to receive a vaccine with more side effects, is less valuable than a less protective but easier to administer vaccine that gets into people's arms.

The real ethical failures of the pandemic have not involved treating people differently or violations of formal equality but, rather, failing to take elementary measures to improve access to protective interventions—even if that access remains unequal. For instance, they have involved sending no vaccines at all to low-income countries initially, and failing to expand access to testing and high-quality masks before the advent of vaccines. It is time for bioethics to de-emphasize charges that health policies that treat individuals or countries differently are unethical—charges that often valorize doing nothing at all or adopting superficially equal approaches like treating vaccinated and unvaccinated people identically. Instead, bioethics should recognize that fairness depends on an effective pandemic response that prevents harm, especially to the least advantaged, and that doing so will often require differential treatment.

Bibliography

Bartlett, N. (2021), 'Does AstraZeneca's COVID vaccine give longer-lasting protection than mRNA shots?' *The Conversation*, https://theconversation.com/does-astrazenecas-covid-vaccine-give-longer-lasting-protection-than-mrna-shots-172609.

Brady, E., Nielsen, M. W., Andersen, J. P., and Oertelt-Prigione, S. (2021), 'Lack of consideration of sex and gender in COVID-19 clinical studies'. *Nature Communications*, 12(1): 1–6.

Chevron USA Inc. v. Echazabal, 536 U.S. 73 (2002), Justia, US Supreme Court, https://supreme.justia.com/cases/federal/us/536/73/.

Childress, J. F., Faden, R. R., Gaare, R. D., Gostin, L. O., Kahn, J., Bonnie, R. J., Kass, N. E, Mastroianni, A. C., Moreno, J. D., and Nieburg, P. (2002), 'Public health ethics: mapping the terrain', *Journal of Law, Medicine & Ethics*, 30(2): 170–8.

Clapham, H. E., and Cook A. R. (2021), 'Face masks help control transmission of COVID-19', *The Lancet Digital Health*, 3(3): e136–7.

Clarke, K. E. (2022), 'Seroprevalence of Infection-Induced SARS-CoV-2 Antibodies—United States, September 2021–February 2022', MMWR. Morbidity and Mortality Weekly Report, 71.

Cloete, J,, Kruger, A., Masha, M., du Plessis, N.M., Mawela, D., Tshukudu, M., Manyane, T., Komane, L., Venter, M., Jassat, W., and Goga, A. (2022), 'Paediatric hospitalisations due to COVID-19 during the first SARS-CoV-2 omicron (B. 1.1. 529) variant wave in South Africa: a multicentre observational study', *The Lancet Child & Adolescent Health*, 6(5): 294–302.

Du, Z., Wang, L., Pandey, A., Lim, W. W., Chinazzi, M., Lau, E. H, Wu, P., Malani, A., Cobey, S., and Cowling, B. J. (2022), 'Modeling comparative cost-effectiveness of SARS-CoV-2 vaccine dose fractionation in India', *Nature Medicine*, 24: 1–5.

Dyer, O. (2022), 'Covid-19: Lockdowns spread in China as omicron tests "zero covid" strategy', *BMJ* (Clinical research ed.), 376: o859.

Feldman, W. B., Avorn, J., Kesselheim, A. S. (2019), 'Potential Medicare savings on inhaler prescriptions through the use of negotiated prices and a defined formulary', *JAMA internal medicine*, 180(3): 454–6.

Frieman, M., Harris, A. D., Herati, R. S., Krammer, F., Mantovani, A., Rescigno, M., Sajadi, M. M., Simon, V. (2021), 'SARS-CoV-2 vaccines for all but a single dose for COVID-19 survivors', *EBioMedicine*, 68.

Gatter, R., Mohapatra, S. (2020), 'COVID-19 and the Conundrum of Mask Requirements', *Washington and Lee University Law Review Online*, 77(1).

Gonsalves, G. (2020), 'We're Never Going Back to Normal', *The Nation*, Oct. 22, 2020, https://www.thenation.com/article/society/covid-surge-winter-biden/.

Gonsalves G. (2022), W'hy Wishful Thinking on Covid Remains As Dangerous as Ever', *The Nation*, Feb. 3, 2022, https://www.thenation.com/article/society/covid-surrender-endemic/. Thrasher S. (2022), 'There Is Nothing Normal about One Million People Dead from COVID', *Scientific American*, Feb. 10, 2022, https://www.scientificamerican.com/article/there-is-nothing-normal-about-one-million-people-dead-from-covid1/.

Guarascio, F., and Rigby, J. (2022), 'COVID vaccine supply for global programme outstrips demand for first time', *Reuters*, Feb. 23, 2022, https://www.reuters.com/business/healthcare-pharmaceuticals/covax-vaccine-supply-outstrips-demand-first-time-2022-02-23/.

Hamel L. (2022), 'KFF COVID-19 Vaccine Monitor: January 2022', https://www.kff. org/coronavirus-covid-19/poll-finding/kff-covid-19-vaccine-monitor-january-2022/.

Monte L. (2021), 'Who Are the Adults Not Vaccinated Against COVID? Dec. 28, 2021', https://www.census.gov/library/stories/2021/12/who-are-the-adults-not-vaccinated-against-covid.html

Hughes, M. T., Auwaerter, P. G., Ehmann, M. R., Garibaldi, B. T., Golden, S. H., Lorigiano, T. J., O'Conor, K. J., Kachalia, A, and Kahn, J. (2021), 'Opinion: The importance of offering vaccine choice in the fight against COVID-19', Proceedings of the National Academy of Sciences, 118(43), 26 Oct, 2021.

Klas, M. Florida Gov. 'DeSantis Signs Bill Banning Vaccine Passports', Government Technology, Health and Human Services, May 3, 2021, https://www.govtech. com/health/florida-gov-desantis-signs-bill-banning-vaccine-passports. Baylis, F., Kofler, N. (2021), 'Vaccination certificates could entrench inequality', Nature, 591(7851): 529–30.

Krishnaratne, S., Littlecott, H., Sell, K., Burns, J., Rabe, J. E., Stratil, J. M., Litwin, T., Kreutz, C., Coenen, M., Geffert, K., Boger, A. H. (2022), 'Measures implemented in the school setting to contain the COVID-19 pandemic: a rapid review', Cochrane Database of Systematic Reviews, 1(1).

Mahase E. (2022), 'Covid-19: Mix and match booster vaccination approach offers best protection, study reports', BMJ (Clinical research ed.), 377: o1052.

Mina, M. J., Andersen, K. G. (2021), 'COVID-19 testing: One size does not fit all', Science, 371/6525: 126–7.

Oliver S. (2021), 'Thrombocytopenic thrombosis after Janssen vaccine: Work Group Interpretation', CDC, Apr. 4, 2021, https://www.cdc.gov/vaccines/acip/meetings/ downloads/slides-2021-04/05-COVID-Oliver-508.pdf.

Osama, T., Razai, M.S., Majeed, A. (2021), 'Covid-19 vaccine passports: access, equity, and ethics', BMJ, 378.

Peel, M., Cameron-Chileshe, J., Pilling, D. (2021), 'G7's vaccine pledge for poor nations branded inadequate by campaigners', Financial Times, June 11, 2021, https://www.ft.com/content/86888591-151c-453d-80ba-49b0b2d1f139.

Persad, G. C., Emanuel, E. J. (2016), 'The ethics of expanding access to cheaper, less effective treatments', The Lancet, 388(10047):9 32–4.

Press Briefing (2021), Press Briefing by White House COVID-19 Response Team and Public Health Officials, Feb. 3, 2021, https://www.whitehouse.gov/briefing-room/ press-briefings/2021/02/03/press-briefing-white-house-covid-19-response-team-and-public-health-officials/.

Quach, C., Deeks, S. (2021), 'COVID-19 vaccination: why extend the interval between doses?' Official Journal of the Association of Medical Microbiology and Infectious Disease Canada, 6(2): 73–8.

Savulescu, J., Cameron, J. (2020), 'Why lockdown of the elderly is not ageist and why levelling down equality is wrong', Journal of Medical Ethics, 46(11): 717–21.

Vannice, K., Wilder-Smith, A., Hombach, J. (2018), 'Fractional-dose yellow fever vaccination—advancing the evidence base', *New England Journal of Medicine*, 379(7): 603–5.

Wallace, M., Moulia, D., Blain, A. E., Ricketts, E. K., Minhaj, F. S., Link-Gelles, R., Curran, K. G., Hadler, S. C., Asif, A., Godfrey, M., and Hall, E. (2022), 'The Advisory Committee on Immunization Practices' Recommendation for Use of Moderna COVID-19 Vaccine in Adults Aged ≥ 18 Years and Considerations for Extended Intervals for Administration of Primary Series Doses of mRNA COVID-19 Vaccines—United States, February 2022. Morbidity and Mortality Weekly Report', 71(11): 416.

Wu, Q., Dudley, M. Z., Chen, X., Bai, X., Dong, K., Zhuang, T., Salmon, D., and Yu, H. (2021), 'Evaluation of the safety profile of COVID-19 vaccines: a rapid review', *BMC Medicine*, 19(1): 1–6.

8

Ethics of Selective Restriction of Liberty in a Pandemic

Julian Savulescu

8.1 Introduction

Restriction of liberty or coercion is an essential response in any pandemic.[1] Measures such as quarantine have been utilized for centuries to prevent the spread of disease (Kass 2001). Other measures include lockdown, mandatory use of health protection measures such as masks, prophylactic treatment, treatment upon exposure, and vaccination. Throughout the COVID-19 pandemic, it was usually applied at a population level. For example, in the UK lockdown applied to everyone equally. There are some exceptions in other countries. Sweden did not close lower secondary and primary schools (Pashakhanlou 2021). Austria and some regions of Russia (TASS 2021) applied selective mandatory vaccination to the elderly. Italy and Greece introduced fines for those over 50 and 60 respectively who were not vaccinated (Joly 2021; Amante, Fonte, and Jones 2022). Another example is Turkey, which selectively locked down 65+-year-olds for an extended period to allow the younger and working population to go out (although they also locked them down on weekends) (Koca-Atabey 2021).

Whilst liberty restriction was generally applied to the population, what was striking about the COVID pandemic was the age stratification of its direct health burdens. It was the elderly who were most at risk of dying from COVID-19, particularly those over the age of 65 (Verity et al. 2020). There were other groups who faced higher risks, including males, the obese, those with co-morbidities, some ethnic minorities, and people with particular disabilities (Williamson et al. 2020). For the purposes of simplicity, I will focus mainly on the aged, though at the end of the chapter I will address the implications for other at-risk groups.

Should those at low risk be subjected to the same liberty restrictions as those at higher risk?

---

[1] This chapter is a development of Cameron et al. (2021). Thanks to Alex Voorhoeve, Walter Sinnott-Armstrong, and Frances Kamm for valuable comments in developing this chapter. Thanks also to the audience of the workshop of the Uehiro-Carnegie-Oxford Conference on Pandemic X, Dec. 2021.

Julian Savulescu, *Ethics of Selective Restriction of Liberty in a Pandemic* In: *Pandemic Ethics: From COVID-19 to Disease X.* Edited by: Dominic Wilkinson and Julian Savulescu, Oxford University Press. © Julian Savulescu 2023. DOI: 10.1093/oso/9780192871688.003.0009

The usual basis for the use of coercion in a pandemic is to prevent transmission. With colleagues, I used the example of a child taking a bottle of toxic bleach to school. The bleach can be taken away from the child not merely because it is a threat to the child but because it is a threat to others (Bambery et al. 2013).

In the COVID-19 pandemic, population-level liberty restriction was said to be justified because everyone was assumed to be capable of transmitting the virus and posing a threat, and everyone was seen to be at some risk. "We are all in this together" was a slogan frequently used to describe this situation. However, I will argue that there are reasons to doubt whether this analogy applies to all groups in a pandemic. As the example of driving shows, we can pose a lethal threat to others provided the threat is reasonable, including that it is proportionate to the individual and collective benefit.

In this chapter I will consider the philosophical arguments for selective restriction of liberty. I will not consider in detail whether the facts justified such selective restrictions of liberty in the COVID-19 pandemic, though I will cite some suggestive evidence. I will not consider public opinion, though this should play some role in formulation of policy (Savulescu, Gyngell, and Kahane 2021).

8.2 The Harm Principle and Liberty Restriction

John Stuart Mill argued that the sole ground for interference in liberty is to prevent harm to others and that harm to self is never a sufficient ground (Mill 1859). This recognizes that people should be free to make their own decisions, including to identify and weigh risks to their own health. The challenge of infectious diseases is that people are not just the victims, they are also the vectors, and so their infection poses a risk of harm to others (Mill 1859). This challenge is amplified in a pandemic, as people pose a risk to others through the potential spread of the disease and by contributing to overwhelming the healthcare system if they become ill.[2]

During the COVID-19 pandemic, a number of liberty-restricting measures were justified on the basis that they would limit the spread of the disease and so prevent the health system from being overwhelmed.[3] Various coercive measures were adopted, including quarantine, isolation, lockdown, and surveillance. Under this framing, the extent to which liberty-restricting measures are justified depends on the level of risk and potential severity of the harm to others (Selgelid 2009).

The problem with this principle is that it does not address the level of liberty restriction which is justified to prevent harm or reduce risk. This could be defined

[2] See, for example, Di Blasi (2020), Ives (2020).   [3] See, for example, BBC News (2020).

in several ways by appealing to the impact on individuals' or groups' rights or the harms to them. In this chapter, I will explore the perspective of non-maleficence as a side-constraint on justice.

Others have noted the problem of quantifying a just liberty restriction. As Verweij identifies, this creates the challenge of delineating between reasonable steps and 'excessive precautions' (Verweij 2005). One popular approach in public health ethics has been the "least restrictive alternative" (Bioethics 2007; Viens, Bensimon, and Upshur 2009). This states that, for a given public health goal, we should adopt the measure which least restricts liberty to achieve that goal.[4] The problem with this is that in many cases greater restrictions on liberty will achieve greater benefits. For example, no social contact with friends and family will save more lives than limited contact. So which policy is justified? If the goal is to prevent deaths in a pandemic, ever increasing liberty restrictions might seem justified and a slippery slope ensues.

Childress et al. (2002) propose five 'justificatory conditions' to proceed with coercive public health measures: effectiveness, proportionality, necessity, least infringement, and public justification. Each of these conditions involves value judgements.

I have elsewhere created and defended an algorithm for when mandatory vaccination is justified (Savulescu 2021), similar to Childress et al.'s conditions. (See Figure 8.1.) This involves evaluating:

1. Gravity of public health emergency.
2. Safety and effectiveness of vaccine.
3. Comparative expected utility compared to less coercive policies.
4. Proportionality of cost associated with refusal to comply with the mandate in relation to 1–3.

In the paper and elsewhere (Giubilini, Savulescu, and Danchin 2022) I consider whether these four conditions are satisfied by COVID vaccinations. In that paper, I described the range of liberty restrictions—from withholding of benefits, or fines, to outright imprisonment. I also described the range of measures that can be employed other than liberty restriction to contain contagion.

For the purposes of this chapter, it is important to point out that this algorithm is typically only applied at a population level. Governments ask: is the cost of coercion justifiable given the safety and effectiveness of the intervention compared to other alternatives, at a population level?

---

[4] For example, Upshur suggests four principles for justifying public health interventions: the harm principle, the least restrictive means principle, the reciprocity principle, and the transparency principle (Upshur 2002).

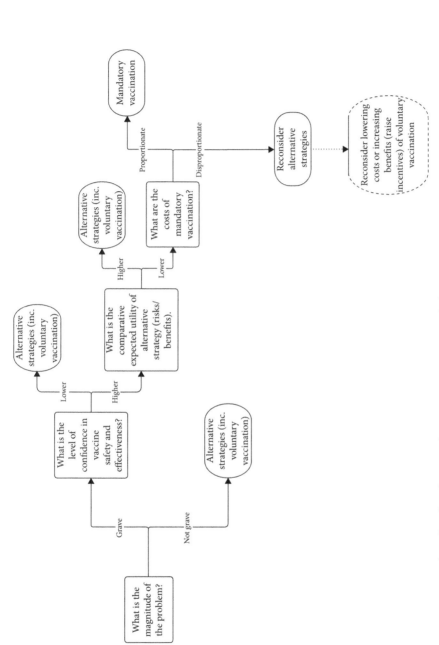

Figure 8.1 An algorithm for when mandatory vaccination is justified.

But given the age stratification of COVID, the vaccines had a favourable risk–benefit profile for one group (the old), but a less favourable profile for another (the young). It was ethically easier to justify a mandatory policy of vaccination for the elderly than it was for children or infants. The elderly clearly benefited from vaccination (and its net expected cost was lower) compared to children who benefited little, if at all. For children, the risks and costs of coercion loomed large.

It might be objected that, while the direct risk posed by COVID to children was low, there were risks to their well-being from an ongoing epidemic (through impact on education, parents' health and income, etc.). If vaccinating all of them reduced these risks to them, then it may be to their advantage that all of them are vaccinated. I will later argue that the "preserve the health system" argument, of which this is a variant, likely failed because it could have been preserved through less restrictive means. In the case of children, the harm of closure of schools was the result of a policy decision, a decision which not every country made—Sweden kept primary schools open.

So it is possible that, if one took an individual or group-specific approach (groups can also be proxies for individuals), mandatory vaccination could have been justified for some individuals or groups, but not others, as some countries like Italy and Greece recognized. If one takes a more individualized or group-oriented approach rather than population-level approach, we should then ask—how much does one group owe another? In a pandemic, we are sometimes addressing the issue of how much expected disutility or harm the government is entitled to cause to one group to benefit or prevent harm to another group.

8.3 Easy Rescue Consequentialism

Another way to approach the question of coercive measures is to ask: how much should governments require their citizens to sacrifice for each other?[5] Or how much should one group be required to sacrifice to benefit a different group? How much harm can the state cause to an individual to benefit another?

According to utilitarianism, very large sacrifices are required. Indeed, provided the utility to another or others is greater than the sacrifice to an individual, that individual ought to make that sacrifice. Thus, if one can eliminate an elderly person's risk of dying of 15% by taking on a 10% chance of dying, one should take the risk. Indeed, a young person should take on a 10% chance of dying even if she

---

[5] Parts of this section on consequentialism are developed from Giubilini et al. (2018b).

only reduced the chance of a group of elderly people dying by 1%, provided that group was larger than 1,000, according to utilitarianism (assuming they would both live as long, though the numbers can be adjusted to yield the same conclusion if they have different life expectancies).

One familiar objection to utilitarianism is that it is too demanding (Wolf 1982). The classic instantiation of this is the Survival Lottery (Harris 1975). In the Survival Lottery, the government randomly picks a healthy individual and kills that individual for their organs. Those organs could save the lives of up to eight individuals. This could be justified on either utilitarian or contractualist grounds (Savulescu 2002). Figure 8.2 is a cartoon of a pandemic version of the Survival Lottery.

Even though this sacrifice might be justified on contractualist or utilitarian grounds, there is a limit to the costs governments should be allowed to impose on individuals to benefit others. This can be called a constraint of non-maleficence which places an upper limit of expected harm to an individual.

Note that this constraint of non-maleficence should apply whatever theory of justice is employed to distribute benefits and burdens. For example, prioritarianism requires giving priority to the worst-off. That is, benefits matter more when they accrue to those who are worse off. However, liberty restriction in a pandemic has winners and losers; it provides benefits and imposes burdens. According to prioritarianism, it could be justifiable to impose large burdens on the well-off for small benefits to the worst-off. Non-maleficence will impose some limit on how much harm can be caused to individuals to bring about the just (or best) outcome.

How great should that limit be? Easy rescue consequentialism provides a plausible answer.

According to easy rescue consequentialism, when I could do something that entails a very small cost to me, and a significant benefit to others, I have a moral obligation to do it. Peter Singer provided the most famous characterization of the duty of easy rescue in his article *Famine, Affluence, and Morality*, through the well-known example of a child drowning in a pond. According to Singer, "if I am walking past a shallow pond and see a child drowning in it, I ought to wade in and pull the child out. This will mean getting my clothes muddy, but this is insignificant, while the death of the child would presumably be a very bad thing" (Singer 1972: 231).

A formulation of the duty of easy rescue has been provided by Scanlon, according to whom, "[i]f we can prevent something very bad from happening to someone by making a slight or even moderate sacrifice, it would be wrong not to do so" (Scanlon 1998: 224).

In *Reasons and Persons*, Derek Parfit extends a principle for attribution of individual moral obligations to contribute to collective effects. Parfit asks us to consider the following collective example:

Epidemic

A highly contagious virus has emerged and is spreading quickly throughout the land. These six people contract it:

You're the doctor who has to treat them.

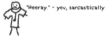
"Hooray." - you, sarcastically

If you do nothing, then five of the six people die.

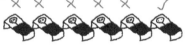

But there's a cure!

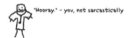
"Hooray." - you, not sarcastically

One of the six has a great immune system and can beat the thing.

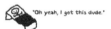
"Oh yeah, I got this dude."

So you can kill him...

"Wait what."

And put his blood in the other five patients.

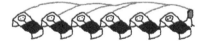

They would survive. Instead of one living and five dying, five live and one dies.

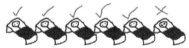

So, you have two options.

Option One, "Inaction," looks like this:

Option Two, "Extraction," looks like this:

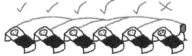

Which option do you choose?

Figure 8.2 A cartoon, *Epidemic*, by artist Dylan Matthews.

a large number of wounded men lie out in the desert, suffering from intense thirst. We are an equally large number of altruists, each of whom has a pint of water. We could pour these pints into a water-cart. This would be driven into the desert, and our water would be shared equally between all these many wounded men. By adding his pint, each of us would enable each wounded man to drink slightly more water – perhaps only an extra drop. Even to a very thirsty man, each of these extra drops would be a very small benefit. The effect on each man might even be imperceptible.   (Parfit 1984: 76)

The principle illustrated in this example is the following:

When (1) the best outcome would be the one in which people are benefited most, and (2) each of the members of some group could act in a certain way, and (3) they would benefit people if *enough* of them act in this way, and (4) they would benefit people *most* if they *all* act in this way, and (5) each of them both knows these facts and believes that enough of them will act in this way, then (6) each of them ought to act in this way (Parfit 1984: 77).

We might call this the principle of "Group Beneficence" (Otsuka 1991). According to this principle, each individual member of the collective has a moral obligation to make her contribution to enable the desired collective effect. But what is absent in this specification of group beneficence is the cost that should be exacted from one individual to benefit the group.

A duty of easy rescue can take a similar collective form which specifies the limits of the cost. I have formalized the collective form of the duty as follows:

If a group of people $(X1 \ldots Xn)$ could all perform some act, V, which would collectively provide a large benefit to Y, then this group $(X1 \ldots Xn)$ ought to V, provided that the cost to each of them of V-ing is small.

(Savulescu 2016: 331)

I call this a duty of "collective easy rescue". While these arguments describe moral obligations, it is plausible that if a government is morally justified in imposing harms on individuals for the benefit of others, it is most justified in imposing those harms when they conform to a duty of easy rescue.

We saw an example of the duty of easy rescue in Parfit's example of the relief of dehydration by those who have plenty of water. The cost to them is small. Vaccination is an example of an action that typically entails at most a small cost to individuals and can significantly benefit others. Vaccines are typically safe and effective, the risks of side effects or iatrogenic diseases is small, and there are typically also significant benefits for the vaccinated individual (Andre et al. 2008). Accordingly, being vaccinated is typically comparable to getting one's clothes muddy in Singer's example (or perhaps, one could argue, even less costly), or giving a pint of water in Parfit's example.

Now one difference between Parfit's example and a pandemic is that harms and benefits are certain in Parfit's example, while a pandemic involves risk and uncertainty. Thus in the case of a pandemic we should consider the *expected* utility or disutility, which is the probability of an outcome multiplied by the value. So where I write harm and benefit in connection with a pandemic, that should strictly be expected utility and expected disutility.

Another difference between Parfit's example and a pandemic is that Parfit's example involves benefiting, whereas in a pandemic we are concerned with one individual not harming another. Of course, for consequentialists, failing to benefit is equivalent to harming. But even for non-consequentialists, the issue is what level of harm or expected disutility can be imposed on one individual to reduce the very small or negligible risk of that individual harming another. The issue of collective rescue becomes, in a pandemic, the issue of collective "not harming".

One difficulty with the collective duty of easy rescue (or not harming) is that it implies that members of the collective X1...Xn could have a duty to V even if their own V-ing would be irrelevant to the production of the benefit to Y because it would be sufficient to produce the benefit that some subset of X1...Xn perform V. Of course, as an individual or group represents a higher risk to others, there is more justification for greater infringement of their liberty (for this reason, those who returned from high-risk areas were subjected to quarantine).

However, in the case we are discussing of the COVID pandemic, we should find the smallest group or the group defined by conditions of fairness, such that it is sufficient to provide the benefit (or prevent the harm to a significant enough degree). In Parfit's case, there is just a group of 1,000 donors. If there had been 10,000 donors, but 9,000 had two pints of water, and 1,000 had five pints, arguably the donation of a pint each should come from those with five pints.

I will now argue that the elderly are, in one way, like those with five pints of water and the young are like those with two pints. While vaccination is an easy rescue for the elderly, it may not be an easy rescue for the young.

8.4 Applying Easy Rescue Consequentialism to the Pandemic

An easy rescue consequentialist approach is preferable to the harm principle because it enables a balancing exercise at a population level that aligns more closely with the aims of public health. Public health aims to protect and promote the health of the population (Selgelid 2009). Public health measures are not simply aimed at ensuring people do not harm others and achieving this in the least restrictive manner. An ethical framework is needed that defines the circumstances in which it would be appropriate to pursue population-wide benefits in light of the costs of doing so. This may be achieved by first considering the consequences of a measure at the population level and then considering the costs to relevant individuals of achieving these benefits. It is necessary to assess the net utility of a measure across the population and the cost to individuals separately, because although the individual may be part of the population, imposing measures on particular individuals may result in disproportionate costs to those individuals. As the Black Lives Matter movement shows, we should consider the costs and benefits to groups, and ultimately individuals. Public health ethics frequently adopts a utilitarian approach which can be insensitive to the impact on individuals.

8.5 Population-Level Consequentialist Assessment

Rather than simply assessing whether there is a sufficient risk of harm to warrant liberty-restricting measures, it is necessary to consider the total utility to the population of a measure and whether the net utility is greater than other available options. Three factors are relevant to this assessment:

- The gravity of the threat to public interest;
- The expected health gains of the measure compared to other measures;
- The extent to which the expected health gains outweigh the restriction of liberty.

At a population level, a measure will be justified if the comparative expected health gain justifies the restriction of liberty. For example, requiring everyone to wear masks might be a reasonable restriction, even if some are unlikely to become ill or pass on the virus. Such an intervention has the potential to reduce disease burden and is a small liberty restriction. It is like requiring motor cyclists to wear helmets.

8.6 Individual Costs

Utility at a population level cannot always be given priority (Selgelid 2005). A key objection to a utilitarian approach is the risk that it will result in utilitarian calculations in which people's liberty and well-being will be sacrificed whenever this would result in a net overall benefit to society. This may mean that particular groups of individuals can be forced to make significant sacrifices in order to achieve marginal social gains or that the burdens of achieving public health aims may continually fall on the same group. This would be unfair. This issue may be overcome by considering the outcomes at an individual level both in terms of well-being and liberty to an individual compared to the benefits to others.

As I have argued, 'If the cost (including foreseeable risk of significant disability or death) to someone of performing an action X (or of refraining from performing an action Y) is sufficiently small to be reasonably bearable, and the resulting benefit to other people (or harm that is prevented) is large relative to the cost, then the agent ought to do X (or not do Y)' (Giubilini et al. 2018a: 186). This is a case of 'easy rescue', and this provides a stronger basis for state intervention to compel the person to perform some action, such as getting vaccinated (Giubilini et al. 2018b).

For example, one modelling exercise conducted by our group in 2020, prior to the introduction of vaccines, suggested that restricting the liberty of those over the age of 50 (while allowing free mixing under the age of 50) would have saved over 400,000 lives in the UK compared to the unmitigated scenario at the height of the pandemic. This would not have saved as many lives as the blanket lockdown of all age groups, the model suggested, but it would have kept mortality at a level experienced at the peak of the pandemic in April and have prevented the collapse of health systems.[6] For an individual over the age of 50, this benefit is achieved at the cost of their liberty. But the liberty restriction also benefits them by preventing their exposure to a disease that poses a particular risk to them. Importantly, this age group is also the most vulnerable to COVID-19 and so the benefit to them is significant. Arguably, it is a net overall benefit to them compared to a policy of no liberty restriction for the over-50s.

At an individual level, whilst the cost of the liberty restriction may be great, this must be weighed against the personal benefit of avoiding the disease. There may even still be a net expected cost to the individual, but this may be outweighed by the benefit to others and reasonable if the net cost is small. For people over the age of 50, this may be a net benefit or at least a case of 'easy rescue', in which the overall cost to the individual of saving others is relatively small, compared to the benefit to others (Giubilini et al. 2018b).

At an individual level, the weighing of costs and benefits for those under the age of 50 is different. This is because imposing liberty restrictions on people under the age of 50 will not directly benefit them in the same way, because COVID-19 does not pose the same risk to them. Despite this reduced personal benefit, those under the age of 50 would still incur the same costs from liberty restrictions as well as costs to their well-being in other ways. For example, the closure of schools during the COVID-19 pandemic significantly harmed children and substantially impacted their development (Christakis, Van Cleve, and Zimmerman 2020). One analysis of the UK's lockdown using the QALY method found that it was likely to have a cost–benefit ratio significantly outside the NHS's standard range (Miles, Stedman, and Heald 2021). As there are fewer benefits for

---

[6] Of course, households mix and care workers have families. The extent to which a selective policy could effectively shield the vulnerable is an open and vexed empirical question.

someone under the age of 50 in being isolated, the relative cost of liberty restrictions may outweigh the potential benefits to others. For those under 50, liberty restrictions may be a more difficult rescue.

Considering the costs and benefits of a measure at both a population and individual level ensures that individuals are not forced to bear disproportionately high costs in terms of either liberty or well-being to achieve marginal social gains and, ideally, benefit from them. It satisfies a constraint of nonmaleficence. An easy rescue consequentialist approach may have supported age-selective liberty restrictions in the COVID-19 pandemic. There are, of course, challenges in identifying relevant costs and benefits and making generalizations across the community about the value of different costs and benefits to individuals (John 2020). For example, the cost of liberty restrictions may vary significantly across individuals, including among people of the same age. But this challenge also arises under the application of the harm principle and least restrictive model. In the assessment of the impact of any policy across a population it is necessary to make generalizations.

One objection is that liberty restriction of those under 50 nonetheless benefits most people because COVID-19 still represents a lethal risk. One could argue that the young giving up certain freedoms still constitutes an easy rescue. This objection ignores other non-COVID-19-related costs to a person's well-being from liberty restrictions.

If COVID-19 did not affect those over the age of 50 at all, but affected those under the age of 50 in the same way, we would not think liberty restrictions were justified in the under-50s. So those liberty restrictions are for the benefit, in the actual case, for those over 50.

Another common objection to selective restriction of liberty is that more utility will be generated by general restriction of liberty (Nix 2022). More lives would be saved by a general lockdown or mandatory vaccination of all in COVID-19. This may well be true. But we should ask whether the additional restriction of liberty represents a case of easy rescue for those adversely affected by it. If the harm to younger people is more than minimal, it may be a difficult rescue.

The key issue is whether moving from a selective liberty restriction to a general restriction of liberty generates enough expected utility to the vulnerable group to justify the costs to the less vulnerable group. According to easy rescue consequentialism, the government can only impose expected harm on the less vulnerable if it were an instance of easy rescue. (Of course, utilitarians would impose costs on the less vulnerable as long as they were even slightly less than the costs to the more vulnerable.) In the case of COVID-19, it is arguable that targeted measures were sufficient to reduce deaths without a generalized liberty restriction, as the experience of Sweden showed: while their nearest neighbours achieved slightly better results through more restrictive measures, the benefits were relatively minor (see Figure 8.3).

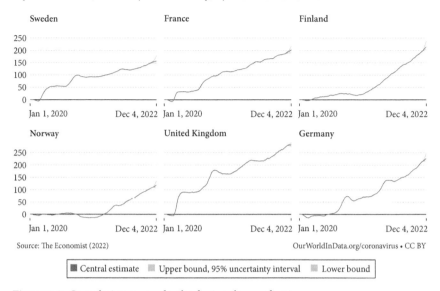

Estimated cumulative excess deaths per 100, 000 people during COVID,
from The Economist

For countries that have not reported all-cause mortality data for a given week, an estimate is shown, with uncertainty interval. If
reported data is available, that value only is shown. on the map, only the central estimate is shown.

Source: The Economist (2022)   OurWorldInData.org/coronavirus • CC BY

Figure 8.3 Cumulative excess deaths during the pandemic.

8.7 Resource Use and Indirect Harm

I will now consider a second argument in favour of selective restriction of liberty
in the case of the COVID-19 pandemic. It is expressed succinctly in the following
two quotes:

"'Lockdown was the only way to stop the NHS being broken'" (Lancaster 2020).

"The single most important action we can all take, in fighting coronavirus, is to
stay at home in order to protect the NHS and save lives" (Guidance 2020).

The commonest justification for general lockdown was that it was necessary to
"flatten the curve", to prevent overwhelming health services such as the NHS. This
was captured in the UK government slogan, "Stay Home, Save the NHS, Save
Lives", which was repeated over and over during the height of the pandemic.

The traditional justification for coercion and liberty restriction is to prevent
transmission to others. This is the harm-to-others justification. However, at the
time of John Stuart Mill there was no national health service or social welfare
state. But with the advent of healthcare, particularly public healthcare, pandemics
cause a second kind of harm—indirect harm. Those who fall ill use limited
healthcare resources and put pressure on health systems.

The stratification of risk in the COVID pandemic means that different groups
are likely to put different pressures on the health system. It was primarily the

elderly, not children, putting the NHS at risk. Of course, if the health system is overwhelmed, everyone is at risk.

Thus the probability of falling ill represents a second kind of harm during a pandemic: it indirectly threatens the health of other people (both the vulnerability to COVID and all other diseases) by consuming limited health resources and threatening the health system.

It is to prevent this harm that coercion could also be justified. But this would only justify coercion of those groups which are likely to put pressure on the health system. In the case of COVID, the group most likely to put pressure on the health system was the elderly. This could justify a selective lockdown or vaccination policy applied only to the elderly (or to other at risk groups) (Savulescu and Cameron 2020).

Now, one immediate objection would be that this argument could apply to using coercion whenever someone is more liable through their behaviour to use health resources. It might be thought that people could be forced to give up smoking, drinking, skiing, overeating, taking drugs, being sedentary, etc. However, we all contribute to the health system in order, partly, to pursue risky lifestyles. And moreover, life involves taking risks. Climbing a mountain or discovering a new habitat involve risks. The difference is that a pandemic represents an extreme and unusual emergency for which the health system is not set up. We as citizens do not contribute sufficient resources to keep a health system running while allowing significant liberty during a pandemic. Thus, as an exception, to keep the system running, we should be able to appeal to indirect harm as a basis for coercion.

It might be objected that we should simply devote more resources to the health system and stop it being overrun. However, there are a number of responses. Firstly, it may not be possible to quickly improve the health system to a sufficient degree. The UK built a number of "Nightingale hospitals", but these failed partly because there were insufficient staff to service them (Marsh and Campbell 2020).

Secondly, resources are limited. Even if they are increased to health, they must be taken from other areas, which will then cause other harms. And at some point, no matter how much is thrown at the problem, a limit will sometimes be reached whereby difficult triage or priority decisions must be made.

Thus, rather than focusing on preventing harm to others through reducing transmission, a consequentialist approach also recognizes that it is possible to limit the harm caused by the disease by focusing on the victim. An individual has limited control over whom they infect, but public health measures may limit the extent to which those most at risk are exposed to the disease. This was called "shielding" the elderly.

Moreover, in COVID-19 the vaccines developed were comparatively better at reducing serious illness than preventing transmission. Current estimates are that they reduce mortality by about 90%, which remains high over time, but that their ability to prevent infection (symptomatic or asymptomatic) wanes sharply, to a lower range estimate of as little as zero by six months after booster (Agency 2022).

When it comes to transmission, one recent study found that "[t]he SARs [secondary attack rates] in household contacts exposed to the delta variant was 25% in vaccinated and 38% in unvaccinated contacts". Moreover, the same study found that "SAR among household contacts exposed to fully vaccinated index cases (25%; 95% CI 15–35) was similar to household contacts exposed to unvaccinated index cases (23%; 15–31)" (Wilder-Smith 2022).

It might be objected that we should give weight to restricting the liberty of those who cause harm rather than their victims. We should not put potential victims of murder in lockdown rather than murderers, even if the this policy were less costly and more successful in stopping harm.[7]

I have discussed one constraint—non-maleficence—on the pursuit of utilitarian or other justice-based public health policies. There may be other constraints, such as human rights, which provide other important considerations.

8.8 Consistency: Compare with Children

Imagine that a future pandemic had the reverse mortality across age groups: young children who contracted Disease X would have a 15% chance of dying and the elderly would have a negligible chance. Society would not hesitate to remove children from school and social interactions and shield them as being vulnerable.

Children cannot consent, whereas the elderly can. But we are discussing non-consensual liberty restriction or coercion. So the autonomy or consent of a group is largely irrelevant.

In the childhood version of Disease X, should society impose a blanket lockdown? It is not immediately obvious that it should—it would depend on whether children could be sufficiently shielded without a blanket lockdown. The default should not be to restrict everyone because of the catastrophic social, economic, and non-pandemic medical effects of general lockdown, as several pandemic plans constructed before the COVID-19 pandemic predicted, including by the WHO (Global Influenza Programme 2019). Yet in the COVID pandemic, such selective restriction of liberty was barely countenanced and, when implemented by Sweden, roundly pilloried.

Generally society adopts a targeted and selective approach towards vaccination. For example, children are vaccinated against meningitis but the elderly are not. This is because children and young people most frequently contract meningitis, and sufficient protection can be obtained for individuals who are vaccinated. Now, older people occasionally develop meningitis and can be a vector. Vaccination of everyone would reduce total deaths. But the incremental benefit is not worth the cost. So a selective approach is adopted.

---

[7] Thanks to Frances Kamm for this objection.

8.9 Objections

8.9.1 Discrimination and the Value of Equality

If these arguments are correct, selective liberty restrictions may be imposed to reduce the disease burden. This leaves the question of whether it would be acceptable to restrict the liberty of a group of people on the basis of particular characteristics in order to reduce the disease burden. For example, age-selective restriction of liberty could be said to be ageist.

The extent to which discrimination is acceptable is identified as a separate consideration because, as Childress et al. identify, moral concerns that justify public health goals, such as producing benefits and preventing harms may conflict with other moral concerns, such as equality (Childress et al. 2002). Equality has value because it demonstrates respect for a person as a distinct individual. Hellman argues that discrimination is wrong when and because it demeans the person affected (Hellman 2011). This is because it reduces them to merely being the particular characteristic that was the ground for discrimination.

While consequentialists such as utilitarians do value equality as equal consideration of interests, selective restriction of liberty may appear to violate Aristotle's principle of equality to treat like cases alike unless there is a morally relevant difference. Failing to treat like cases alike constitutes unjust discrimination.

8.9.2 Relevant Differences

However, there *can* be relevant differences that can form the basis of a selective liberty restriction policy without constituting unjust discrimination. During the pandemic, people returning from high-risk areas were routinely required to quarantine on the basis of being at higher risk of infecting others. This is not discrimination against these people because the feature—return from a high-risk area—tracks a relevant feature associated with elevated risk of carrying COVID-19.

In a similar way, those who are at higher risk of becoming ill and placing pressure on the health system could be required to "shield" or selectively self-isolate. If the aim of a measure is to reduce disease burden, it may be acceptable to differentiate between people based on their risk as a relevant criterion. In the case of COVID-19, there was a clear correlation between age and risk of death. The risk of a 20–24-year-old dying as a result of an episode of infection with SARS-CoV-2 was estimated to be 4/100,000 or 0.004% (O'Driscoll et al. 2021), which is lower than the yearly risk of dying in a car accident in the United States (Levin et al. 2020). Considered in isolation, this risk does not warrant liberty-restricting measures. But the risk of a person over the age of 85 dying was estimated at 7%

(Levin et al. 2020). This is a significant risk of death that may warrant liberty-restricting measures. What the age-based mitigation strategy highlights is that it is not necessary to impose the same restrictions on the whole population in order to avoid this risk. Instead, measures may focus on preventing those most at risk from contracting the virus. This would mean restricting the liberty of those who face a 7% risk of death, but not those who face a 0.004% risk.

Restricting everyone's liberty to avoid the same risk is levelling-down equality (Savulescu and Cameron 2020). People at significant risk of death from a pandemic disease are likely to need to submit to liberty restrictions in order to avoid this risk, but this does not necessarily mean that everyone should be subjected to the same liberty restrictions. It is common for governments to impose liberty-restricting measures on particularly vulnerable groups for paternalistic reasons, but it is also preventing harm to others through use of limited hospital resources.

Implementing such measures every time a particular group was identified as posing a risk to others would significantly undermine equality. The issue is when such discrimination is justified.

As I have pointed out, the annual risk of dying in a car accident for someone under 30 is about the same as dying of an episode of COVID-19 (Schaefer et al. 2020). Now, the risk of other groups dying in car accidents is much higher: those who are drunk, abusing drugs, have epilepsy, or other underlying medical conditions, and the elderly. However, the response is not to ban all driving of cars because some groups have a higher chance of dying or being injured in a car accident. The response is to ban those at a *sufficiently* higher risk.

There is one obvious disanalogy between driving and COVID-19. In the case of driving, those at higher risk are both a higher risk to themselves and to others. This is not the case for most of the lower-risk age groups in relation to COVID-19—they are not at a significantly higher risk of harming themselves, but do put others at higher risk. On this basis, everyone's liberty should be restricted because everyone is at an elevated risk of harming others.

This is an important point, but there is a relevant response. In both COVID-19 and driving, there are two kinds of harm that may be caused. The first is the direct harm: colliding in a car or passing on the virus. The second is using limited health resources for hospital care following a not-immediately-fatal incident. Generally, we allow people to take risks that expose them to utilizing health resources. Healthcare is there to facilitate people realizing their plans of the good life, which may require driving a car. But, unlike driving, as I have pointed out, a pandemic is an extreme emergency. In such a situation, the state is entitled to restrict freedom to prevent overwhelming of the health system in order to ensure people can continue to access healthcare. This is not the case in ordinary driving, where no extreme emergency exists.

So while we don't normally take "use of limited health resources" to be a decisive factor in restricting liberty, in a pandemic I assert that it can sometimes be. And it is on this ground that those who are more at risk (the over-50s) present a kind of harm that others who are under 50 do not present (even if both present the same risk of spreading the virus). And it is on this ground that their liberty can be restricted, just as in the driving case. Age is different, in one way, to "drunk-driving". It is a characteristic of a person over which that person has no control or responsibility. It is also a characteristic that is protected by law (Equality Act, 2010), which prevents discrimination on the basis of age, sex, race, gender orientation, etc.

But being young also falls under "age". The young expect to gain far less from general liberty restriction than the old, and may lose a lot. This is to discriminate, in one way, against the young. An egalitarian application of liberty restriction should aim to distribute expected benefits and burdens equally or fairly across age groups.

8.9.3 Reinforcing Structural Injustice and Further Disadvantaging the Worst-Off

The argument outlined so far could be extended to justify selective restriction of liberty of those with other COVID-19 risk factors, such as those who are immunosuppressed, males, the obese, and certain ethnic groups. Gostin and Berkman argue that "in the exercise of compulsory powers, distributive justice requires a fair allocation so as not to burden unduly particularly vulnerable populations" (Gostin and Berkman 2007). One objection to a policy of selective restriction of liberty is that those at increased risk may be at increased risk as a result of pre-existing structural injustice. This is particularly the case for racial, ethnic minorities, those in lower socio-economic groups, and, to a lesser degree, the aged.

The flip side of this is that the most vulnerable, for example the aged, would be better off if there was blanket, rather than selective, liberty restriction. Prioritarianism, or giving priority to the worst-off, requires general liberty restriction.

There are several responses to these arguments.

Firstly, although it may be true that it is better for those who are vulnerable to COVID for there to be blanket restrictions, it is far from clear that it is better for other vulnerable people, e.g. those with cancer, for there to be a blanket restriction of liberty. And many of the most disadvantaged were hardest hit by the socio-economic and health effects of lockdowns (Palomino, Rodríguez, and Sebastian 2020).

Secondly, even if it were the case that it is better for the most vulnerable to have a blanket lockdown or other coercive policy, as I have argued before, we must ask whether it is worth the incremental utility compared to a selective approach. Indeed, although prioritarianism requires giving some priority to the worst-off, it doesn't require giving *absolute* priority. To take an extreme example, if moving from selective to blanket lockdown saved a hundred 85-year-old lives for one year, would it be worth 20,000 cases of severe depression, or £10 billion, or twenty suicides of young people, etc.? The issue of proportionality looms large.

8.9.4 Historically Wrong Discrimination and Symbolic Value of Equality

In discussions about quarantine and other coercive measures to limit the spread of an infectious disease, concern about past practices has encouraged a focus on equality. Fairchild et al. explain: "One way to understand the past approach to disease and containment is to read it in a story of blame and social division" (Fairchild, Gostin, and Bayer 2020). For example, the suspicion of a plague-related death in Chinatown in San Francisco in 1900 led to the evacuation of white residents, while Chinese residents were blockaded within the district (Fairchild, Gostin, and Bayer 2020). Such treatment is plainly wrong. People were treated differently on the basis of their ethnicity, even though this had no effect on the spread of the disease.

These historic wrongs have justifiably encouraged a focus on equality. For example, Selgelid (2009) argues that liberty-restricting measures must be used in an equitable manner. Selgelid suggests this may be achieved by avoiding applying such measures in a discriminatory manner against marginalized groups or by requiring that such measures are only used in a discriminatory manner when there is strong justification. This would recognize that some members of society require special protection. Viens et al. argue that if liberty-restricting measures are employed in a discriminatory fashion, this will violate a state's obligation not to discriminate and so is unjustifiable (Viens, Bensimon, and Upshur 2009). They suggest this is the case "even if restrictive measures are implemented in a way that makes them measurably successful overall in containing the contagion" (Viens, Bensimon, and Upshur 2009).

These broad statements appear to overstate the extent to which it is wrong to implement measures that treat people differently. Discrimination on the basis of a particular characteristic may be morally permissible when that characteristic correlates with a morally relevant difference. For example, during the COVID-19 pandemic, people living in the Australian state of Victoria faced significantly harsher restrictions on their movement than the rest of Australia (Victoria, Australia 2020a and 2020b). This was not unjust discrimination against Victorians but, rather, reflected the fact that the virus was more prevalent in the state, such that it was appropriate to differentiate on the basis of geographic location. If other states had experienced similar rates, similar restrictions would have been justified.

Differential treatment on the basis of relevant differences is not just permissible, but is necessary to achieve equitable outcomes. Universally applied social distancing measures during COVID-19 created a superficial equality, but the impact of the measures was 'profoundly unequal'.[8] Restrictions on when it is acceptable to leave home have a different impact on someone who has a stable home environment and has the option to work from home, compared with someone who has neither. Just as there are relevant differences in assessing the impact of liberty restrictions on particular groups, there are also relevant differences in assessing the risks of particular groups contracting the disease.

Nonetheless, segregating a group risks stigmatizing that group, sending the (wrong) message that some groups are less deserving of liberty than others. This is particularly egregious if applied to racial or ethnic minorities who have seen liberty unjustifiably restricted in the past. Some would argue that the symbolic value of equality is worth its costs. Indeed, returning to structural injustice, it is doubly egregious if a group's vulnerability is the result of past injustice and that group now experiences greater liberty restriction.

There are, as usual, possible responses to these objections. Firstly, measures should be taken to "send the right message" about why selective restriction of liberty is being employed and to promote the interests of those who lose their liberty in other ways, perhaps even through financial compensation.

Secondly, this may be a good argument against selective restriction of liberty of some racial groups. But age is different to race (and other risk factors, such as being male or obese). We will all be old one day, if we are lucky. This is a feature of all of our lives, generally. Yet we cannot change our race (unless one believes these categories are socially constructed). And even if we could change race, we would not all share the common feature of being in one racial group, in the way we do with older age. There may be reasons to treat some groups differently to others, and there may be a reason to treat age differently. The old have been young, but the young have not been old.

Elsewhere I have shown widespread support for the use of age in allocating ventilators and vaccines when these are limited resources (Wilkinson et al. 2020), and this has been demonstrated in other trade-off situations (Savulescu, Kahane, and Gyngell 2019). Indeed, giving a lower priority to age is supported by both utilitarianism and contractualism. From behind a veil of ignorance (where one does not know who in society one will be), it would be rational to prefer priority to be given to the young in allocation of life-saving resources because each of us would stand to live longer. There is weaker utilitarian or contractualist support for using other protected characteristics like sex or race (Savulescu, Gyngell, and Kahane 2021). Indeed, the public support for using such characteristics is much weaker than for using age (Kappes et al. 2022).

---

[8] European Institute for Gender Equality, EIGE-2021 Gender Equality Index 2021 Report: Health https://eige.europa.eu/publications/gender-equality-index-2021-report/covid-19-pandemic-aggravates-and-brings-forth-health-inequalities.

Another reason is that age is necessarily associated with some degree of vulnerability and that vulnerability is not entirely socially constructed. As we age, our body slowly deteriorates and dies. That is what makes the aged vulnerable. It will happen to all of us at some point if we live long enough. This is different to the vulnerabilities associated with race, ethnic minority, and lower socioeconomic class, which are in part, or large part, socially constructed.

So while concerns about the symbolic value of equality, expressivism, reinforcing past injustice, and disadvantaging the worst-off have some force, they apply less to age than to other risk factors.

8.9.5 Proportionality

The identification of higher-risk groups is not necessarily a sufficient basis to discriminate. It will always be possible to identify a particular group that is at higher risk from an infectious disease, and accepting liberty restrictions in each of these cases would significantly undermine equality. The issue is identifying when the difference is significant enough to warrant discrimination. This may be understood in terms of proportionality. When would discrimination be a proportionate response?

Human rights law recognizes that a human right may be limited when this would be proportionate. The tests developed under human rights law to determine whether the limitation of a right is proportionate may provide practical guidance in determining when a discriminatory measure is appropriate. Human rights instruments such as the European Convention on Human Rights recognize the right to equal enjoyment of human rights, including the right to freedom of movement, and so are relevant to discriminatory liberty-restricting measures.[9] There are a number of variations of the proportionality test, but the four-limb test developed in the UK is discussed here (Bjorge and Williams 2016; Ramshaw 2019).[10] This suggests that a measure will be proportionate if:

1. the objective was sufficiently important to justify limiting a fundamental right;
2. the measure designed to meet the objective was rationally connected to it;

---

[9] *Convention for the Protection of Human Rights and Fundamental Freedoms*, open for signature 4 November 1950, 213 UNTS 221 (entered into force 3 September 1953), articles 2 and 14. This is not intended to be a legal analysis of the application and discussion of proportionality tests applied under human rights law. As the concept of proportionality has been developed under human rights law and been the subject of significant debate, the test is discussed here to determine whether they may provide normative guidance for policymakers during a pandemic.

[10] *Bank Mellat v HM Treasury (No 2)* [2014] AC 7000, [20].

3. the means used to impair the right or freedom were no more than is necessary to accomplish the objective; and
4. the measure strikes a fair balance between the rights of the individual and the interests of the community.

If these tests are applied to the historic instances of discrimination discussed above (such as the Chinatown example), it is clear they would fail on the second and third limb. This is because there was no rational connection between ethnicity and those diseases and because it was no more necessary to restrict the liberty of these groups than others. However, this does not mean that it will never be proportionate to discriminate.

The measures proposed in the age-selective liberty restriction may be proportionate under this test. Limiting the number of deaths that occur during a pandemic may be sufficiently important to justify limiting the right to equality and so may fulfil the first limb. Under the second limb the disease modelling described previously demonstrates that there may be a rational connection between restricting the liberty of one group of people and limiting the negative impacts of a pandemic.

The application of the third limb raises a number of issues. If the objective is to limit morbidity and mortality, an age-selective restriction strategy is not strictly necessary, as there are a range of other options, such as non-selective strategies. But each of these options also has negative effects and conflicts with other moral concerns.

The fourth limb is the broadest and may create some ambiguity, as the relevant 'interests of the community' are undefined. In relation to the age-based mitigation strategy, this would achieve substantial benefits in reducing morbidity and mortality and preventing the health system from being overwhelmed.

The proportionality test may provide guidance about the acceptability of future discriminatory liberty-restricting measures. The measure may be acceptable if:

1. The objective is to limit the disease burden.
2. The measure is designed to prevent those who are most at risk from contracting the disease.
3. The liberty restrictions imposed must be no more than are necessary to limit exposure to the virus.
4. Liberty-restricting measures on high-risk groups would significantly reduce the utilization of limited health resources and the mortality rate of the disease, which would otherwise result in a large number of deaths.

This test recognizes the value of equality and that the issue should not be reduced to a question of health benefits versus liberty restrictions. It is important that each person is respected as an individual and that they are not arbitrarily discriminated against.

8.10 An Algorithm for Decision-Making

Below is an algorithm (Figure 8.4) which captures these considerations for determining when liberty-restricting measures may be acceptable. This recognizes that liberty-restricting measures should only be implemented when the threat posed is sufficiently grave, that the costs and benefits must be weighed at the community and individual level, and that discriminatory measures should only be imposed if they would be a proportionate response.

8.11 Conclusion

In this chapter I have not sought to decisively argue that selective restriction of liberty should have been employed in the COVID-19 pandemic. Rather, I have created a framework where selective restriction of liberty could be justified in a future Pandemic X. Whether it is, or not, will depend on the relevant empirical facts. There are no doubt other arguments (some based on intergenerational desert and justice arguments) that would support age-selective liberty restrictions, but in this chapter I have concentrated on when consequentialist considerations could justify selective restriction of personal liberty, particularly age-selective liberty restrictions. I have also considered the extension of such arguments to other at-risk groups, such as males, the immunosuppressed, the obese, and ethnic minorities. I did not consider the implications for those who were infected prior to vaccination, but the arguments presented here would justify selective restriction of liberty of the non-immune and immunity passports (Brown et al. 2020 and 2021).

In order to identify appropriate responses to a pandemic, governments should adopt a consequentialist approach with the aim of reducing the disease burden to an acceptable level of harm. What constitutes an acceptable level of harm will depend on a range of factors, including the morbidity/mortality impact of an unmitigated epidemic, the extent to which this harm could be reduced with selective measures, the extent to which the disease has spread already in a population, the political and geographic features that impact the ability to eliminate and prevent reintroduction of the virus, the harms of countermeasures, and the resources available to the government. Selective restriction of liberty is justified when the problem is grave, the expected utility of the liberty restriction is high and significantly greater than the alternatives, and the costs of the liberty restriction are relatively small at an individual level. That is, when the need for liberty restriction is considered an 'easy rescue'. Discrimination can be justified under

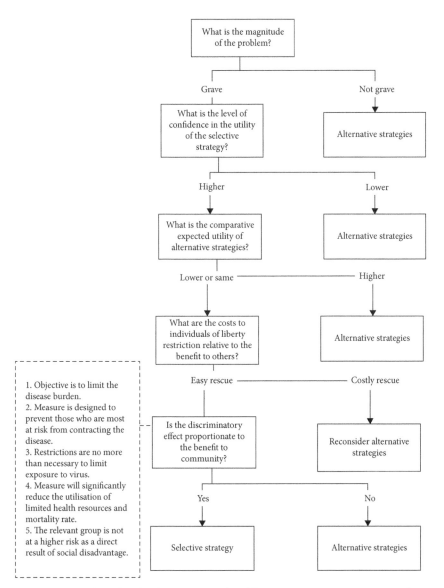

Figure 8.4 An algorithm for determining when liberty-restricting measures may be acceptable.

these conditions when it is proportionate and limited to a very specific public health challenge.

I have outlined easy rescue consequentialism as a basis for just liberty restriction in a pandemic and set the constraint of non-maleficence at a low level: only small costs should be imposed. However, the key is proportionality—in a very grave emergency large costs might be placed on individuals to bring about very large benefits, as the cartoon of the epidemic (Figure 8.2) illustrates. But COVID-19 is not an extremely grave emergency: Sweden (which imposed few liberty restrictions) found that in 2020, COVID-19 "caused life expectancy levels to revert back to those observed in 2018 for women and in 2017 for men", and, for further context, had experienced an unusually steep drop in mortality in 2019 (Kolk et al. 2022). However, if COVID-19 had been as lethal as Ebola, then much more significant liberty restrictions would have been justified.

What level of harm can be imposed on individuals for the sake of public health is a deep ethical, not scientific, question. We ought to begin with the least demanding requirement of easy rescue consequentialism: when the harm imposed on individuals is small, and the benefits to others are great, liberty should be restricted. This satisfies a constraint of non-maleficence.

This would have implications outside of pandemics. For example, it would justify opt-out or even mandatory blood or posthumous organ "donation". It would justify the use of data for research purposes for public health without consent. A collective duty of easy rescue would have significant implications for public policy generally.

In the Introduction to this volume, we considered a version of Pandemic X. It was H7N9 avian influenza with human-to-human spread (bird flu). It had high mortality in people in their twenties, like Spanish flu. Whose liberty should be restricted in such a pandemic through lockdown, quarantine, mandatory vaccination, or other coercive measures will be determined by how transmissible such a virus is, how much reduction in transmission is achieved by coercive measures, whether those who are vulnerable can be protected without liberty restriction of others, how likely an individual who contracts the virus is to require hospitalization, and the capacity of the health system. We require both ethics and science to decide whether liberty restriction should be general or selective.

Bibliography

Agency (UK Health Security) (2022). COVID-19 Vaccine Surveillance Report: Week 24, 16 June 2022.

Amante, Angelo, Giuseppe Fonte, and Gavin Jones (2022). 'Italy extends COVID vaccine mandate to everyone over 50', *Reuters*, 6 Jan. 2022.

Andre F. E., Booy R., Bock H. L., Clemens J., Datta S. K., John T. J., Lee B. W., Lolekha S., Peltola H., Ruff T. A., Santosham M., Schmitt H. J. (2008). 'Vaccination greatly reduces disease, disability, death and inequity worldwide', *Bulletin of the World Health Organization* 86(2): 140–6.

Bambery, Ben, Michael Selgelid, Hannah Maslen, Andrew J. Pollard, and Julian Savulescu (2013). 'The case for mandatory flu vaccination of children', *American Journal of Bioethics* 13(9): 38–40.

BBC News, (2020). 'Johnson orders UK to 'stay home' to protect NHS from coronavirus', 23 Mar. 2020.

Bioethics, Nuffield Council on (2007). 'Public health: Ethical issues', 13 Nov. 2007.

Bjorge, Eirik, and Jack R. Williams (2016). 'The protean principle of proportionality: How different Is proportionality in EU contexts?' *Cambridge Law Journal* 75(2): 186–9.

Brown, Rebecca C. H., Julian Savulescu, Bridget Williams, and Dominic Wilkinson (2020). 'Passport to freedom? Immunity passports for COVID-19', *Journal of Medical Ethics* 46(10): 652.

Brown, Rebecca C. H., Dominic Kelly, Dominic Wilkinson, and Julian Savulescu (2021). 'The scientific and ethical feasibility of immunity passports', *The Lancet Infectious Diseases* 2 (3): e58–e63.

Cameron, James, Bridget Williams, Romain Ragonnet, Ben Marais, James Trauer, and Julian Savulescu (2021). 'Ethics of selective restriction of liberty in a pandemic', *Journal of Medical Ethics* 47(8): 553–62.

Childress, James F., Ruth R. Faden, Ruth D. Gaare, Lawrence O. Gostin, Jeffrey Kahn, Richard J. Bonnie, Nancy E. Kass, Anna C. Mastroianni, Jonathan D. Moreno, and Phillip Nieburg (2002). 'Public health ethics: Mapping the terrain', *Journal of Law, Medicine & Ethics* 30(2): 170–8.

Christakis, Dimitri A., Wil Van Cleve, and Frederick J. Zimmerman (2020). 'Estimation of US children's educational attainment and years of life lost associated with primary school closures during the coronavirus disease 2019 pandemic', *JAMA Network Open* 3 (11): e2028786.

Di Blasi, Erica (2020). 'Italians over 80 'will be left to die' as country overwhelmed by coronavirus', *The Telegraph*, 14 Mar. 2020 (accessed 4 July 2022).

Fairchild, Amy, Lawrence Gostin, and Ronald Bayer (2020). 'Vexing, veiled, and inequitable: Social distancing and the 'rights' divide in the age of COVID-19', *American Journal of Bioethics* 20(7): 55–61.

Giubilini, Alberto, Thomas Douglas, Hannah Maslen, and Julian Savulescu (2018a). 'Quarantine, isolation and the duty of easy rescue in public health', *Developing World Bioethics* 18(2): 182–9.

Giubilini, Alberto, Thomas Douglas, and Julian Savulescu (2018b). 'The moral obligation to be vaccinated: utilitarianism, contractualism, and collective easy rescue', *Medical Health Care Philosophy* 21(4): 547–60.

Giubilini, Alberto, Julian Savulescu, and Margie Danchin (2022). 'Reply', *Journal of Pediatrics* 240: 319–20.

Global Influenza Programme (2019). 'Non-pharmaceutical public health measures for mitigating the risk and impact of epidemic and pandemic influenza, World Health Organization, 19 Sept. 2019.

Gostin, Lawrence O., and Benjamin E. Berkman (2007). 'Pandemic influenza: Ethics, law, and the public's health', *Georgetown Law Faculty Publications and Other Works* 449.

Guidance (GOV.UK) (2020). published 23 March 2020, https://www.gov.uk/government/publications/full-guidance-on-staying-at-home-and-away-from-others/ (accessed 5 July 2022).

Harris, John (1975). 'The survival lottery', *Philosophy* 50(191): 81–7.

Hellman, Deborah (2011). *When is Discrimination Wrong?* (Cambridge, MA: Harvard University Press).

Ives, Jonathan (2020). 'Coronavirus may force UK doctors to decide who they'll save', *The Guardian,* 11 Mar. 2020 (accessed 4 July 2022).

John, Stephen (2020). 'The ethics of lockdown: Communication, consequences, and the separateness of persons', *Kennedy Institute of Ethics Journal* 30(3): 265–89.

Joly, Josephine (2021). 'COVID in Europe: Greece begins fining those over 60 who are unvaccinated', *Euronews*.

Kappes, Andreas, Hazem Zohny, Julian Savulescu, Ilina Singh, Walter Sinnott-Armstrong, and Dominic Wilkinson (2022). 'Race and resource allocation: an online survey of US and UK adults' attitudes toward COVID-19 ventilator and vaccine distribution', *BMJ Open* 12: e062561.

Kass, Nancy (2001). 'An ethics framework for public health', *Public Health Matters* 91(11): 1776–82.

Koca-Atabey, Müjde (2021). 'Disability and old age: The COVID-19 pandemic in Turkey', *Disability & Society* 36(5): 834–9.

Kolk, Martin, Sven Drefahl, Matthew Wallace and Gunnar Andersson (2022). 'Excess mortality and COVID-19 in Sweden in 2020: A demographic account', *Vienna Yearbook of Population Research* 20(1): 1-32.

Lancaster, Chancellor of the Duchy of (2020). 'Lockdown was the only way to stop the NHS being broken', *The Times*, 28 Nov. 2020.

Levin, Andrew T., William P. Hanage, Nana Owusu-Boaitey, Kensington B. Cochran, Seamus P. Walsh, and Gideon Meyerowitz-Katz (2020). 'Assessing the age specificity of infection fatality rates for COVID-19: Systematic review, meta-analysis, and public policy implications', *European Journal of Epidemiology* 35(12): 1123–38.

Marsh, Sarah, and Denis Campbell (2020). 'Nurse shortage causes Nightingale hospital to turn away patients', *The Guardian*. https://www.theguardian.com/world/2020/apr/21/nurse-shortage-causes-nightingale-hospital-to-turn-away-patients.

Miles, David K., Michael Stedman, and Adrian H. Heald (2021). "Stay at Home, Protect the National Health Service, Save Lives': A cost benefit analysis of the lockdown in the United Kingdom', *International Journal of Clinical Practice* 75(3): e13674.

Mill, John Stuart (1859). *On Liberty* (London: John W. Parker & Son).

Nix, Hayden P. (2022). 'Canadian perspective on ageism and selective lockdown: a response to Savulescu and Cameron', *Journal of Medical Ethics* 48(4): 268.

O'Driscoll, Megan, Gabriel Ribeiro Dos Santos, Lin Wang, Derek A. T. Cummings, Andrew S. Azman, Juliette Paireau, Arnaud Fontanet, Simon Cauchemez, and

Henrik Salje (2021). 'Age-specific mortality and immunity patterns of SARS-CoV-2', *Nature* 590: 140–5.

Otsuka, Michael (1991). 'The paradox of group beneficence', *Philosophy and Public Affairs* 20(2): 132–149.

Palomino, Juan C., Juan G. Rodríguez, and Raquel Sebastian (2020). 'Wage inequality and poverty effects of lockdown and social distancing in Europe', *European Economics Review* 129: 103564.

Parfit, Derek (1984). *Reasons and Persons* (Oxford: Oxford University Press).

Pashakhanlou, Arash Heydarian (2021). 'Sweden's coronavirus strategy: The Public Health Agency and the sites of controversy', *World Medical Health Policy* 14(3): 507–27.

Ramshaw, Adam (2019). 'The case for replicable structured full proportionality analysis in all cases concerning fundamental rights', *Legal Studies* 39(1): 120–42.

Savulescu, Julian (2002). 'The embryonic stem cell lottery and the cannibalization of human beings', *Bioethics* 16(6): 508–29.

Savulescu, Julian (2013). 'Winchester Lectures: Kamm's trolleyology and is there a morally relevant difference between killing and letting die?' *Practical Ethics in the News*, 23 Oct. 2013.

Savulescu, Julian (2016). 'Concise argument—wellbeing, collective responsibility and ethical capitalism', *Journal of Medical Ethics* 42: 331–33.

Savulescu, Julian (2021). 'Good reasons to vaccinate: mandatory or payment for risk?' *Journal of Medical Ethics* 47(2): 78–85.

Savulescu, Julian, and James Cameron (2020). 'Why lockdown of the elderly is not ageist and why levelling down equality is wrong', *Journal of Medical Ethics* 46(11): 717.

Savulescu, J., C. Gyngell, and G. Kahane (2021). 'Collective Reflective Equilibrium in Practice (CREP) and controversial novel technologies', *Bioethics* 35(7): 652–63.

Savulescu, Julian, Guy Kahane, and Christopher Gyngell (2019). 'From public preferences to ethical policy', *Nature Human Behaviour* 3(12): 1241–3.

Scanlon, Tim (1998). *What We Owe to Each Other* (Cambridge, MA: Harvard University Press).

Schaefer, G. Owen, Clarence C. Tam, Julian Savulescu, and Teck Chuan Voo (2020). 'COVID-19 vaccine development: Time to consider SARS-CoV-2 challenge studies?' *Vaccine* 38(33): 5085–8.

Selgelid, Michael J. (2005). 'Ethics and infectious disease', *Bioethics* 19(3): 272–89.

Selgelid, Michael J. (2009). 'Pandethics', *Public Health* 123(3): 255–9.

Singer, Peter (1972). 'Famine, affluence, and morality', *Philosophy and Public Affairs* 1(3): 229–43.

TASS (2021). 'Twelve Russian regions introduce mandatory vaccination for residents over 60', *TASS Russian News Agency*, 11 Nov. 2021.

Upshur, R. E. G. (2002). 'Principles for the justification of public health intervention', *Canadian Journal of Public Health* 93(2): 101–3.

Verity, Robert, Lucy C. Okell, Ilaria Dorigatti, Peter Winskill, Charles Whittaker, Natsuko Imai, Gina Cuomo-Dannenburg, Hayley Thompson, Patrick G. T. Walker, Han Fu, Amy Dighe, Jamie T. Griffin, Marc Baguelin, Sangeeta Bhatia, Adhiratha Boonyasiri, Anne Cori, Zulma Cucunubá, Rich FitzJohn, Katy Gaythorpe, Will Green, Arran Hamlet, Wes Hinsley, Daniel Laydon, Gemma Nedjati-Gilani, Steven Riley, Sabine van Elsland, Erik Volz, Haowei Wang, Yuanrong Wang, Xiaoyue Xi, Christl A. Donnelly, Azra C. Ghani, and Neil M. Ferguson (2020). 'Estimates of the severity of coronavirus disease 2019: a model-based analysis', *The Lancet Infectious Diseases* 20(6): 669–77.

Verweij, Marcel (2005). 'Obligatory precautions against infection', *Bioethics* 19(4): 323–35.

Victoria (2020a). Stay at Home Directions (Non-Melbourne) (NO 4), Public Health and Wellbeing Act 2008 (VIC), section 200, (27 August 2020).

Victoria (2020b). Stay at Home Directions (Restricted Areas) (No 14). Public Health and Wellbeing Act 2008 (VIC), section 200, (27 August 2020).

Viens, Adrian M., Cécile M. Bensimon, and Ross E. G. Upshur (2009). 'Your liberty or your life: Reciprocity in the use of restrictive measures in contexts of contagion', *Journal of Bioethical Inquiry* 6: 207–17.

Wilder-Smith, Annelies (2022). 'What is the vaccine effect on reducing transmission in the context of the SARS-CoV-2 delta variant?' *The Lancet Infectious Diseases* 22(2): 152–3.

Wilkinson, Dominic, Hazem Zohny, Andreas Kappes, Walter Sinnott-Armstrong, and Julian Savulescu (2020). 'Which factors should be included in triage? An online survey of the attitudes of the UK general public to pandemic triage dilemmas', *BMJ Open* 10(12): e045593.

Williamson, Elizabeth J., Alex J. Walker, Krishnan Bhaskaran, Seb Bacon, Chris Bates, Caroline E. Morton, Helen J. Curtis, Amir Mehrkar, David Evans, Peter Inglesby, Jonathan Cockburn, Helen I. McDonald, Brian MacKenna, Laurie Tomlinson, Ian J. Douglas, Christopher T. Rentsch, Rohini Mathur, Angel Y. S. Wong, Richard Grieve, David Harrison, Harriet Forbes, Anna Schultze, Richard Croker, John Parry, Frank Hester, Sam Harper, Rafael Perera, Stephen J. W. Evans, Liam Smeeth, and Ben Goldacre (2020). 'Factors associated with COVID-19-related death using OpenSAFELY', *Nature* 584: 430–6.

Wolf, Susan (1982). 'Moral saints', *Journal of Philosophy* 79(8): 419–39.

PART III
BALANCING ETHICAL VALUES

9

How to Balance Lives and Livelihoods in a Pandemic

Matthew Adler, Richard Bradley, Maddalena Ferranna, Marc Fleurbaey, James Hammitt, Rémi Turquier, and Alex Voorhoeve

9.1 Introduction

Control measures, such as "lockdowns", have been widely used to suppress the COVID-19 pandemic. Under some conditions, they prevent illness and save lives. But they also exact an economic toll. How should we balance the impact of such policies on individual lives and livelihoods (and other dimensions of concern) to determine which is best? A widely used method of policy evaluation, benefit–cost analysis (BCA), answers these questions by converting all the effects of a policy into monetary equivalents and then summing them up. A different method, social welfare analysis, proceeds by determining the effects of a policy on individual wellbeing and then applying an aggregation formula to them to evaluate the overall effects of a policy. In this chapter, we survey these methods and argue that social welfare analysis has important advantages. One crucial advantage is that it enables ethical considerations relating to the impact of policies on individual wellbeing and its distribution to be incorporated into policy assessments in a transparent way. We illustrate this with a simple numerical model for evaluating pandemic policies that vary in terms of the stringency of the controls that they impose on individual behaviour, showing how the evaluation depends on the ethical significance accorded to their impact on the wellbeing of different age and income groups.

9.2 Benefit–Cost Analysis

Benefit–cost analysis of policies that seek to reduce the mortality risks imposed on individuals by a pandemic involves assigning a monetary value to the consequent reduction of the number of people that die. The monetary measure of the value of saving lives most widely used is the Value of a Statistical Life (VSL).

Matthew Adler, Richard Bradley, Maddalena Ferranna, Marc Fleurbaey, James Hammitt, Rémi Turquier, and Alex Voorhoeve, *How to Balance Lives and Livelihoods in a Pandemic* In: *Pandemic Ethics: From COVID-19 to Disease X*. Edited by: Dominic Wilkinson and Julian Savulescu, Oxford University Press. © Oxford University Press 2023. DOI: 10.1093/oso/9780192871688.003.0010

When the individuals whose lives would be saved are not known, each of the people at risk would be willing to pay some money to increase their chance of survival. VSLs describe the monetary values that individuals attribute to a reduction in their own mortality risk. To be precise, these monetary values are derived from the rate at which people are willing to trade off small changes in their income against small changes in their risk of death. This, in turn, is estimated from individuals' reported preferences or from those that they reveal in workplace and consumption behaviour, such as the choices they make amongst jobs involving different levels of risk or their purchases of risk-reducing equipment. For example, if someone would accept a pay cut of $1,000 per year to reduce their annual risk of mortality by 0.1% (but would not accept a larger pay cut), then we say that the monetary value of their statistical life is $1,000,000. Note that this is not the same as saying that they would be willing to accept $1,000,000 in return for certain death or would pay this amount to guarantee their survival. Rather, it means that each of 1,000 people, identical in all relevant ways, would, considering their self-interest alone, be willing to pay an equal share of a $1,000,000 cost for something that reduces the number of them expected to die in the year by one. In this simple example, in a binary choice between (a) implementing a policy that reduced the risk of death in a year for each of 1,000 people by 0.1% and (b) not undertaking any such risk reduction policy, benefit–cost analysis would recommend implementing the risk reduction policy if and only if the aggregated monetary cost of doing so was less than $1,000,000.

A person's VSL can depend on characteristics such as their age, their income and wealth, or the overall level of risk they face. This can have unacceptable consequences for evaluating policies. In particular, the fact that someone who is well off is likely to place a higher monetary value on risk reduction than someone who is less well off implies that if individual-specific VSLs are used in a benefit–cost analysis of policies, the interests of the well-off will count for more than those of the less-well-off (because the monetary value the better-off place on reducing their risk of death is higher).

By using a single VSL, such as the population average rather than individual-specific ones, this problem is avoided. But others are then created. In particular, it seems reasonable to treat people in different age groups differently when assessing policies. Death is commonly considered a more serious loss from the societal and ethical perspective when it occurs earlier in life. Reasoning in terms of life years preserved rather than lives saved appears to better take account of this widespread sentiment. The skewed age distribution of COVID-19 fatalities makes this problem especially pressing.

A common solution is to use a different measure for policy evaluation: the Value of a Statistical Life Year (VSLY). The VSLY is obtained by dividing the average VSL of the population by the average life expectancy remaining (an individual's current life expectancy remaining is the number of additional years she can be expected to live, if she doesn't die now). The value of saving the life of someone in any particular age cohort is then given by the product of the VSLY and the life expectancy remaining for the cohort. This yields a value of life saving that varies by age.

One criticism of both VSL and VSLY measures is that they do not take into account quality of life. Many people would not regard a year of life spent bedridden as equivalent to a year of life in excellent health, for instance. Quality-Adjusted Life Years (QALYs) are a way of allowing the value attributed to a life saved to depend on both its remaining length and its quality. The value of living in an impaired health state—say, with diminished lung function due to COVID-19—is derived from people's preferences. These preferences may be elicited in a number of ways. Individuals may simply be asked to assign a numerical value to life in a particular health state in comparison to both death and life in full health. Alternatively, they may be asked how they would balance a longer life in an impaired state against a shorter, healthier life, or asked what risk of death they would be willing to run in order to be fully cured of their impaired health. These preference-based assessments can be questioned (Hausman 2015). For example, there is evidence that healthy people are poor predictors of what life would be like in states of impaired health (Dolan and Kahneman 2008, Walasek et al. 2019). Nonetheless, even rough indicators of the quality of life in impaired health states can be better than measures that neglect quality altogether. This is particularly clear in the pandemic, in which it is important to take into account the effects of contracting the illness on those who do not die from it. For this reason, the use of QALYs in public health to determine resource allocation is widespread.

It is also controversial. One key concern is that, when it comes to life extension, the use of QALYs regards as more valuable the life years gained by people who would, if saved, be in good health than the life years gained by people who would, if saved, live with disabilities or in poor health, because extending the lives of the former would generate higher health-related quality of life (National Council on Disability 2019). Arguably, this objection is best addressed not by rejecting the use of QALYs but by assigning special value to improvements in the quality (and length) of life of those who are worse off (John, Millum, and Wasserman 2017).

Estimates of VSL and VSLY vary considerably between countries. Part of this variation is due to differences in income per capita. For example, Robinson et al. (2019) recommend estimating a VSL for a country by adjusting estimates for the USA for the difference in income, and a VSLY by dividing the VSL by the average remaining years of life. For the USA, the typical VSL is around $10,000,000, and the VSLY a little over $300,000 (see also Kniesner and Viscusi forthcoming). By way of illustration, for a country with per capita income of $10,000, a VSL of around $1,650,000 and a VSLY of around $50,000 are suggested by this approach. (These quantities are in international dollars, that is, corrected for differences in purchasing power between different countries.)

A similar variation is observed in the monetary costs that public actors regard as reasonable to incur to gain one QALY. One approach is to estimate the value of a QALY by dividing the VSL by the average remaining QALYs (Hirth et al. 2000). This produces values modestly larger than the VSLY. By contrast, the World Health Organization (WHO) has suggested that interventions that generate a QALY for less than 1 times per capita income are good value for money and that interventions that generate a QALY for up to 3 times per capita income may be worth the cost (Bertram et al. 2016). These values are much smaller. The ranking of policies to deal with the pandemic based on benefit–cost analysis may well depend on which values are adopted. It is therefore critical that attention be given to the justification of any particular choice.

9.3 Social Welfare Analysis

An alternative approach to BCA, social welfare analysis, proceeds by measuring the joint health and economic impact of policies on individual wellbeing and then aggregating individual wellbeing gains and losses to yield an overall measure of how beneficial a policy is. This method has a singular advantage over BCA. Unlike population-average VSLs, the individual-specific wellbeing values that social welfare analysis uses are sensitive to individuals' characteristics, such as their age and income. And while the individual-specific VSLs, VSLYs, and values of QALYs of the well-off are inflated, relative to those of less well-off individuals, by the fact that money has relatively lower marginal value for the well-off, this is not true of individual wellbeing or social welfare values. So, the aforementioned bias in favour of the well-off that the use of individual-specific monetary values introduces into BCA does not plague social welfare analysis.

There are three basic elements to any social welfare analysis of a policy: (1) a measure of the level of wellbeing associated with different possible lives, determined by bundles of the goods that matter to individuals—income, health, longevity, and so on; (2) a representation of the effects of the policy in question on the wellbeing so measured of different individuals at different times; and (3) an assignment of a value to the policy on the basis of these effects (the social welfare function).

Many different methods are used to obtain an interpersonally comparable measure of wellbeing (for a comprehensive review, see Adler and Fleurbaey 2016). Subjective wellbeing approaches draw on individuals' reports of their mental and emotional state to identify their current wellbeing or on lifetime satisfaction scores to identify the determinants of their wellbeing (Clark et al. 2018). Preference-based approaches derive a wellbeing measure from individuals' preferences, on the basis of an ethically grounded normalization of levels of satisfaction. One such approach (Adler 2019) relies on preferences between probability distributions (lotteries) over alternative possible lives, normalizing wellbeing to equal zero and one at two benchmark lives. The equivalent income approach, by contrast, uses income or wealth, corrected for the value of non-market aspects of life, such as longevity, on the basis of individuals' preferences over these aspects (Fleurbaey and Blanchet 2013). Finally, in the capability approach, wellbeing is associated with the attainment of functionings—states and activities recognized to be of value—and with the opportunities to achieve them (Sen 1999).

In social welfare analysis, a policy is modelled as a probability distribution over the comprehensive wellbeing outcomes that it induces. A reduction in a risk to an individual brought about by a policy will be marked by the increase in the expected lifespan (longevity) of the individuals and, taking into account the costs associated with it, the probability of achieving different levels of wellbeing in the future (relative to not enacting the policy). Policies then have to be evaluated against these effects across the entire population. The effect of a policy that reduces the risk of contracting COVID-19 by some percentage and at some financial cost, for instance, can be modelled by the shift in the probability distribution of population wellbeing levels generated by the bundles of longevity, health, and income mentioned above. Since this shift captures not just the impact of the policy on individuals' longevity and health but also how these factors, together with income, co-determine changes in individuals' wellbeing, it provides all the information required for a comprehensive analysis of the overall effects of implementing the policy.

To determine these effects of a policy, social welfare analysis proceeds by aggregating the set of individual wellbeing values achieved by implementing this policy. It does so by means of a social welfare function (SWF) that assigns to each distribution of individual wellbeing a measure of social value. A commonly used SWF is the utilitarian one, which assigns to each set of individual wellbeing values the total (or the average) of the values. This way of aggregating individuals' wellbeing allows for sensitivity to inequalities in the population in the distribution of the bundle of goods determining individuals' wellbeing, but it is insensitive to inequalities in the distribution of wellbeing itself. In other words, it is indifferent to whether a given increment in wellbeing accrues to a well-off or a badly off person. In this respect, it is in tension with the common conception that policymakers should be inequality-averse, i.e. should favour policies that, *ceteris paribus*, result in less unequal distributions of wellbeing.

This limitation can be addressed by using distribution-sensitive SWFs that prefer policies that produce more equal distributions over those that produce more unequal ones. Different kinds of such SWFs reflect different moral views about what is at stake. Egalitarian SWFs commonly care about both inequality and total wellbeing. On these SWFs, a gain to a worse-off person is especially valuable because it reduces inequality (Atkinson 1970). Prioritarian SWFs, in contrast, treat a given improvement in the wellbeing of the worse-off as mattering more than the same improvement to the well-off, *not* because this reduces inequality but on the grounds that the former improves a person's wellbeing from a lower absolute level (Adler 2019). In numerical implementations, the two approaches often involve the same functional forms, especially the additive function popularized by Atkinson (1970). Because of this commonality in functional form (despite the difference in rationale), the literature often follows Atkinson (1970) in using the terms "inequality aversion" and "priority for the worse off" interchangeably. We do so here too.

SWFs that show special concern for the worse-off are divided on the question of whether, in circumstances in which policy outcomes are uncertain, what matters is the expected social value of the distribution of wellbeing that individuals will end up with once a policy has been implemented (the *ex post* approach) or the social value of the individuals' *expected* wellbeing levels associated with the policy (the *ex ante* approach).[1]

The choice of SWF is fundamentally an ethical one, as it requires balancing the wellbeing losses and gains of (classes) individuals with different characteristics. It is important to note that the implications of a choice of SWF for aggregating wellbeing also depends on the underlying measure of wellbeing, so such ethical evaluation has to include all aspects of the analysis. In our opinion, this is a second important advantage of social welfare analysis: it allows for unavoidable ethical choices to be made much more explicitly and transparently than does BCA.

To illustrate how social welfare analysis can be applied to the assessment of policy responses to the pandemic, we develop a numerical model which allows us to explore in some detail the impact on different age groups of various policy responses to the pandemic and the sensitivity of the assessment of policies to the disvalue attached to inequalities. In developing the model, one very important simplifying assumption is that we assume away any uncertainty about pandemic parameters (e.g. emerging variants of the virus, or the effectiveness of lockdowns on the spread of disease) that policymakers actually face. One further important limitation of our numerical analyses is that policy parameters are assumed to remain constant throughout the pandemic, whereas in practice adjustment of these parameters depending on the state of immunization of the population is likely to be recommended.

We also make two important ethical choices. Firstly, we adopt an *ex post* approach, that is, we focus on the anonymized final distribution of individual

---

[1] To illustrate the difference, consider a simple case in which two individuals, Ann and Bea, face death unless they are offered a vaccine, which would ensure they live in full health for a normal lifespan. Unfortunately, only one vaccine dose is available. Suppose that death would be equally bad for Ann and Bea, and Ann's wellbeing if vaccinated would be equal to Bea's wellbeing if she were vaccinated instead. Suppose we can either give the vaccine to Ann outright or instead flip a fair coin. An *ex post* approach would be concerned solely with how individuals end up. Hence, it would be indifferent to these two distribution methods (supposing that the method itself had no effects on Ann and Bea's final wellbeing). In contrast, an *ex ante* approach that was concerned with improving the prospects of those with worse prospects would strictly prefer the coin flip.

wellbeing. In doing so, we rely on the fact that when the pandemic's parameters are given, there is no uncertainty about this distribution. Secondly, we follow the "equivalent income" approach in using a monetary measure of lifetime wellbeing. This approach measures an individual's actual lifetime wellbeing by the annual income they would require in a benchmark situation with a guaranteed longevity of a hundred years in good health, in order to be as well off in their own estimation as they currently are. (For example, suppose that Charles would after careful deliberation be indifferent between his actual situation, in which he will live in good health and with an annual income of $70,000 until the age of 65, at which point he will die, and a hypothetical situation in which he lives in good health until the benchmark age of 100 with an annual income of $40,000. Then his equivalent income is $40,000.) This measure of wellbeing mimics BCA when social welfare is simply the sum of equivalent incomes, i.e. when inequality aversion in equivalent income is zero in the social welfare function, but departs from it when the social welfare function incorporates a special concern for the less-well-off. Jointly, these choices imply that the modelled inequality aversion reflects a concern with the inequalities in equivalent income that in fact arise from the implementation of a policy (once uncertainty has been resolved). Other preference-based measures of wellbeing (as in Ferranna et al. 2022) incorporate diminishing marginal value of income at the individual level, so that social welfare analysis with such measures is very similar to social welfare analysis with equivalent incomes and greater inequality aversion. For instance, utilitarianism in Ferranna et al. (2022) corresponds to a form of prioritarianism over equivalent incomes. The conclusions that we draw about the implications of different SWFs (in particular, the contrast between results obtained for various degrees of inequality aversion) need to be understood with this in mind. Evidently, the exercise could be done with different choices and with potentially different conclusions. Since our analysis here is not meant to provide policy prescriptions but rather to illustrate the proposed approach to policy evaluation based on a social welfare function rather than VSL, we will here review the sensitivity of policy evaluation only for a limited range of value judgments *within* the *ex post*, equivalent income framework. However, one lesson we emphasize is that policy evaluation should also involve an analysis of the robustness of conclusions with respect to variations in these aspects of the framework, e.g. to a different choice of wellbeing measure.

9.4 Evaluating Policies: a Numerical Illustration

The model we develop here draws on the prior work of Ferranna et al. (2022) and Adler et al. (2020). The former makes a comparison of three approaches to policy evaluation in the context of the pandemic: benefit–cost analysis, utilitarianism, and prioritarianism. They simulate a scenario without any policy intervention and compute the cost that society would be willing to bear to completely avoid the pandemic as depicted in this scenario. The larger this willingness to pay, the more willing the policymaker should be to implement stringent control policies to suppress the pandemic. In order to evaluate effects on inequalities, they introduce two age groups (young and old) and five income groups (quintiles) and assume that the COVID-19 mortality risk increases with age and decreases with income. They show, in particular, that BCA implies a greater social willingness to pay to avoid the pandemic, because the other two approaches are sensitive to inequalities (inequalities in income for utilitarianism, inequalities in wellbeing for prioritarianism) and because pandemic suppression policies would impose costs on low-income groups which loom large in social welfare. They observe that, among the worst-off groups (i.e. the young and poor who die prematurely), the *ex post* distribution of welfare pits the potential victims of the pandemic who would survive due to pandemic suppression against those who would not benefit from suppression and would die whether or not suppression was practised (from COVID-19 or other causes). They note that, perhaps surprisingly, a strong priority to the worse-off may reduce the social willingness to pay to avoid the health impacts of the pandemic, since the very-worst-off—the people who would die at a relatively young age during the pandemic of other causes or of the pandemic despite any measures to control it—would bear the cost of such a policy (i.e. a loss of income due to lockdown) without reaping any benefit. However, they also observe that, independently of the value framework, a redistribution of the policy costs towards the richer (e.g. through the implementation of unemployment benefits and other COVID-19-related public transfers) increases the social willingness to pay to avoid the pandemic. One message of their analysis is that concern for the less-well-off can motivate strong support for suppression policies when the costs of these policies on the incomes of the poorest are substantially mitigated but may not do so otherwise.

The exercise in Ferranna et al. (2022) highlights the importance of both inequalities and ethical evaluation of these inequalities in the evaluation of COVID-19 control policies. In particular, it points to a careful consideration of the cost side of the policies, and the identification of which individuals are likely to experience larger net benefits from the policy. However, the framework is too simple to allow inferences about the ideal policy to control the pandemic. For example, should we aim at a strict control policy that completely suppresses the pandemic or at a laxer policy that mitigates the consequences of the pandemic without completely suppressing it? In addition, even though the willingness to pay to avoid the pandemic decreases with the degree of priority to the worst-off, this willingness to pay might still be higher than the willingness to pay to mitigate the pandemic without suppressing it. In other words, the framework in Ferranna et al. (2022) is not informative about the ranking of alternative COVID-19 control policies. Nor does it permit us to explore how that ranking varies according to the adopted value framework.

Here we expand their numerical model in two directions. First, we examine a range of policy parameters through scenarios of policy interventions taking the form of repeated lockdowns. We focus on two policy dimensions that would be involved in such a policy. The first is the reduction of contacts through lockdowns. This reflects how "tight" the lockdowns are, e.g. the number of businesses and individuals that are affected, or the extent of indoor capacity restrictions (e.g. the number of people allowed in a restaurant). The second policy dimension involves the strictness of the thresholds of the impact on population health for triggering (and then eventually ending) lockdown episodes. We assume that the occupancy rate of intensive care units (ICUs) would be used to determine when to start and end a lockdown, with a higher threshold for the start of a lockdown and a lower one for ending it. The population is more often under a lockdown when these thresholds are lower. We can then compare the outcomes of policies that are more or less stringent in terms of both the tightness of lockdowns and the strictness of the trigger thresholds.

The second direction in which the illustration is extended beyond Ferranna et al. (2022) concerns the description of inequalities. We introduce eight age groups (rather than two) and attempt to compute their lifetime wellbeing in a way that takes account of macroeconomic growth and the usual profile of income through the life cycle. This may be quite an important matter in order to analyse the relative priority of different age-income groups in the pandemic context. Indeed, a suppression policy is generally thought to oppose the self-interest of younger groups who suffer from income losses in the economy to the self-interest of the elderly, who are much more vulnerable to COVID-19 and who stand to benefit much more from the health effects of the policy. However, the picture may actually be more complex. First, the young victims of COVID-19, even if their numbers are small, lose a lot because their premature death deprives them of many more years of life than the older individuals. Second, past and (likely) future economic growth implies that the lifetime living standard of the young cohorts is (likely to be) much higher than the older cohorts' living standards.

As in Ferranna et al. (2022), the US population is used to simulate the various scenarios. The model of the pandemic is similar to their model as well as the model in Adler et al. (2020), with a few changes.[2] Contagion through contacts is modelled with a variant of the susceptible-infected-recovered (SIR) model, which takes account of the fact that at high levels of infection the contagion is less than

[2] Details of the model and the dataset construction are available from the authors. We thank Siméon Campos for help in building the data set.

proportional to the number of infected people,[3] and that people spontaneously reduce their contacts when contaminations rise. The economic slowdown is assumed to be directly proportional to the reduction in contacts (which is partly spontaneous and is reinforced by lockdown measures). Lifetime wellbeing is computed on the basis of past growth rates for previous periods, and a growth rate of 2% per year in real income is assumed for the remainder of the century. The pandemic is assumed to fade out after two years and policy is thus tested only over this time span (2020–1). The infection rate and infection-fatality rate are kept at levels estimated for the initial variants of the COVID-19 virus. Some simulations for a milder but more contagious virus like the Omicron variant are presented at the end of this section.

In the simulations, a permanent testing policy is assumed to be implemented throughout the period, in which symptomatic people are tested and isolated if positive, with the accuracy of the testing process assumed to be 70%.[4] The contact reduction due to lockdown that we consider ranges from 50% to 90% and refers to the number of people that anyone meets, not to the frequency of going out.[5] Regarding the lockdown trigger threshold, we will restrict attention to two policies. Our "strict" policy triggers a lockdown when 30% of ICU capacity is occupied by those ill with COVID-19 and ends it when this level of occupancy falls to 20%. Our "lax" policy has a starting threshold of 70% of ICU capacity being so occupied, and a stopping threshold of 60%.

Individuals are divided into different age-income-longevity groups depending on their current age, their income group,[6] and the longevity they ultimately realize. As we take an *ex post* approach to policy evaluation, what matters is the realized longevity of individuals, not their life expectancy. Thus, a 60-year-old individual in the lowest income group who dies at age 70 ends up in a different category, for social welfare, than a 60-year-old individual in the lowest income group who dies at age 80. Individual lifetime wellbeing is computed as the undiscounted sum of a power utility function including an additive term representing a critical level of income below which utility is negative.[7] As already explained,

---

[3] This is because the probability of avoiding becoming infected is the product of the probabilities, for each contact with another person, of not becoming infected as a result of the contact. This product is not linear in the proportion of infected people.

[4] This includes the precision of the test and the compliance with the testing request for symptomatic people.

[5] This means that no specific assumption is made about the technology of contacts (quadratic or otherwise). When people go out to meet other people in a public place, reducing the frequency of going out by half divides the number of people anyone meets by four, a quadratic relation. In contrast, when people go out to meet specific people, cutting visits by half reduces contacts by half, a linear relation. Our modelling parameter is the number of contacts, not the frequency of going out.

[6] We assume that there is no social mobility, i.e. individuals remain in the same income group throughout their entire life (although income increases over time).

[7] Specifically, the per-period (one year) utility is $u(c) = \dfrac{c^{1-\gamma}}{1-\gamma} - \dfrac{c_0^{1-\gamma}}{1-\gamma}$, where $\gamma = 1.25$ and $c_0 = \$1,000$. The parameter γ is taken from Becker et al. (2005), but c_0 is taken to be greater than their \$353 value, which is very low for the USA.

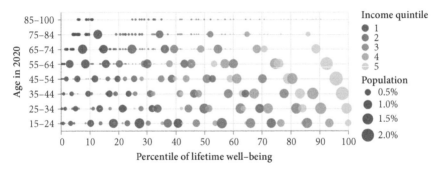

Figure 9.1 Distribution of the various age-income-longevity groups. Note: Each bullet represents an age-income-longevity group. Grey hues depict the income quintile to which the group belongs. Bullet sizes reflects the size of the group in percentage of the total population. For each age group, the rightward spread of bullets of the same shade of grey reveals the overall wellbeing induced by greater longevity within an income group. (For example, among the 15–24-year-olds in the lowest income quintile—the dark grey bullets along the bottom horizontal line—the shortest-lived will be in the lowest centile of lifetime wellbeing, and the longest-lived in the 40th centile.) This graph is made under a stringent policy.

wellbeing is measured not in "utils" but in money-metric terms as the annual income that, received every year over a 100-year lifetime, would yield the same lifetime utility as the contemplated income-longevity profile of any individual. This measuring rod (equivalent income) yields the same ranking of wellbeing in different age-income-longevity groups as the common utility function.

The inequalities in the population can be described in terms of where the different age-income-longevity groups are spread over the distribution of lifetime wellbeing (Figure 9.1). To focus on one group in particular: the elderly appear everywhere in the distribution, including among the most disadvantaged, but neither at the very bottom nor at the very top. This is due to the fact that they enjoy the benefit of longevity, but their life has been spent mostly in poorer times.

Let us first briefly review the macro-scale health and economic consequences of a suppression policy, for the different policy parameter values. Figure 9.2 depicts the total number of deaths over the two years of the pandemic as a function of how tight the lockdown is in terms of percentage of contact reduction (x-axis) and of its ICU thresholds (different lines for the "strict" 30%–20% start–stop thresholds and the "lax" 70%–60% thresholds). Three main observations can be made. First, by and large, a more stringent policy (tighter and more readily triggered lockdowns) reduces fatalities. Second, there are exceptions for the tightness of lockdown, because, for example, an 80% reduction in contacts, compared to 60%, may crush a first wave more effectively but also keep the population more vulnerable to a second wave (see the dashed line). Third, there are complementarities between tightness and more readily triggered lockdowns, as the more readily triggered lockdowns reduce fatalities more markedly when they are tighter.

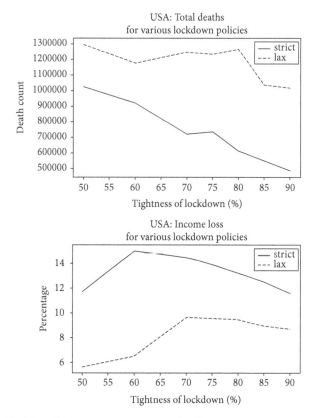

Figure 9.2 Health and income consequences of policy parameters.

In Figure 9.2, the lower panel shows an interesting inverse U-shape for the economic impact. While a minimally restrictive policy (relatively loose lockdown and lax triggering thresholds, i.e. the dashed line bottom left) implies moderate costs (which occur mostly due to spontaneous reduction in contacts and economic activity undertaken by people), a very restrictive policy (in particular, tightening lockdowns when they occur) can also moderate the economic costs by enabling economic activity to restart after very substantially suppressing the pandemic. Together, the two graphs suggest that middle-of-the-road policies (e.g. relatively loose lockdowns) may be particularly ineffective, as they fail to produce good health outcomes and nevertheless induce the highest economic costs.

How do these patterns of health and income effects combine to determine social welfare when inequalities are taken into account? Figure 9.3 shows social welfare levels for the same policies as the previous figure, but under different degrees of priority to the less-well-off (inequality aversion), with a moderate degree of priority modelled in the upper panel, and a larger degree modelled in the lower panel.

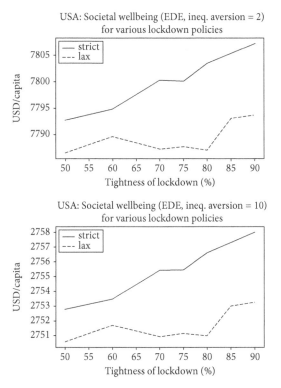

Figure 9.3 Social welfare impact of various policies. Note: Social welfare is measured here as the equally-distributed equivalent (EDE) of the distribution of wellbeing. The EDE is the level of wellbeing that, if equally enjoyed by all the population, would yield the same level of social welfare as the contemplated situation. A degree of inequality aversion equal to x means that increasing the level of wellbeing of a person who is half as well off as another is 2^x times more valuable.

Comparing Figure 9.3 to Figure 9.2 reveals that health outcomes loom large in our social welfare analysis. A stricter policy for triggering lockdowns generates higher social welfare because the health gains outweigh the losses in income. Together with the fact that both lines reach their highest point when lockdowns are at their most tight (in terms of contact limitation) this indicates that, despite being relatively more expensive, the most stringent policies prevent sufficiently more deaths to make them more beneficial from a societal point of view. We note, however, that in line with the results reported in Figure 9.2, if a laxer threshold for triggering lockdown is used, as indicated by the lower, dashed line, then tightening lockdowns from low to moderate is not, on balance, advantageous, because over time it does little to lower deaths, but it does have higher economic costs.

It is noteworthy that the social welfare analysis of policies in our model is not very sensitive to changes in the degree of priority for the worse-off (i.e. the degree of inequality aversion). Indeed, the ranking of policies seems barely affected by the coefficient of inequality aversion. It is interesting to compare this finding to that of Ferranna et al. (2022).[8] They find that an increase in inequality aversion reduces somewhat society's maximum willingness to pay to eliminate the pandemic. For example, in a scenario with a regressive distribution of both the deaths from COVID-19 and the costs of lockdown, they find that a utilitarian SWF (zero inequality aversion) is willing to incur up to a 15% reduction in GDP to avoid the loss in health induced by the pandemic, while a prioritarian SWF with inequality aversion equal to 2 is willing to incur no more than an 11% reduction.[9] The differing effects of inequality aversion as between the current exercise and Ferranna et al. (2022) are not, on reflection, very surprising. Ferranna et al. (2022) seek to identify a precise cut-off value: the maximum GDP reduction that is no worse than an uncontrolled pandemic. By contrast, Figure 9.3 shows the ranking of lax versus strict lockdown triggers for different levels of lockdown tightness. While increasing inequality aversion does change (somewhat) the Ferranna et al. (2022) cut-off, it does not change the ordinal ranking of the different types of policies. Another difference is that Ferranna et al. (2022) ignore the influence of income growth over a lifetime, which this chapter does take into account. As a consequence, in Ferranna et al. (2022) older individuals represent a greater share of the better-off than they do in our chapter, which has a greater share of the elderly among the less-well-off because they experienced poverty when they were young. Because in our analysis a more substantial share of the older population is ranked low in the distribution of lifetime wellbeing, the benefit of reducing their mortality looms larger. This comparative finding therefore brings home the importance of the choice of lifetime wellbeing as a metric of concern, as well as of taking full account of the hardships endured by older generations when incomes were much lower than they are now.

We can now compare these results with what would be obtained with a more conventional benefit–cost analysis based on the value of a statistical life (VSL), multiplied by the number of COVID-19 fatalities to assess the total value of health loss, and also adding up the total loss of income over the two years. The results are depicted in the upper panel of Figure 9.4. As should be expected, the analysis yields similar results as the social welfare analysis with zero inequality aversion over equivalent incomes. (The latter is not shown here, but the shape of

---

[8]   In making such comparison, one must account for the fact that they employ a somewhat different metric of individual wellbeing, on which equivalent income (which is our metric) has diminishing marginal wellbeing impact. But, fortunately, our study and Ferranna et al. (2022) are fully comparable if one relates a coefficient of inequality aversion of x in this chapter with a coefficient of $x+1.25$ in Ferranna et al. (2022).

[9]   To be precise, Ferranna et al. (2022) find an 11.1% maximum GDP reduction for ex post prioritarianism, and a 10.6% maximum GDP reduction for ex ante prioritarianism. Recall that utilitarianism (resp., prioritarianism) in Ferranna et al. (2022) corresponds to inequality aversion around 1.25 (resp., 3.25) over equivalent incomes.

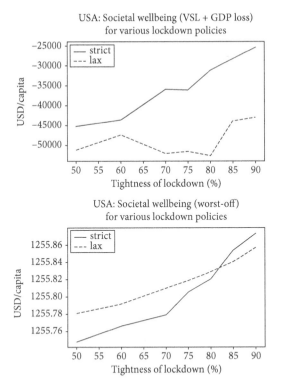

Figure 9.4 Cost-benefit analysis of policy options, based on VSL (left) or the worst-off (right).

the graphs is virtually identical and displays a similar pattern to the upper panel in Figure 9.3.)

Going to the other extreme of inequality aversion, the lower panel of Figure 9.4 displays an evaluation based on the situation of the very-worst-off in the population, i.e. the youngest who die at the end of the first year of the pandemic. Their situation is determined solely by the economic costs in the first year, since, *ex post*, they do not benefit from the reduction in mortality rates. The curves are thus quite different, making strict trigger thresholds appear undesirable for moderate tightness levels of lockdown. Nonetheless, making lockdowns tighter is always preferable in the model. This is because tightening them when they do occur means they can last less long, which generates economic benefits for the worse-off.

There remains an interesting question about how the net benefits and burdens of policies are distributed among the young and old as well as among the poor and the rich, and extent to which their interests align. To investigate it, one can compute the average level of equivalent income for age-income groups under different policies. This averaging operation ignores the *ex post* inequalities induced by the random distribution of sickness and death across the population during the pandemic and focuses on the average wellbeing offered by the policies to these various age-income groups. Consider three policies: a lenient policy (with lockdown bringing a mere 50% contact reduction and start–stop thresholds for lockdowns of 70% and 60% of ICU capacity, respectively), a middling policy (70% contact reduction during lockdown, with start–stop thresholds of 50% and 40%), and a stringent policy (90% contact reduction during lockdown and thresholds of 30% and 20%).

Figure 9.5 depicts who gains or loses (negative signs in cells mark losing sub-groups, all others gain) and the relative gain or loss in average equivalent income (grey hues) for each group, when moving from the lenient to the middling policy in the left panel, and from the middling to the stringent policy in the right panel. It shows that the younger and poorer groups suffer from the implementation of a middling policy compared to a lenient policy, which confirms the widespread perception in many countries in which a middle-of-the-road policy has been implemented. In contrast, all groups gain when moving from a middling to a stringent policy. In both cases, the relative gains are concentrated among the rich elderly (right-hand panel, darker squares indicate concentrated gains).

These results are obtained under the assumption that the distribution of fatalities and economic costs is unfair, with fatality rates and the ratio of economic costs to income being lower for richer groups.[10] If measures were taken to guarantee that fatality rates from the pandemic were independent of income and

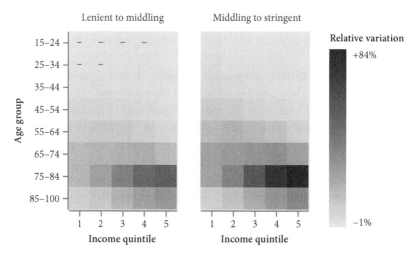

Figure 9.5 Gains and losses from lockdown policy for the various age-income groups.

[10] To be precise: fatality rates are assumed to be inversely proportional to the square root of income, and costs are assumed to be proportional to the square root of income.

costs were distributed in a progressive fashion, then the gains of policy would be even more concentrated on the rich, because they would benefit more from health outcomes in both moves, and more from the improvement in economic outcomes when moving from middling to stringent policies, due to their greater share in the benefit of a reduced macroeconomic cost. However, only the very youngest and poorest group would lose when moving from the lenient to the middling policy.

Finally, we briefly examine how policies compare under a pandemic which is more like the Omicron variant, i.e. with three-times greater contagion rate and three-times lower infection-fatality and hospitalization rates, and with a contagion rate for recovered patients that is no longer zero but similar to the contagion rate of the initial virus for susceptible patients. This makes for a quicker succession of waves over the considered time horizon (two years), with a greater number of total fatalities due to many more cases. Figure 9.6 shows the main results, which still display a preference for tighter lockdowns but no longer so clearly for more stringent ICU thresholds, especially when high priority is put on the worse-off populations. (Importantly, these results should not be considered directly relevant to the case of a late variant that, like Omicron, emerges after a significant proportion of the population has been immunized or has antibodies from earlier variants; they merely illustrate how trade-offs depend on some key non-policy parameters of pandemics.)

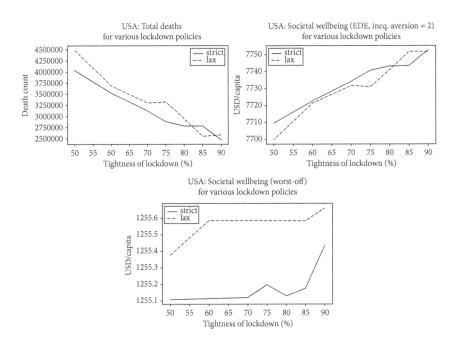

Figure 9.6 Policy evaluation under a pandemic that is like Omicron from the start.

9.5 Conclusion

Roughly speaking, the COVID-19 crisis involves a trade-off between lives and livelihoods. Lockdown or other control measures to limit the uncontrolled spread of the virus reduce deaths, but they come with an economic cost. This statement is imprecise in three ways, however. First, a laissez-faire policy of doing nothing to combat the pandemic may itself have net economic costs, relative to some control policy, insofar as laissez-faire induces individuals to reduce their risks via uncoordinated efforts at social isolation, with consequent economic costs.

Second, governments have many options to combat a pandemic other than the extreme options of laissez-faire and a maximally stringent lockdown. It is quite possible that a given policy intervention P^* is actually a "win/win" relative to another policy intervention P: that P^* not only reduces deaths relative to P but also reduces economic costs. This possibility is demonstrated by our numerical illustration. A policy of implementing a tight lockdown under a sufficiently strict ICU threshold leads not only to fewer deaths but also to lower costs, relative to a policy of a moderately contact-reducing lockdown for the same threshold (see Figure 9.2).

Third, the impact of policies on individuals' fatality rates and incomes, and the overall effect on individuals' wellbeing, may well differ for different population groups. For example, Figure 9.5 shows that younger and poorer individuals lose on balance in moving from a lenient policy to a middling policy, while other groups benefit.

One general lesson is therefore that evaluating pandemic policies requires careful efforts to model the effect of policies on different groups. Of course, such modelling is itself costly and yields uncertain results, but it would seem that reasonable modelling efforts would at least differentiate individuals by both age and income—as in our numerical simulation. Different age groups differed dramatically with respect to the fatality costs of COVID-19: older individuals faced a much higher risk of dying if infected but would lose less life expectancy if they did die. The costs of lockdown tended to fall more heavily on people with lower income who cannot work from home, but these costs can be reallocated toward richer individuals through taxes and government assistance.

Evaluating COVID-19 policies also requires an evaluation methodology, which permits an assessment of the policies once modelled. This chapter has argued in favour of the social-welfare-function approach, as opposed to valuing life-saving with VSL, VSLY, or QALYs. As explained, VSL and VSLY measures do not take account of quality of life, and these measures also overweight the interests of the rich relative to others because the rich are willing to pay more for risk reduction. Meanwhile, a policy assessment based on simple cost-per-QALY places a greater weight on life extension for those in better health and ignores the distribution of income—problems which can be avoided by using a measure of wellbeing that takes account of both health and income and a social welfare function that assigns extra weight to the worse-off.

The social welfare methodology requires normative choices of two kinds. We need to specify a procedure for wellbeing measurement—so as to assign a numerical value to a given individual bundle of whichever attributes are being modelled as the source of wellbeing (income, longevity, health, etc.). We then need to specify the type of social welfare function. In this chapter, we have focused on social welfare functions which differ in their degree of priority to the worse-off. There is, however, one kind of case in which this degree of priority does not matter: if all groups are better off with one policy than a second, any SWF which respects the Pareto principle will favour the first policy regardless of the priority assigned to the worse-off.[11] In short, the level of priority to the worse-off matters only in determining how to trade off wellbeing gains to one group against losses to another.

Even when there are such trade-offs, the level of priority to the worse-off need not matter very much. This will depend on the specifics of the policies being compared. For example, our numerical illustration found that the ranking of policies that impose very tight restrictions on people's contact during lockdowns versus policies that have looser restrictions during lockdowns was independent of the degree of priority for the worse-off. A policy recommendation that is invariant to both changes in the degree of special concern for the worse-off and the choice of wellbeing measure is especially robust. Conversely, to the extent that the recommendations of the SWF framework depend upon these moral judgments, the framework makes transparent just where normative deliberation needs to occur.

The next pandemic will be different from the COVID-19 pandemic. But the types of interventions that may be useful to moderate it will likely be similar in that they will involve trade-offs between economic costs and health benefits, and in that these costs and benefits will be distributed unequally in the population. When we face such trade-offs, social welfare analysis provides a valuable framework for evaluating which of the many possible policy responses are most consistent with a concern for greater wellbeing and its fairer distribution.

Acknowledgements

Alex Voorhoeve's work on this chapter was supported through the Bergen Center for Ethics and Priority Setting's project 'Decision Support for Universal Health Coverage', funded by NORAD grant RAF-18/0009. Drafts of this chapter were presented at Cambridge University, the Hebrew University of Jerusalem, the Uehiro Conference on Pandemic Ethics, and Utrecht University. We are grateful for comments from audience members and from Julian Savulescu, Dominic Wilkinson, and an anonymous reviewer.

[11] The Pareto principle is that if everyone is at least as well off under policy P* as under policy P, then P* is at least as good as P.

Bibliography

Adler, Matthew D. (2019), *Measuring Social Welfare: An Introduction* (Oxford: Oxford University Press, 2019).

Adler, Matthew D., Richard Bradley, Maddalena Ferranna, Marc Fleurbaey, James K. Hammitt, and Alex Voorhoeve (2020), 'Assessing the Wellbeing Impacts of the COVID-19 Pandemic and Three Policy Types: Suppression, Control, and Uncontrolled Spread', T20 Policy Brief, https://www.g20-insights.org/policy_briefs/assessing-the-wellbeing-impacts-of-the-covid-19-pandemic-and-three-policy-types-suppression-control-and-uncontrolled-spread/.

Adler, Matthew D., and Marc Fleurbaey (2016), *Oxford Handbook of Wellbeing and Public Policy* (Oxford: Oxford University Press, 2016).

Atkinson, Anthony B. (1970), 'On the Measurement of Inequality', *Journal of Economic Theory* 2(3): 244–63.

Becker, Gary, Tomas J. Philipson, and Rodrigo R. Soares (2005), 'The Quantity and Quality of Life and the Evolution of World Inequality', *American Economic Review* 95: 277–91.

Bertram, Melanie, Jeremy Lauer, Kees De Jonckheere, Tessa Edejer, Raymond Hutubessy, Marie-Paule Kieny, and Suzanne Hill (2016), 'Cost–Effectiveness Thresholds: Pros and Cons', *Bulletin of the World Health Organization* 94: 925–30, doi: http://dx.doi.org/10.2471/BLT.15.164418.

Clark, Andrew, Sarah Flèche, Richard Layard, Nattavudh Powdthavee, and George Ward (2018), *The Origins of Happiness: The Science of Wellbeing over the Life-Course* (Princeton NJ: Princeton University Press, 2018).

Dolan, Paul, and Daniel Kahneman (2008), 'Interpretations of Wellbeing and Their Implications for the Valuation of Health', *The Economic Journal.* 118(525): 215–34.

Ferranna, Maddalena, J. P. Sevilla, and David E. Bloom (2022), 'Prioritarianism and the COVID-19 Pandemic', in M. D. Adler and O. Norheim (eds.), *Prioritarianism in Practice* (Oxford: Oxford University Press, 2022).

Fleurbaey, Marc, and Didier Blanchet (2013), *Beyond GDP: Measuring Welfare and Assessing Sustainability* (Oxford: Oxford University Press, 2013).

Hausman, Daniel (2015), *Valuing Health* (Oxford: Oxford University Press, 2015).

Hirth, Richard, Michael Chernew, Edward Miller, Mark Fendrick, and William Weissert (2000), 'Willingness to Pay for a Quality-Adjusted Life Year: In Search of a Standard', *Medical Decision-Making* 20(3): 332–42, doi:10.1177/0272989X0002000310.

John, Tyler, Joseph Millum, and David Wasserman (2017), 'How to Allocate Scarce Health Resources without Discriminating against People with Disabilities', *Economics and Philosophy* 33(2): 161–86.

Kniesner, Thomas J., and W. Kip Viscusi (forthcoming), 'The Value of a Statistical Life', *Oxford Research Encyclopedia of Economics and Finance.* Vanderbilt Law Research Paper No. 19–15.

National Council on Disability (2019), *Quality-Adjusted Life Years and the Devaluation of Life with Disability.* National Council on Disability, Washington, DC.

Robinson, Lisa, James K. Hammitt, and Lucy O'Keeffe (2019), 'Valuing Mortality Risk Reductions in Global Benefit–cost Analysis', *Journal of Benefit–cost Analysis* 10(S1), 15–50, doi:10.1017/bca.2018.26.

Sen, Amartya K. (1999), *Commodities and Capabilities* (Oxford: Oxford University Press, 1999).

Walasek, Lukasz, Gordon D. Brown, and Gordon D. Ovens (2019), 'Subjective Wellbeing and Valuation of Future Health States: Discrepancies between Anticipated and Experienced Life Satisfaction.' *Journal of Applied Social Psychology* 49(12): 746–54.

10

Pluralism and Allocation of Limited Resources

Vaccines and Ventilators

Dominic Wilkinson

10.1 Conflicting Values, Conflicting Choices

10.1.1 Problems

The defining feature of a pandemic is its scale. An infectious disease that acutely spreads affecting a large number of individuals in multiple different countries across the world will necessarily have a very large human impact. It will also, almost inevitably, lead to intense pressure on a range of medical resources and a need to make difficult decisions about how to allocate them.

Depending on the specific country, and depending on the time point, different resources have been in short supply during the coronavirus pandemic. These have ranged from personal protective equipment to novel therapeutic agents, oxygen to continuous positive pressure devices, ambulances, care staff, medical appointments, hospital beds, petrol, and even toilet paper. For this chapter I will focus on two key resources that have been scarce and needed to be prioritized during the pandemic: ventilators and vaccines. While these specific resources may or may not be relevant in future pandemics, they are useful to examine. First, these are life-saving resources—decisions about how we allocate them in a pandemic could affect not only who lives or dies but also how many live or die. Second, both are examples of perennially scarce medical resources. Investment might reduce the problem of demand exceeding supply, but it cannot avoid the problem. Even in high-income countries in non-pandemic times there are challenges in making ventilators available to all patients who might benefit from them. They are expensive to purchase and maintain, but, even more importantly, such equipment requires highly specialized, trained medical and nursing staff. Novel vaccines take time to develop and then to produce in bulk. Notwithstanding the unprecedented pace of development and distribution of a vaccine against COVID-19, there have been inevitable delays in scaling up production once they had been shown to be effective and safe. Third, these two resources epitomize two different types of

Dominic Wilkinson, *Pluralism and Allocation of Limited Resources: Vaccines and Ventilators* In: *Pandemic Ethics: From COVID-19 to Disease X*. Edited by: Dominic Wilkinson and Julian Savulescu, Oxford University Press.
© Dominic Wilkinson 2023. DOI: 10.1093/oso/9780192871688.003.0011

medical response to a pandemic. Vaccines are a preventative intervention. They are relatively low-cost but are given to a very large number of people. For example, the whole global population might benefit from vaccination if Disease X were to pose a serious threat to all (regardless of age and underlying medical condition). Ventilators are a life-saving supportive intervention. They are relevant to a smaller number of individuals but are resource-intensive in terms of money, equipment, supplies, companion treatments (for example, sedation/anaesthetic agents), and especially staff. As I note in Section 10.4, because of the different nature of these two interventions, they have different ethical implications for allocation.

10.1.2 Choices

One striking feature of the coronavirus pandemic has been the variation between countries in their approaches to a range of different questions. That has perhaps been most evident in the approach to lockdowns and restrictions of liberty (Cameron et al. 2021), but it has also been seen in very different approaches to allocation of ventilators and vaccines.

There are multiple factors that have affected countries' choice of resource allocation policy—including the different circumstances of the country (for example, the prior resources of the country, the severity of the pandemic wave), different scientific advice (or interpretations thereof), and different legal or political frameworks. However, one key factor reflects the weight given to different ethical values that are relevant to allocation.

While there are multiple values that might be drawn on (Giubilini et al. 2021), broadly speaking there are several key ethical values that are crucial to allocation of scarce medical resources (Emanuel et al. 2020). The first of these is the value of promoting wellbeing through medical benefit (in particular prevention of death, avoidance or relief of medical illness or morbidity). The second value is that of treating people equally (or equitably). A third (overlapping) value relates to treating those who are most disadvantaged or worst off. A fourth commonly cited value is that of caring for those providing healthcare. (This could be ethically justified in straightforward utilitarian terms—i.e. because of their instrumental importance in achieving the greatest benefit overall. Or it could be justified as a form of recompense for risks undertaken in the service of others.) Depending on its ethical and legal framework, a country might prioritize one of these values over the other. For example, a utilitarian approach would pursue whichever policy would maximize utility (wellbeing) (Savulescu et al. 2020a). An egalitarian policy would potentially focus on equality of access to treatment. A prioritarian approach would prioritize those who are worst off. One challenging element of resource allocation is that these ethical values necessarily conflict in a setting of scarcity. It is usually not possible to promote greatest medical benefit, greatest equality, and attention to greatest need/disadvantage simultaneously. Decisions must be made.

Some of the different policy choices seen in relation to ventilator and vaccine allocation appear to reflect different weights given to these ethical values. For example, guidelines from the French anaesthesia and intensive care society explicitly endorsed that the aim of ventilator allocation should be to maximize numbers of deaths avoided and the number of life years saved (Société Française d'Anesthésie-Réanimation 2020).[1] In contrast, Belgian guidelines concentrated on medical urgency and contemplated a lottery for deciding between patients with similar urgency (Jöbges et al. 2020).[2] Some US triage guidelines recommended that triage officers be blinded to all patient factors other than acute illness severity and intubation status, while others prohibited consideration of disability or age in allocation, giving more apparent weight to equality (Antommaria et al. 2020). For vaccines, the UK approach concentrated primarily on the risk of severe COVID-19, giving priority first to residents of (and workers in) care homes for older adults, then other frontline healthcare workers and older adults in descending order of age (with some listed medical conditions giving extra priority). This was based on a desire in the first phase to protect those at highest risk of dying from COVID-19 (in the second phase, it was based on prevention of hospitalization) (COVID-19 green book 2021). Other countries had a less stratified approach. For example, in February 2021, in San Luis Obispo County in California, all those eligible for the vaccine over the age of 65 were able to register online and were put in a lottery to receive a vaccine appointment (Health Agency, County of San Luis Obispo 2021). In India, free-of-cost vaccines were made available to healthcare workers and all those over the age of 45, with younger patients a lower priority (National Expert Group on Vaccine Administration for COVID-19 2021). A different approach was taken by Indonesia, which elected (at least in the initial phase) to prioritize vaccination for younger adults (aged 19–59) ahead of the elderly (Fuady et al. 2021).

10.1.3 Public Values

Different countries may place greater or lesser weight on competing ethical values because members of those communities or the politicians representing them see those values as more or less important. There is some interesting evidence

---

[1] "The principal challenge is to minimise the number of deaths and secondarily to maximise the total number of years of life saved. Each decision must thus aim to maximise the chance of survival – not only of each individual patient, but also and especially of the greatest total number of patients" (p. 3).

[2] The idea of using first come, first served or a lottery was removed in a later version of the Belgian guidance (Ehni et al. 2021).

relating to shared and diverging views on vaccine allocation between countries. A large international survey and conjoint analysis of competing factors in allocation, involving more than 15,000 respondents in thirteen countries, found that healthcare and those with "high risk of COVID-19 death" were more likely to be allocated vaccine in all thirteen countries (Duch et al. 2021). However, while there was evidence of significant apparent consensus, there were some differences. Respondents from China were less likely to allocate the vaccine to older recipients. (The authors speculated that this may have reflected a concern about giving a new vaccine to older individuals. However, it might also have reflected a greater ethical weight placed on saving the lives of those who are younger.) Those who identified as having a left/centre political ideology were less likely to allocate the vaccine to recipients in the highest income bracket (compared with those identifying with a right-of-centre political ideology). In another study, over 80% of a US representative sample indicated strong support for allocating vaccines to those with the highest risk of severe illness (Gollust et al. 2020). A US Gallup/COVID Collaborative survey found that 74–85% of respondents supported giving priority for vaccine access to Black, Hispanic, and Native Americans (Persad et al. 2020). We surveyed more than 2,500 members of the general public in the US and UK, and found very similar apparent ethical values between the countries (Kappes et al. 2022). Most respondents allocated scarce vaccines in a way that would avoid the most cases of severe illness from COVID (i.e. consistently prioritizing those who were at higher risk of severe COVID). In that survey we specifically explored how much weight respondents gave to perceived social injustice and race compared with risk of severe COVID. In scenarios involving recipients otherwise equivalent in risk, respondents were more likely to allocate a vaccine to a patient from a racial minority. However, race was not given more weight in resource allocation than other risk factors such as sex and obesity. Significantly, respondents did not prioritize race over risk of severe COVID.

There is also some evidence about public views on allocation of ventilators in the pandemic. In a survey of the UK public, we found that a majority prioritized patients who would have a higher chance of survival, had longer life expectancy, required shorter duration of treatment, were younger, or were less frail. Where there was a small difference between two patients, a larger proportion elected to toss a coin to decide which patient to treat (Wilkinson et al. 2020). Our survey findings were somewhat different from another general public surveys conducted during the COVID-19 pandemic. Buckwalter and Peterson conducted an online survey with US respondents. Participants indicated support for triage policies that aimed to save the most lives ("utilitarian" policy) or treat the sickest patients (labelled "prioritizing the worst off"), but disagreed with policies that treated patients in order of arrival ("egalitarian") or prioritized based on social importance (Buckwalter and Peterson 2020). They also appeared to support policies that would mitigate disadvantage for people of colour. A German study prior to the pandemic did not find support for age as a criterion relevant to prioritizing healthcare, (Diederich et al. 2011), while a US study during the pandemic found that respondents allocated more ventilators to younger patients (Huseynov et al. 2020). Similar to our findings in relation to vaccines, in our survey examining the relevance of perceived social injustice on allocation US and UK respondents did not give additional priority to patients from a racial minority (Kappes et al 2022).

10.2 Pluralism in Pandemics

In determining how we respond to a pandemic threat like coronavirus or the future Disease X, one "monistic" philosophical response to the diversity of opinions is to attempt to determine which view is correct and to apply that to policy. For example, we could try to defend and apply a consistently utilitarian approach to allocation (Savulescu et al. 2020a). In contrast, philosophical *pluralism* endorses or accepts that there may be a range of different answers without it being always possible to decide between them. There are different forms of pluralism. For the purposes of this discussion I will draw on two: value pluralism and political pluralism (Galston 1999). The former is the view that there is more than one moral value at stake in decisions. The latter refers to the idea that within any society there will be a diversity of value systems, and a diversity of views about how to live. As a consequence, negotiation, tolerance, and compromise are necessary.

It is beyond the scope of this chapter to give a detailed history or exposition of political pluralism, but it is worth briefly outlining its relevance for debates about medical treatment.

The starting point is an empirical observation—within contemporary societies we encounter diversity. John Rawls, in his book *Political Liberalism*, noted that democracies are "always marked by a diversity of opposing and irreconcilable religious, philosophical and moral doctrines" (Rawls 1993). Rawls saw such diversity as arising from incompatible beliefs about the ultimate purpose and meaning of human life but also from the limits of the human capacity to reason and evaluate. How should we respond to such diversity? Rawls, Berlin, and others have suggested that the most appropriate response is a liberal one—that as far as possible we should allow people to live their lives according to their own values. In particular, we should avoid imposing the values of the majority on all. However, in thinking about allocation of resources, a simple liberal approach is not sufficient. In such situations, where it is necessary to decide on a uniform law or policy, compromise may be needed, but this should respect and tolerate a range of different viewpoints where possible.

Political pluralism can be based on value pluralism. If there are multiple incommensurable values at stake, it is understandable if different individuals weigh these differently in their lives and reach different conclusions, for example about when medical treatment should cease. Yet political pluralism can be based more simply on humility in the face of moral uncertainty. We cannot be sure that our view is the correct one and should take into account the possibility that others are right. However, it is important to note that pluralism is distinct from relativism (Berlin 1998). Allocation policies do not need to take into account all values that might be espoused, nor do they necessarily need to give equal weight to different values.

Prior to the coronavirus pandemic, and during it, various authors have sought to develop approaches that incorporate more than one ethical value. For example, in an influential paper published in *The Lancet* in 2009, Persad, Wertheimer, and Emanuel evaluated eight allocation principles. These reflected the three ethical values summarized above (and also considered social usefulness). They reviewed some existing approaches, including the United Network for Organ Sharing (UNOS) points system used for organ allocation, and ultimately recommended a different multi-principle allocation system (Persad et al. 2009). Early in the COVID-19 pandemic, Emanuel along with other colleagues drew on the same underlying value pluralism to propose some pragmatic recommendations for allocation of treatment in the impending crisis. They recommended, for example, that:

1. Maximizing benefits (both saving lives and maximizing life years) should be most important;
2. Frontline healthcare workers (and others vital to keep critical infrastructure running) should receive priority;
3. Random allocation (but not first come, first served) could be used to allocate between those with similar prognosis (Emanuel et al. 2020).

A somewhat similar multi-principle approach was incorporated into guidance developed by White and colleagues at the University of Pittsburgh and applied in various US states, including Pennsylvania and Minnesota (White and Lo 2020). That approach recommended prioritizing first based on short-term prognosis (chance of survival, based on acute severity of illness), while also giving lower priority to patients likely to die within the near term (<5 years) even if they recovered from COVID. It also considered giving additional priority to those vital to the public health response, and (as a tiebreaker) patients from younger age groups.

As noted in Section 10.1, many countries' vaccine allocation schemes have included priority both for those at higher risk of COVID and for healthcare/care home workers. This might plausibly reflect giving ethical weight both to securing greatest medical benefit and to social instrumental value (i.e. healthcare workers are prioritized in order to enable ongoing medical care provision and reduce nosocomial spread). But some have argued that vaccine priority in a crisis should be given preferentially to groups who have been structurally and historically disadvantaged, even if it would result in fewer lives being saved (Schmidt 2020). Schmidt argued in favour of a weighted lottery incorporating the Area Deprivation Index to give residents of historically disadvantaged neighbourhoods a higher chance of receiving a vaccine. Others have also endorsed a weighted lottery as a way of balancing competing ethical values for allocation of vaccines and other scarce medication (Jansen and Wall 2021).

I have focused in this chapter on vaccine allocation within countries, but some similar issues have arisen when allocating vaccines between countries. The international COVAX initiative aimed to equitably allocate vaccines between countries on an "equal proportional share" principle, wherein in the first phase each participating country receives enough doses to vaccinate 20% of their population. However, this appears to give a great deal of weight to equality at the cost of health benefit. In another paper, Emanuel pointed out that this plan would give equal number of doses to Malaysia and Peru, though Peru had experienced by early 2021 seven times more cases and more than sixty times as many deaths as Malaysia (Emanuel et al. 2021). Emanuel proposed a modified allocation scheme that would give countries in greater need (i.e. at highest risk of premature deaths) more vaccine doses initially.

10.3 Challenges to Developing Pluralistic Resource Allocation in a Pandemic

Faced with Disease X, there are good reasons to adopt a pluralist approach to resource allocation. It is clear that more than one ethical value is relevant to these decisions. Moreover, within the community there are different views about how to balance these values. I have noted some significant overlap in views based on empirical studies of the views of the public during the pandemic (I will return to the significance of this in Section 10.4.2). However, there also appear to be some key areas of disagreement. That particularly applies to the incorporation of certain characteristics such as age or disability into decisions. Our survey relating to ventilator allocation found that the majority of respondents chose to allocate the last remaining ventilator to a younger patient rather than to someone elderly (other factors were equal). However, approximately 20% elected to toss a coin to decide between patients fifteen years apart in age (Wilkinson et al. 2020). This was more marked in relation to pre-existing disability, where in several scenarios approximately 40% of respondents elected to toss a coin to decide between patients, one of whom had a greater degree of physical or cognitive disability. In the UK, early in the pandemic, national guidance that recommended clinicians take into account the degree of patient frailty when deciding about admission to intensive care was subject to legal challenge on the basis that it discriminated against those with underlying disability (Hodge Jones and Allen 2020).[3]

There are several challenges to a pluralistic approach that have been particularly apparent in the coronavirus pandemic. It will be important to consider these for Disease X.

10.3.1 Epistemic Challenges

One difficulty in thinking about an approach that takes into account different ethical values is to know how much weight to give to them. The multi-principle allocation schemes proposed by Emanuel and White both give greatest weight to maximizing benefit, while others have criticized this emphasis, citing concerns about equality or fairness (Kerr and Schmidt 2021; Supady et al. 2021). Although surveys cannot (on their own) resolve ethical questions, one potential way of helping to determine how much weight to give to a particular value would be to evaluate the views of the wider community. That could help to identify areas of common ground as well as ethical diversity. In a democracy, such a process could provide a legitimate basis for giving greater weight to those ethical values that are most widely or most deeply supported by the community.

Some work on this had occurred prior to the coronavirus pandemic. For example, the University of Pittsburgh framework was influenced by public engagement work including community engagement forums focused on pandemic resource allocation that had taken place in the state of Maryland in the preceding two decades (Daugherty Biddison et al. 2014; Daugherty Biddison et al. 2017; Daugherty Biddison et al. 2018). When the Maryland forums were replicated in Texas, a greater emphasis was placed on the significance of family (Schoch-Spana et al. 2020). This suggests that it may be inappropriate to extrapolate from the values obtained in other countries, or even in other regions within a country. Furthermore, it should be questioned whether the views of the community obtained in relation to a hypothetical future pandemic would necessarily correspond to those at the time of a crisis. Some have speculated that the brutal reality of a pandemic would lead to greater emphasis on achieving the most benefit overall from scarce resources(Savulescu et al. 2020a), while others hypothesized that community fears might lead to greater concern for individual rights (Antoniou et al. 2021). The lack of relevant information about the values of the community prompted a number of researchers to perform community surveys

---

[3] Ironically, one of the responses to this criticism was to recommend that the clinical frailty scale not be used for patients under the age of 65. In doing so, the policy became explicitly ageist (Wilkinson 2020).

during the coronavirus pandemic. Those studies provide some valuable insights, as noted in Section 10.1.3. However, they also highlight serious limitations. Firstly, such surveys took considerable time to set up, perform, analyse, and publish. Two of the earliest COVID pandemic studies on ventilator allocation (Buckwalter and Peterson 2020; Wilkinson et al. 2020) were published as preprints in late June and early October 2020, and in a journal in November and December the same year. However, this meant that contemporaneous data was too late to be of any value for the first wave of the pandemic (March–May) when many health systems were most concerned about the risk of intensive care capacity being overwhelmed, and were actively attempting to generate policies and guidance. Secondly, the sort of data that was obtained during the pandemic was quite different from that obtained in the Maryland deliberative democratic forums. Those forums had comprised a series of full-day in-person meetings. However, the studies occurring during the pandemic had largely involved relatively short online surveys. Such methods allow quantitative data from large groups that are somewhat representative of the wider community. However, they potentially yield only immediate intuitive responses to short focused questions or scenarios. The insights gained might be thought to be superficial or highly context-specific. It is often difficult to know why certain views were held, what the participants' understanding was, and whether their answers represent considered reflection. A small deliberative study, undertaken in the UK at a similar time to the previously mentioned online surveys (but published in March 2021), found some endorsement of a utilitarian approach to triage (maximizing chance of survival), but tempered with equality and priority (vulnerability) concerns (Kuylen et al. 2021). Framing of problems may be influential. For example, when US participants were asked about policy choices, they appeared to give significant weight to social justice (as well as utility). Researchers found less support for triage allocation approaches focused on saving most lives, if that would disadvantage people of colour (Buckwalter and Peterson 2020). In contrast, our study from US residents indicated that, given specific dilemmas of having to choose to allocate a single remaining ventilator, respondents overwhelmingly chose to direct treatment solely based on which patient had the higher chance of survival (regardless of race) (Kappes et al. 2022). Finally, those members of the community most likely to be adversely affected by a pandemic are often under-represented in surveys relating to the views of the public about triage (Kerr and Schmidt 2021). That may be even more likely to be the case during a crisis.

10.3.2 Normative Challenges

If we have reliable, applicable data on the values of the community, there remains a challenge in knowing how to use that in developing pluralistic policy.

Identifying values that are held by the majority of the community provides support for incorporating those into resource allocation approaches. Yet, as already noted, such empirical evidence does not resolve ethical questions. There may be some values that are held by a majority in the community that should not be included in allocation because views are based on ignorance, forgetfulness, inattention, bias, or the influence of powerful emotions (Sinnott-Armstrong and Skorburg 2021). On the other hand, if we are political pluralists, the fact that a particular ethical value is supported by only a minority of the community does not mean that it can necessarily be ignored. As long as it has some reasonable basis, we should attempt to respect it and reflect it in policy if we can.

Furthermore, there is a particular challenge in knowing how much weight to give to different values and then in how to translate that into specific decisions. Providing a ventilator or a vaccine is necessarily a binary decision (patients cannot have only part of a ventilator). Individual patients or patient groups may have some ethical factors favouring allocation (better prognosis, more life years), and others not in their favour (prior socio-demographic advantage, not a frontline worker). Should some ethical values be given lexical priority and, if so, which? Can some values be traded against others and, if so, how?

10.3.3 Political Challenges

Many countries had undertaken preparations for a possible pandemic, including developing approaches to the allocation of ventilators or vaccines. And yet, at the start of the coronavirus pandemic there seemed to be, in many parts of the world, a sense of being caught out. There was considerable political sensitivity about endorsing triage policies, even where these had been prepared. Some professional guidance, developed early in the crisis, was rapidly withdrawn in response to criticism, or perceived criticism. For example, the Italian Society of Anesthesia, Analgesia, Resuscitation and Intensive Care produced guidelines in March 2020, after the relatively well-resourced intensive care facilities in northern Italy were overwhelmed by the early first wave of COVID (Craxì et al. 2020; Vergano et al. 2020). The guideline noted that age, comorbidities, and functional status should be evaluated as part of a decision about admitting to intensive care, and noted that an age limit might need to be considered if there were severe shortages (Vergano et al. 2020). It was greeted with an outcry in Italy, and it was accused of being ageist, discriminatory, and unconstitutional (Craxì et al. 2020). Draft clinical guidance was developed in the UK in late March 2020; it was designed to provide a practical, consistent approach to decision-making in the event of hospitals reaching capacity. Yet the guidance was never published, ostensibly because of a lack of need; many suspected that this reflected a political unwillingness to be associated with an explicit rationing policy (Orfali 2021; Wilkinson 2020).

Kristina Orfali, comparing the response to the pandemic in the United States to countries in Europe noted a striking lack of willingness in European countries with large publicly funded healthcare systems to openly support rationing policies in the pandemic. "[F]ew countries will acknowledge that any triage has taken place for fear of being held responsible for the lack of health care resources or for the failures to provide an efficient response to the crisis"(Orfali 2021). It appeared in retrospect clear that de facto rationing had occurred in both France and the UK (particularly in relation to transfer to hospital); however, there was no official policy, and politicians and officials denied that this had occurred.

10.4 Disease X

This book is focused on identifying how the experience of the COVID pandemic could help to improve the ethical response to future pandemics. In terms of a pluralistic ethical response to allocating scarce resources like ventilators and vaccines, there are several key lessons.

10.4.1 Preparation

For ethical guidance to be pluralistic, it needs to reflect the (multiple) values of those in the community. However, the epistemic, normative, and political challenges in creating such guidance mean that attempting to do so when the crisis has arrived may be impossible. Orfali speculated that the lack of prior engagement with the community in Europe impeded pandemic preparation, compared with the extensive public discussions that had occurred in the US (Orfali 2021). It also meant that public debate about the issues during the pandemic was limited, and as a consequence public trust was threatened.

Some of the research performed during this pandemic in relation to public values may be helpful for future pandemic planning—even though it was not able to inform the response this time. But there will be a need to build on that body of work to ensure that the picture gained is sufficiently fine-grained to be reliable. Some of the technological developments and expertise arising during the pandemic might be able to facilitate community engagement. For example, the use of online public engagement might broaden the group of individuals able to participate. This could address concerns about under-representation of disadvantaged groups.

I mentioned one concern, that values obtained prior to a pandemic might be different from those obtained during the crisis (or might even shift over time during a prolonged crisis). Some of the evidence about public values obtained during the coronavirus pandemic is relatively reassuring on this front. One study gave a group of approximately 130 older adults in the US in 2014, and a second group in early 2020, a set of hypothetical moral dilemmas (Antoniou et al. 2021). The researchers found no difference in their overall utilitarian responses. However, they did find that compared with the earlier group the cohort recruited during the pandemic gave a slightly smaller number of utilitarian responses in dilemmas involving a clash between personal rights and overall benefit.[4] Our own study of ethical response to ventilator triage during the pandemic yielded very similar responses to a prior survey (which had focused on a related set of choices in relation to newborns) (Arora et al. 2016; Wilkinson et al. 2020). We also found very similar patterns of response (strong endorsement of prioritizing ventilators to those at highest risk of surviving) among UK respondents completing a survey in June 2020 and those completing a second survey in December 2020 (Kappes et al. 2022).

Preparation may also help to address political concerns about the acceptability of triage frameworks. That can be by identifying broad community support for a particular approach to allocation of resources like ventilators or vaccines (for example, as summarized in Section 10.1.3). It may also be less acutely sensitive. Development and approval in advance of a hypothetical allocation framework may be able to be endorsed by politicians because it will be implemented at some future time point (and thus is politically less risky). There is also the possibility that later use of a pre-approved framework could also be less politically sensitive, since any faults can be attributed to predecessors!

10.4.2 Ethical Convergence

Pandemic preparation doesn't necessarily make any easier the normative challenge of reconciling or balancing conflicting ethical values. However, one possibility is that analysis and debate may identify areas of ethical convergence, where it is possible to identify key elements for allocation frameworks.

One way of thinking about ethical values (or reasons) in a pluralistic approach is that each identified value represents a vector (Savulescu and Protopapadakis 2019). These values have a direction and a strength. Where the vectors all pull in different directions simultaneously, we may find ourselves at a standstill. However, sometimes on reflection it becomes clear that some of the vectors are stronger than others. In other situations, we find that several different vectors pull in the same direction. Then it becomes clear that, notwithstanding our commitment to pluralism, there is most reason to take one approach over another. (See Figure 10.1.)

---

[4] Respondents gave utilitarian answers in approximately six out of eight scenarios in 2014, five out of eight in 2020.

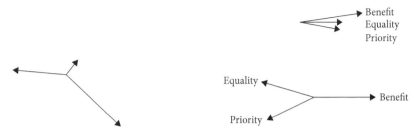

Figure 10.1 Ethical vectors: A. Values have directions and strength. B. Different number choices (key values converge). C. Same number choices (values diverge).

One example of ethical convergence might be the principle of saving the most lives. When we are allocating scarce medical resources there are two different types of choice. One sort of choice involves saving more or fewer lives. This is a *different number* choice (Wilkinson and Savulescu 2018). For example, a much-discussed philosophical thought experiment involves choosing to send a lifeboat in one direction to save five people at risk of drowning, or in the other direction to save a single person (Arora et al. 2016; Taurek 1977). At first glance, this dilemma appears to be a choice between a utilitarian or egalitarian approach. Value pluralism might mean that we could make either choice. However, further analysis yields the conclusion that both egalitarians and utilitarians should support a policy that would send the boat to save the five (Arora et al. 2016; Wilkinson and Savulescu 2018). This would give equal weight to the value of each life (Broome 1994). It would be fair to save the greater number (and, of course, this would also maximize benefit). Indeed, on the assumption that two patients who will die without treatment are equally badly off, a prioritarian approach could also support this allocation. This conclusion is obviously significant for our approach to allocation of vaccines or ventilators. For vaccines, it would lead to prioritization of those at highest risk of serious illness. For ventilators, it would support prioritization on the basis of probability of survival and expected duration of treatment. Prioritization of patients expected to require a shorter duration of treatment would mean that more patients could be treated on ventilators in intensive care. The use of time-limited trials of treatment (with subsequent withdrawal) would facilitate treatment where there is uncertainty about duration of treatment. (Patients who are unwilling to agree to a time-limited trial would have a lower priority for treatment.)

The other sort of allocation choice could be called a *same number* choice. It involves choosing between groups of patients, or individual patients where there are equivalent numbers who would be saved, but they differ in some relevant characteristic. For example, choosing to allocate a vaccine to patients with or without prior disadvantage—of older or younger age, expected to live for a longer or shorter time, or with a higher or lower quality of life—would be a same number choice. In such decisions, values of equality or priority would potentially lead in opposite directions from securing greatest benefit, and there is a need to choose between values.

However, it is worth highlighting that the conflict between values may be more or less troublesome depending on the specific decision. Here, there is a significant difference between allocation of ventilators and allocation of vaccines.[5] For ventilators, if there is a choice between two patients, one of whom is older, has prior disadvantage, perhaps has more co-morbidities and is more frail, prioritarianism might direct treatment to the more unwell, older patient, while a utilitarian approach would often prioritize the younger patient since they are more likely to survive, but also likely to survive for longer, and perhaps with a higher quality of life. (The value of equality might suggest that each patient should have an equal chance of receiving the treatment.) In contrast, for allocating *preventative interventions* like vaccines, giving priority to older, sicker, more frail patients would give priority to the most vulnerable, but also potentially save the most lives/life years. Models suggest that vaccine allocation would yield the greatest number of quality-adjusted life years (i.e. the greatest overall benefit) by allocating based on descending age and medical vulnerability (Moore et al. 2021). In that case, we would get the same answer from both prioritarian and utilitarian approaches.

10.4.3 Collective Reflective Equilibrium

Where values do diverge, information about the views of the public could be used to support the development of policy approaches. For example, Julian Savulescu has described and applied a process that he refers to as Collective Reflective Equilibrium in Practice (Savulescu et al. 2021). This builds on a Rawlsian decision procedure and seeks coherence between considered moral judgements, moral principles and values, and relevant background theories. The idea is that data on public intuitions is scrutinized and screened for bias, reliability, understanding, and generalizability. It is then used, not to resolve theoretical disagreement (i.e. whether utilitarians, egalitarians, or prioritarians are correct in their view about allocation of resources), but rather to identify a legitimate, ethically justified policy (Savulescu et al. 2021).

---

[5] This supports the recommendation by Emanuel et al. that approaches to prioritization should vary by intervention (Emanuel et al. 2020).

Using such a process, the evidence on the views of the public summarized in Section 10.1.3 could be combined with theoretical analysis and considered judgement to yield policies on vaccine and ventilator allocation. For example, it appears clear that there is very strong public support for allocating vaccines preferentially to those at highest risk and to health workers (Duch et al. 2021; Persad et al. 2020). That would align with key ethical values and the arguments summarized above that for this sort of intervention there is ethical convergence. However, there appears to be somewhat less support for allocating vaccines preferentially to those from disadvantaged socio-demographic groups. The large international survey suggests relative priority to those in the lowest income groups (Duch et al. 2021). This might plausibly reflect awareness that during the pandemic such individuals have often been at higher risk of exposure to the virus because of types of dwelling and work, and least able to self-isolate. A US survey, similarly, found support for giving priority to those in racial/ethnic communities who had been disproportionately affected during the pandemic (Persad et al. 2020). However, neither evaluated how this should be weighed against other considerations. In our study of US/UK attitudes to inclusion of race in prioritization, there was very little support for prioritization ahead of others at higher (medical) risk of severe COVID (Kappes et al. 2022). This would support a policy using this factor as a "tiebreaker" consideration. It might be that, within age bands, those from disadvantaged backgrounds have priority access. Alternatively, there might be special efforts to make available the vaccine to members of such communities when they become eligible to receive the vaccine. (Whether this would be successful is a separate question. Perhaps paradoxically, vaccine uptake has often been lowest in some socio-demographic subgroups within the community at higher risk of severe illness from COVID.)

For ventilators, surveys appear to show strong support for prioritization of those individuals most likely to survive (as well as those likely to receive treatment for a shorter period of time) (Wilkinson et al. 2020). As noted in Section 10.4.2, this would line up with ethical convergence in allocating treatment in order to save the most lives. The more challenging choices relate to same-number-type decisions, including factors such as patient age or quality of life into triage. One factor that has been incorporated into a number of triage guidelines in the coronavirus pandemic is that of patient frailty (Wilkinson 2020). This is an ethically complex factor to include in triage since it simultaneously is associated with several different elements of prognosis that might (or might not) be relevant to allocation. For example, more frail patients who need intensive care are less likely to survive, but also likely to survive for a shorter period of time, with reduced quality of life. However, that might be an advantage from the point of view of ethical convergence. Few studies have evaluated the public's attitudes towards including frailty in intensive care triage, and that may merit further, more detailed evaluation. In one study that has evaluated this, members of the UK general public strongly supported prioritization of less frail patients in the setting of pandemic triage and critically scarce resources (Wilkinson et al. 2020). (A small deliberative study also found support for this [Kuylen et al. 2021].)

10.4.4 Dissensus and Parity

Convergence and consensus may be possible. But they will not resolve all dilemmas. What should we do then?

One way of balancing two of the ethical values in allocation (benefit and equality) would be to draw on the concept of parity (Wilkinson and Savulescu 2018). This is the idea that patients who differ to some degree in a characteristic relevant to allocation may nevertheless be treated similarly. For example, if one of two patients has a slightly higher predicted chance of survival, it might be warranted to nevertheless give them both equal chances of receiving treatment. This would reflect consideration of inevitable uncertainties in prognostication. However, it would also give some weight to the value of equality. The greater our degree of uncertainty in predicting outcome, and/or the greater the weight that we give to equality, the broader the group of patients who will be treated as equivalent for allocation. When we asked members of the general public their views on ventilator triage dilemmas, they elected to toss a coin to decide only when patients were very similar in their estimated chance of survival. However, in other (same number) scenarios—where patients differed in degree of disability or in age—there was more apparent willingness to give patients equal chances. This suggests that we could potentially include some more controversial characteristics for ventilator allocation (for example, age and disability). This might, for example, mean that advanced age or severe disability could be incorporated into triage where resources are limited, but lesser degrees of age or disability would not be (even if they were associated with prognosis). That would give some weight to the value of equality, but be balanced against benefit.

Where there is clear divergence in the values endorsed by different members of the community or between the community and the results of ethical analysis, it may not be clear how to reconcile these. There may be more than one ethically justified legitimate policy option, and different communities may reach different conclusions (Savulescu et al. 2020b). Perhaps we should accept the inevitability of ethical dissensus (Wilkinson et al. 2016). Ultimately, that may itself be useful, since it could represent a form of natural experiment and make it possible (afterwards) to review the impact and acceptability of different approaches taken. (To some degree, this book represents just such an endeavour to evaluate the strategies adopted for the COVID pandemic.)

10.4.5 AI ethics

Finally, and more speculatively, it is possible that lessons from the COVID pandemic might lead us to a more radically different allocation approach for Disease X.

Machine learning and artificial intelligence (AI) is being actively explored for a wide range of different applications where the limits of human capacities significantly constrain our ability to make important decisions. That applies to various important areas of science relevant to Disease X (for example, forecasting infection dynamics, early detection of flu-like illness, monitoring of response to existing and novel treatments) (Syrowatka et al. 2021). However, it also applies to some of the ethical elements of resource allocation (Sinnott-Armstrong and Skorburg 2021).

AI could play an important role in identifying and assessing the values of the community as they relate to allocation of resources. It might thus help with some of the epistemic problem of identifying and weighing the values that are relevant to pluralistic allocation. It might help in modelling and evaluating different allocation frameworks. And it could be used to provide a sophisticated way of yielding decisions about allocation of scarce treatments that could incorporate both different patients factors and ethical values. For example, some authors have proposed the use of weighted lotteries to allocate scarce novel therapeutic agents in the setting of the COVID pandemic (White and Angus 2020). Such lotteries are designed to allow centralized, consistent, procedurally fair allocation that incorporates strong commitment to equality alongside some adjustment to priority for benefit (or disadvantage). However, it would be possible for AI-based allocation to use more sophisticated models that would incorporate a range of patient factors as well as different ethical values, identifying when priority should be given, when some form of randomization might be justified (for example, when patients fall into a "parity" group), and when treatment should not be allocated.

The use of AI in allocation raises other issues beyond the scope of this chapter. AI-based allocation may be perceived as lacking ethical transparency (Durán and Jongsma 2021), or subject to bias in the data or assumptions incorporated into programming. (Though such concerns potentially apply even more strongly to conventional "human" resource allocation.) There is important empirical work to be done to assess the acceptability of such an approach, particularly given that in the past the public has been strongly sceptical about the use of lotteries for allocation (Grover et al. 2020; Krütli et al. 2016; Schoch-Spana et al. 2020).

10.5 Conclusions

Balancing competing ethical values in a pluralistic approach to allocation is difficult. However, realistically there is no alternative, and this will be essential for our response to future pandemics. I have outlined some of the practical and normative challenges evident from the coronavirus pandemic in vaccine and ventilator allocation. I have also identified some potential learning points. There appear to be significant areas of agreement within and between countries about which values might be given most weight in allocation. There are also some important points of ethical convergence. Through a process of practical collective reflective equilibrium we may be able to develop in advance pandemic allocation plans that could be adopted or adapted for Disease X.

Bibliography

Antommaria, A. H., et al. (2020), 'Ventilator Triage Policies During the COVID-19 Pandemic at U.S. Hospitals Associated With Members of the Association of Bioethics Program Directors', *Annals of Internal Medicine*, 173/3: 188–94.

Antoniou, Rea, et al. (2021), 'Reduced utilitarian willingness to violate personal rights during the COVID-19 pandemic', *PLOS ONE*, 16/10: e0259110.

Arora, C., et al. (2016), 'The Intensive Care Lifeboat: a survey of lay attitudes to rationing dilemmas in neonatal intensive care', *BMC Medical Ethics*, 17/69.

Berlin, I (1998), 'On pluralism', *New York Review of Books*, XLV/8.

Broome, J (1994), 'Fairness versus doing the most good', *The Hastings Center Report*, 24/4: 36–9.

Buckwalter, Wesley, and Peterson, Andrew (2020), 'Public attitudes toward allocating scarce resources in the COVID-19 pandemic', *PLOS ONE*, 15/11: e0240651.

Cameron, James, et al. (2021), 'Ethics of selective restriction of liberty in a pandemic', *Journal of Medical Ethics*, 47/8: 553–62.

COVID-19 green book (2021), 'Chapter 14a: COVID-19-Sars-CoV-2', in Mary Ramsay (ed.), *Immunisation against infectious disease* (UK Health Security Agency).

Craxì, Lucia, et al. (2020), 'Rationing in a Pandemic: Lessons from Italy', *Asian Bioethics Review*, 12/3: 325–30.

Daugherty Biddison, E. Lee, et al. (2014), 'The community speaks: understanding ethical values in allocation of scarce lifesaving resources during disasters', *Annals of the American Thoracic Society*, 11/5: 777–83.

Daugherty Biddison, E. Lee, et al. (2017), 'Scarce Resource Allocation During Disasters: A Mixed-Method Community Engagement Study', *Chest*, 153/1: 187–95.

Daugherty Biddison, E. Lee, et al. (2018), 'Too Many Patients…A Framework to Guide Statewide Allocation of Scarce Mechanical Ventilation During Disasters', *Chest*, 155/4: 848–54.

Diederich, A., Winkelhage, J., and Wirsik, N. (2011), 'Age as a criterion for setting priorities in health care? A survey of the German public view', *PLOS ONE*, 6/8: e23930.

Duch, Raymond, et al. (2021), 'Citizens from 13 countries share similar preferences for COVID-19 vaccine allocation priorities', *Proceedings of the National Academy of Sciences*, 118/38: e2026382118.

Durán, Juan Manuel, and Jongsma, Karin Rolanda (2021), 'Who is afraid of black box algorithms? On the epistemological and ethical basis of trust in medical AI', *Journal of Medical Ethics*, 47/5: 329–35.

Ehni, Hans-Jörg, Wiesing, Urban, and Ranisch, Robert (2021), 'Saving the most lives – A comparison of European triage guidelines in the context of the COVID-19 pandemic', *Bioethics*, 35/2: 125–34.

Emanuel, Ezekiel J., et al. (2020), 'Fair Allocation of Scarce Medical Resources in the Time of Covid-19', *New England Journal of Medicine*, 382/21: 2049–55.

Emanuel, Ezekiel J., et al. (2021), 'Enhancing the WHO's Proposed Framework for Distributing COVID-19 Vaccines Among Countries', *American Journal of Public Health*, 111/3: 371–3.

Fuady, Ahmad, et al. (2021), 'Targeted Vaccine Allocation Could Increase the COVID-19 Vaccine Benefits Amidst Its Lack of Availability: A Mathematical Modeling Study in Indonesia', *Vaccines*, 9/5.

Galston, William A (1999), 'Value pluralism and liberal political theory', *American Political Science Review*, 93/4: 769–78.

Giubilini, A., Savulescu, J., and Wilkinson, D. (2021), 'Queue questions: Ethics of COVID-19 vaccine prioritization', *Bioethics*, 35/4: 348–55.

Gollust, Sarah E., et al. (2020), 'US Adults' Preferences for Public Allocation of a Vaccine for Coronavirus Disease 2019', *JAMA Network Open*, 3/9: e2023020-e20.

Grover, Simmy, McClelland, Alastair, and Furnham, Adrian (2020), 'Preferences for scarce medical resource allocation: Differences between experts and the general public and implications for the COVID-19 pandemic', *British Journal of Health Psychology*, 25/4: 889–901.

Health Agency, County of San Luis Obispo (2021), 'Anyone Eligible for First Dose of COVID-19 Vaccine Can Register for Appointment Lottery', https://www.slocounty.ca.gov/ (accessed 3 Nov. 2021).

Hodge Jones and Allen (2020), 'NICE amends Covid-19 critical care guideline after judicial review challenge' (updated 31 Mar. 2020), https://www.hja.net/press-releases/nice-amends-covid-19-critical-care-guideline-after-judicial-review-challenge/ (accessed 16 June 2020).

Huseynov, Samir, Palma, Marco A., and Nayga, Rodolfo M. (2020), 'General Public Preferences for Allocating Scarce Medical Resources During COVID-19', *Frontiers in Public Health*, 8/928.

Jansen, Lynn A., and Wall, Steven (2021), 'Weighted Lotteries and the Allocation of Scarce Medications for Covid-19', *Hastings Center Report*, 51/1: 39–46.

Jöbges, Susanne, et al. (2020), 'Recommendations on COVID-19 triage: international comparison and ethical analysis', *Bioethics*, 34/9: 948–59.

Kappes, A., H. Zohny, J. Savulescu, I. Singh, W. Sinnott-Armstrong, and D. Wilkinson, (2022), 'Public attitudes towards race and resource allocation in a pandemic', *BMJ Open*, 12:e062561. doi: 10.1136/bmjopen-2022-062561.

Kerr, Whitney, and Schmidt, Harald (2021), 'COVID-19 ventilator rationing protocols: why we need to know more about the views of those with most to lose', *Journal of Medical Ethics*, 47/3: 133–6.

Krütli, P., et al. (2016), 'How to Fairly Allocate Scarce Medical Resources: Ethical Argumentation under Scrutiny by Health Professionals and Lay People', *PLOS ONE*, 11/7: e0159086.

Kuylen, Margot N. I., et al. (2021), 'Should age matter in COVID-19 triage? A deliberative study', *Journal of Medical Ethics*, 47/5: 291.

Moore, Sam, et al. (2021), 'Modelling optimal vaccination strategy for SARS-CoV-2 in the UK', *PLOS Computational Biology*, 17/5: e1008849.

National Expert Group on Vaccine Administration for COVID-19 (2021), 'Revised Guidelines for implementation of National COVID Vaccination Program', https://www.mohfw.gov.in/pdf/RevisedVaccinationGuidelines.pdf (accessed 3 Nov. 2021).

Orfali, Kristina (2021), 'Getting to the Truth: Ethics, Trust, and Triage in the United States versus Europe during the Covid-19 Pandemic', *Hastings Center Report*, 51/1: 16–22.

Persad, G., Wertheimer, A., and Emanuel, E. J. (2009), 'Principles for allocation of scarce medical interventions', *Lancet*, 373/9661: 423–31.

Persad, Govind, Peek, Monica E., and Emanuel, Ezekiel J. (2020), 'Fairly Prioritizing Groups for Access to COVID-19 Vaccines', *JAMA*, 324/16: 1601–2.

Rawls, John (1993), *Political Liberalism* (New York: Columbia University Press).

Savulescu, J., and Protopapadakis, E. (2019), ' "Ethical Minefields" and the Voice of Common Sense: A Discussion with Julian Savulescu', *Conatus Journal of Philosophy*, 4/1.

Savulescu, Julian, Persson, Ingmar, and Wilkinson, Dominic (2020a), 'Utilitarianism and the pandemic', *Bioethics*, 34/6: 620–32.

Savulescu, Julian, Cameron, James, and Wilkinson, Dominic (2020b), 'Equality or utility? Ethics and law of rationing ventilators', *British Journal of Anaesthesia*, 125/1: 10–15.

Savulescu, Julian, Gyngell, Christopher, and Kahane, Guy (2021), 'Collective Reflective Equilibrium in Practice (CREP) and controversial novel technologies', *Bioethics*, 35/7: 652–63.

Schmidt, Harald (2020), 'Vaccine Rationing and the Urgency of Social Justice in the Covid-19 Response', *Hastings Center Report*, 50/3: 46–9.

Schoch-Spana, Monica, et al. (2020), 'Influence of community and culture in the ethical allocation of scarce medical resources in a pandemic situation: Deliberative democracy study', *Journal of Participatory Medicine*, 12/1: e18272.

Sinnott-Armstrong, W., and Skorburg, J. A. (2021), 'How AI Can Aid Bioethics', *Journal of Practical Ethics*, 9/1.

Société Française d'Anesthésie-Réanimation (2020), 'Priorisation des traitements de réanimation pour les patients en état critique en situation d'épidémie de COVID-19 avec capacités limitées', (updated April 3 2020) https://sfar.org/priorisation-des-traitements-de-reanimation-pour-les-patients-en-etat-critique-en-situation-depidemie-de-covid-19-avec-capacites-limitees/ (accessed 3 Nov. 2021).

Supady, Alexander, et al. (2021), 'Allocating scarce intensive care resources during the COVID-19 pandemic: practical challenges to theoretical frameworks', *Lancet Respiratory Medicine*, 9/4: 430–4.

Syrowatka, Ania, et al. (2021), 'Leveraging artificial intelligence for pandemic preparedness and response: a scoping review to identify key use cases', *npj Digital Medicine*, 4/1: 96.

Taurek, J (1977), 'Should the numbers count?', *Philosophy and Public Affairs*, 6/4: 293–316.

Vergano, Marco, et al. (2020), 'SIAARTI recommendations for the allocation of intensive care treatments in exceptional, resource-limited circumstances', *Minerva Anestesiologica*, 86.

White, Douglas B., and Angus, Derek C. (2020), 'A Proposed Lottery System to Allocate Scarce COVID-19 Medications: Promoting Fairness and Generating Knowledge', *JAMA*, 324/4: 329–30.

White, Douglas B., and Lo, Bernard (2020), 'A Framework for Rationing Ventilators and Critical Care Beds During the COVID-19 Pandemic', *JAMA*, 323/18: 1773–4.

Wilkinson, Dominic J. C. (2020), 'Frailty Triage: Is Rationing Intensive Medical Treatment on the Grounds of Frailty Ethical?', *American Journal of Bioethics*, 21/11: 48–63.

Wilkinson, Dominic, et al. (2020), 'Which factors should be included in triage? An online survey of the attitudes of the UK general public to pandemic triage dilemmas', *BMJ Open*, 10/12: e045593.

Wilkinson, D., and Savulescu, J. (2018), 'Prioritisation and parity: which disabled infants should be candidates for scarce life-saving treatment', in D. Wasserman and A. Cureton (eds.), *Oxford Handbook of Philosophy and Disability* (Oxford: Oxford University Press).

Wilkinson, D., Truog, R., and Savulescu, J. (2016), 'In Favour of Medical Dissensus: Why We Should Agree to Disagree About End-of-Life Decisions', *Bioethics*, 30/2: 109–18.

11

Fairly and Pragmatically Prioritizing Global Allocation of Scarce Vaccines during a Pandemic

G. Owen Schaefer

11.1 Background

The COVID-19 pandemic has been, of course, a crisis of massive scale, devastating in both the direct impact of the virus on human health but also the indirect effects of public health restrictions taken to contain and minimize the virus's spread. The combined toll has caused, according to one estimate, over 20 million years of life lost (Pifarré i Arolas et al. 2021); according to another estimate, the pandemic caused almost 100 million people to enter into extreme poverty in 2020 (Mahler et al. 2021). This crisis has, unfortunately, also been marked by widespread moral failure. Some of this has manifested in certain governments' unwillingness to enact necessary and proportionate public health measures—for example, the Brazilian Senate found President Bolsonaro's conduct so egregious as to constitute a crime against humanity (Reeves 2021). And at the international level, this failure has manifested itself most distressingly in the form of narrow-minded nationalism, according to which countries have strictly prioritized the needs of their own peoples over those abroad, even when the differences in need are massive (Eaton 2021).

The ill effects of vaccine nationalism are most evident from the inequitable distribution of life-saving, safe, and effective COVID-19 vaccines around the world. To be sure, some degree of national priority may be reasonable, on a variety of grounds: countries are best placed to promote the rights and interests of their own residents; coercive enforcement of laws on residents requires reciprocal promotion of those residents' interests; and associative ties generate special obligations to co-nationals that countries can justifiably reflect in their policies. However, there are limits on the justifiable limits of national prioritization, insofar as countries and/or their citizens also owe duties to the rest of the world in virtue of their humanity. A robust ethical response would seek to strike a reasonable balance between a country's obligations towards its own residents and obligations towards

G. Owen Schaefer, *Fairly and Pragmatically Prioritizing Global Allocation of Scarce Vaccines during a Pandemic* In: *Pandemic Ethics: From COVID-19 to Disease X*. Edited by: Dominic Wilkinson and Julian Savulescu, Oxford University Press.
© Oxford University Press 2023. DOI: 10.1093/oso/9780192871688.003.0012

the global community (Beaton et al. 2021; Emanuel, Buchanan, et al. 2021; Ferguson and Caplan 2020).

Yet nations seem unconstrained by any significant ethical limits on their behavior, only willing to share vaccines abroad when they have secured sufficient supply for their entire domestic population, plus excess stockpiles for boosters and populations who may become eligible for vaccinations in the future, irrespective of the comparatively massive need for those same vaccines abroad (Bariyo and Steinhauser 2021). The wages of such inequity are paid through the preventable infections and deaths of millions around the world (Chinazzi et al. 2020; Wagner et al. 2021). This is perhaps not surprising, given existing trends in international aid and health expenditure, but normalcy does not attenuate or excuse the degree of moral failing.

Nevertheless, the situation has not been entirely bleak. Countries have devoted some limited supplies and funds to international distribution efforts. This has manifested itself most prominently through COVAX, a vaccine program that is a component of the Access to COVID Tools Accelerator. COVAX, which is co-led by Gavi, the Vaccine Alliance; the Coalition for Epidemic Preparedness Innovations; and the World Health Organization, had the ambition to be a central global hub for COVID-19 vaccines, from development and production through distribution. The lofty ideal was for countries to 'buy in' to COVAX, which would use those funds to sponsor research, development, and production of novel vaccines, then distribute those vaccines in an equitable manner to all participating countries (Kupferschmidt 2020).

COVAX has fallen far short of its ideal (Usher 2021a). Early on, it became evident that vaccine development and manufacture would be primarily led by direct national funding and private pharmaceutical company investment. So COVAX shifted to primarily emphasize vaccine distribution. In this area, it has made meaningful contributions, distributing 400 million doses of vaccines internationally by October 2021 (Mancini et al. 2021). Yet this was far fewer than initial projections and goals, which had to be periodically scaled back as the pandemic progressed (Usher 2021b).

Because COVAX was not substantially invested in the development and manufacture of vaccines, and has been chronically underfunded, it had only limited ability to secure early contracts to procure vaccine supply. The vast majority of stock was snapped up through bilateral deals by wealthy nations. Some of that excess stock was subsequently distributed internationally, including through COVAX, but it took some time for sufficient supply to become available to adequately supply the most underserved global populations. And even when supply became no longer constrained, or when supply became no longer the main constraining factor, the damage of inequitable distribution over at least a year cannot be undone.

This severe supply crunch meant the way in which international efforts like COVAX allocated limited vaccine supply played a crucial role in the outcomes of the distribution. Sending 1 million doses to country A meant those doses cannot be sent to Countries B, C, D, etc. Because of the crunch, those countries had to wait a considerable amount of time before they received their own share. In other words, under conditions of scarcity, distribution is a zero-sum game. Principles of prioritization are required to determine who will get that limited supply, and in what order.

Some have suggested an apparent way out of dilemmas of allocation would be to alleviate the supply crunch by ramping up production, facilitated by waivers of intellectual property rights and technology transfers (Gonsalves and Yamey 2021). Discussion of such approaches is largely outside the scope of this chapter, but I will just note that waivers themselves are likely to have little effect in terms of near-term relief of supply shortages; Moderna has consistently declined to enforce its patents, yet production of its vaccine remains limited to facilities it is partnering with due in part to the complexities of the mRNA manufacturing process involved (Santos Rutschman and Barnes-Weise 2021).

The remainder of this chapter is primarily concerned with exploring the most ethically defensible approach to prioritization of vaccines under such conditions of absolute scarcity in a global pandemic. This will be naturally contextualized to the COVID-19 pandemic, but is also meant to be forward-looking. COVID-19 will not be the last global pandemic, nor the last time global supplies of crucial tools like vaccines are scarce and thus allocation principles are needed. Principles of prioritization are essential for organizations like COVAX, as well as individual countries or other coalitions distributing limited supply internationally.

After summarizing two leading contenders for ethical allocation schemes, I will propose a compromise approach that uses proportion of population as a baseline for distribution, then substantially weight that proportion based on individual countries' needs. This would lead to countries seemingly in the most desperate need for vaccines receiving less supply than they would under a purely needs-based approach. But this is acceptable because we cannot be very confident that people in those countries would really benefit more from the vaccines compared with other populations.

11.1.1 The Proportional Allocation Scheme

COVAX at least initially opted for a Proportional Allocation Scheme (PAS) that provided supply to countries in direct proportion to their population, irrespective of the degree of severity of the COVID-19 outbreak in their country or ability to procure vaccines on their own. The initial goal was to ensure each country had supply to vaccinate 3% of its population, with subsequent tranches ramping up in phases until each country had supply sufficient for 20% of its population. At that 20% threshold, COVAX would enter into a new phase where an alternative scheme would be used that more resembles the needs-based Fair Priority Model (FPM) described below (World Health Organization 2020).

PAS is predicated largely on a certain interpretation of the value of equality. Given a fixed pie, PAS aims to distribute the pieces as evenly as possible across the global population. Indeed, in other contexts, proportionality can serve as a form or instantiation of equality, for example in regard to proportional representation. A legislature may be designed to ensure each representative covers roughly the same number of constituents, thereby ensuring roughly equal indirect voting power for each citizen. That is to say, everyone's vote has roughly the same degree of proportionate influence on the composition of the legislature to roughly the same extent (van der Hout and McGann 2009). Similarly, central governments distributing funds to regions proportionally based on those regions' populations ensures roughly equal distribution of funds per individual.

In addition to this ethical justification, PAS has two pragmatic considerations in its favor that I will analyze in greater detail below. Firstly, needs-based frameworks like FPM rely on ascertaining which populations would benefit most from being provided a given supply of vaccines. However, there is a high degree of uncertainty concerning that question, compared with fairly robust population measures of PAS. Metrics like degree of burden of disease or mortality outcomes are challenging to reliably ascertain, particularly in low-income countries that presently see the lowest vaccination rates. COVID-19 progression and spread has proven difficult to reliably model, international hotspots shift rapidly, epidemiological vaccination uptake rates are variable, and supply of vaccination from other sources like bilateral deals can regularly shift.

Secondly, political considerations may favor an international approach like COVAX using PAS, since arguably PAS is much more likely to secure international funding than a needs-based approach because PAS guarantees richer funding countries return on their investment in terms of vaccine supplies proportionate to their population. In this way, choice of allocation approach might in turn enlarge the supply of vaccines that programs have to allocate, eclipsing any marginal benefit of FPM over PAS.

11.1.2 The Fair Priority Model

As elaborated in greater length elsewhere, the Fair Priority Model (FPM) for vaccine allocation is an alternative to PAS that is predicated on three values: benefiting people and limiting harm, prioritizing the disadvantaged, and equal moral concern (Emanuel, Persad, Kern, et al. 2020). These values have wide appeal, particularly among international stakeholders who must make allocation decisions as part of programs like COVAX. In some cases, there may be tensions between those values, but the Fair Priority Model is a proposal that is meant to promote all three. In this context, targeting countries that would benefit most from vaccination not only would (in theory) prevent the most harm from COVID-19 but also would naturally lead to prioritizing the disadvantaged in a way that does not unequally privilege some populations on the basis of irrelevant moral considerations like their wealth or political standing.

Challenges for FPM quickly emerge when we attempt to specify which countries would benefit more from vaccination. The original model proposed that, during the most acute phase of the global pandemic (which, at this point of writing, is still unfortunately ongoing), this should be determined based on how many Standard Expected Years of Life Lost (SEYLLs) would be prevented through allocation of a given supply. SEYLLs were chosen because death, as the most severe outcome of COVID-19, is reasonably the most important outcome from COVID to minimize and mitigate. It is also a proxy for other ill effects of COVID, such as hospitalization, long-term effects and the indirect effects of public health measures that are often taken in order to prevent further deaths (Emanuel, Persad, Kern, et al. 2020). The use of this metric has come under criticism on various grounds (Harris 2021; Jecker et al. 2021), but for the purpose of this chapter those objections will be set aside. Whether SEYLLs, lives saved, hospitalizations due to COVID, or other metrics are used, they all share a similar flaw discussed below: relative uncertainty and unreliability, as compared with a pure population estimate. As such, my proposed approach will be applicable, no matter which metrics are ultimately decided upon.

Yet, bracketing for a moment those practical challenges, FPM is at the theoretical level ethically dominant over the most prominently deployed alternative of PAS. As noted above, PAS appears to prioritize equality as a value. This, however, is not entirely accurate. Countries are not strictly speaking treated equally: larger countries receive more vaccines.

Nor are vaccines distributed equally to individuals under PAS. Under conditions of scarcity, some in the population will receive doses and some will not. If a country has 1 million people and is allocated 1,000 doses of vaccines, each individual does not get an equal 0.1% of a vaccine dose. Rather, 0.1% of the population are given one full dose; the result is in some ways a form of massive inequality, more unequal in one way than a scenario where no one gets any doses. As such, proportional allocation does not promote the value of equality.

This failure to promote strict equality in allocation may not be ethically troublesome. After all, a responsible country will ensure that doses are not allocated randomly or by lottery to their domestic population (which would arguably be the purest form of equality, giving all residents equal ex ante chances of being vaccinated), but given to those who need vaccines the most, are most critical to maintaining public health and well-being, and/or are at most risk of spreading the virus to others (Emanuel, Persad, Upshur, et al. 2020). Yet adducing all those considerations to justify prioritization at the domestic level only highlights how priorities such as alleviating need or minimizing disease burden, rather than enforcing strict equality, are the most pressing. Similar considerations should obtain at the international level, which are better reflected by FPM's need sensitivity than PAS's insensitivity to need.

Another consideration in favor of PAS over FPM may be that it spreads vaccine supply more evenly across countries, such that vaccines do not end up getting primarily distributed to a small number of very high-need countries. This concern, though, presumes all doses would be allocated in one single tranche to the highest-needs countries. A more robust application of FPM would disburse vaccines in small tranches, and each tranche would account for the effect on need from the previous tranche, such that a country previously in greatest need might no longer be so after receiving a certain amount of vaccines. A finely tuned application of FPM, then, can ensure that a small number of countries do not completely dominate receipt of vaccine supplies.

It is often emphasized that equity, rather than strict equality, is what really matters: treating people differentially, based on factors that are morally relevant. It is standard practice, including in domestic healthcare expenditure and international aid, to expend more resources on those who are in greater need of those resources. This is the essence of the FPM value of equal moral concern. Everyone's interests matter equally, but some people's interests may be advanced more substantially through devotion of the same amount of resources. PAS, by contrast, is insensitive to differential need, and therefore does not properly advance the value of equity (Herzog et al. 2021).

For these reasons, FPM is a more ethically defensible model than PAS, at least at the level of ethical assessment.

11.2 Pragmatic Challenges

Theory and practice should theoretically be the same, so the saying goes, but in practice they are not. This is applicable to vaccine allocation, where the most persuasive arguments for PAS are pragmatic in nature. Two such arguments will be entertained here, one relating to uncertainty and the other relating to political acceptability. While both could hypothetically be relevant, only the former is ultimately persuasive given the actual way the COVID-19 crisis has played out, and, in light of that, how we may expect future pandemic responses to progress.

11.2.1 Uncertainty

If we could ascertain with absolute certainty the degree to which people in certain countries would benefit from a given supply of vaccines, FPM would be straightforward to apply and there would be little reason to opt for a purely proportional approach. Unfortunately, the reality of the situation is quite different. Uncertainty over who would benefit most exists at a number of points of analysis, which compounds to ultimately give one limited confidence in the claims of FPM's potential benefits. Sources of uncertainty include: whether a given metric accurately captures the reality on the ground; reliability of medium-term projections of COVID-19 outcomes within and between countries; efficiency with which vaccines distributed to a given country will actually be deployed; and degree of efficacy of a given vaccine in a particular population.

Let us first consider the most basic issue of measuring a population's current degree of need for a COVID-19 vaccine. There is a high degree of variability in different countries' ability to conduct COVID-19 surveillance, that is to accurately measure their true burden of disease. Some LMICs are under-resourced, and/or have greater priorities to attend to than tracking COVID cases (Ibrahim 2020). And even HICs like the US have encountered challenges to surveillance (Brown and Walensky 2020). This in turn may lead to under-reporting of deaths from COVID, as many may die without a diagnosis. Using alternative metrics of excess deaths (deaths over and above what is normally expected) may somewhat ameliorate this, and also help account for the ethically relevant indirect effects of COVID through, for example, disruption to the economy or healthcare systems. But measurements of excess deaths are themselves not always reliable, or easily comparable between countries. Countries are variable in reporting this data, with many countries' information lagging months behind others (Kiang et al. 2020).

This in turn raises the issue of dynamism: hotspots of large number of cases or deaths may emerge over the course of a few weeks or months, and disappear as quickly. For example, India went from around 700 COVID-19 deaths daily in early March 2021 to around 26,000 daily deaths in early May 2021, then down to 6,000 daily deaths in early July 2021 (World Health Organization 2021). At the same time, vaccine allocation is not instant: after identifying a country as a target for allocation, arrangements for shipping, importation, storage, and distribution must be made. And even once the first inoculations are made, it will typically be several weeks hence before a second dose can be given to provide the most protective effect. By the time full protection is given, it may well be that what was once a desperate situation has been greatly attenuated. At the same time, other global hotspots are likely to accrue—places where, if vaccines had been more evenly distributed, people would have benefited more as compared with locations recently recovering from a surge.

Additionally, different countries will have different capacities to make efficient use of vaccine supply that cannot be easily anticipated. As of this writing, mRNA vaccines require super-cold storage that will be less feasible in LMICs, but are also more effective at preventing disease and death from COVID-19 (Kim et al. 2021). There might be some wastage in distributing mRNA vaccines to LMICs, yet if they are more protective than alternatives and certain LMICs are in desperate need, that wastage could ultimately be acceptable. At the same time, estimates of such a risk of wastage may be overstated (James 2021). Even with other vaccines that do not require super-cold storage, countries may encounter unanticipated logistical challenges in distributing supplies effectively. Similarly, vaccine uptake rates are variable between countries in ways that are difficult to predict (Wouters et al. 2021). The upshot is that, even if country A appears to be in greater need of vaccines than country B, the actual distribution of vaccines in country B may be better tuned to that country's needs, and alleviate need more effectively, than if doses had been given to country A.

A final area of uncertainty to consider is that variants of concern have emerged that appear to mitigate the protective effects of vaccines. Uncertainty here comes in two interrelated forms: estimation of the loss of protection due to a given variant from a given vaccine, and current or projected degree of spread of a given variant in a given population. Estimations for the loss of protection from variants such as Delta have varied wildly across different studies, which will partly be due to much of this data coming from real-world evidence of spread (Baraniuk 2021; Puranik et al. 2021). Relatedly, just as surveillance of COVID-19 cases is of limited reliability in some settings, ability to detect different variant prevalence in different countries will also vary substantially (Robishaw et al. 2021). The result is that it will be unclear whether and to what extent the existence of a given variant in a given population will affect estimations of which populations would benefit most from limited vaccine supply.

This paper will not attempt to quantify the cumulative effect of the preceding forms of uncertainty, but it will suffice to say that these are substantially greater than the simple measure of a country's total population, which is the only piece of information needed according to PAS.

Nevertheless, uncertainty would not justify the purely proportional approach of COVAX during its first phase of distribution (World Health Organization 2020). That would only be the case if we were not able to justify any claims about which populations might benefit more from receiving a given supply of vaccine than others. The above compounded uncertainty substantially weakens the evidence base concerning need, but does not eliminate our ability to justify the (weakened) claim that some countries need doses more than others. Hotspots do not uniformly emerge or disappear, and epidemiological models are not completely useless at projecting likely future cases or deaths. Ignoring this evidence in allocation would do a disservice to the values of the FPM, where the information, however imperfect, can be used to save lives, target underserved populations, and effectively promote global health.

How exactly to move forward in light of this uncertainty will be discussed in greater detail below, but first we must consider a different pragmatic objection to FPM that is primarily political.

11.2.2 Political Appeal

In public statements, WHO chief scientist Soumya Swaminathan has emphasized that PAS was chosen in part because it is more attractive to potential funders of COVAX than FPM. Swaminathan points out that "[t]here's a big, big risk that if you propose a very idealistic model, you may be left with nothing" (Samuel 2020). This is not because some countries ideologically oppose something like FPM or have a conception of justice that more closely aligns with PAS. Rather, COVAX was designed to appeal to the self-interest of rich and poor countries alike: all would 'buy in' to the facility, to pool resources and make distribution more efficient. In turn, vaccines would be distributed proportionally to participants. Everyone gets a payout, so to speak. But under FPM, some wealthy funders may balk because they risk getting very little from COVAX if they manage to get COVID under control through public health measures or other means.

Taking up this argument, Sharma, Kawa, and Gomber have argued that PAS can be projected to live up to the ideals of the FPM better than FPM itself (Sharma et al. 2021). This is because, even if FPM is much more effective in itself at getting a given supply of vaccines to those who need it most, the probability that FPM will scuttle the whole project and we will be left with no multilateral distributive effort (which is much worse for meeting global need than either FPM or PAS allocation) would swamp any marginal benefits of FPM or PAS. While Sharma, Kawa, and Gomber overstate their case by claiming FPM would be as bad as nothing—this presumes COVAX is an all-or-nothing endeavor, where in fact it is able to distribute vaccines in direct proportion to its funding—the broader point still holds that political considerations could make PAS a more pragmatic approach.

At the time these arguments were made, they may have been persuasive because there was still hope that COVAX could effectively serve as a global hub of vaccine distribution. But as it turns out, even with PAS, COVAX failed to achieve this goal. Wealthy countries pursued bilateral agreements aggressively, with limited and delayed funding support for COVAX. This was a regrettable but unsurprising turn of events, given nationalistic tendencies. Indeed, as Swaminathan has pointed out, vaccine nationalism also dominated the response to the 2009 swine flu pandemic (Samuel 2020). Countries could maximize their own supply of vaccines by ignoring collective global interests in vaccinating the world (including indirect benefits to countries of reducing spread abroad that may blow back domestically) and focus on securing favorable bilateral deals with pharmaceutical companies. This is in part because, even with COVAX's attempt to have wealth countries self-pay for their own supply in the scheme, their funding would partly cross-subsidize LMICs in COVAX. A given dollar would go less far in COVAX than it would in a purely bilateral deal. In addition, countries are able to directly negotiate contracts in bilateral deals that are strongly in their national interest, rather than rely on COVAX's negotiation, which may be slower and not focused on any one country's particular interests.

COVAX has, in fact, now abandoned the aim of distributing some of its procured supply to self-paying high-income countries, given that almost all those countries have secured much greater vaccine supply through bilateral deals than COVAX would be able to distribute to them (Guarascio 2021). So for the COVID pandemic this political rationale does not apply; any funding appeals will be based on global solidarity or altruism, and wealthy countries' own supply would be untouched whether PAS or FPM are used for allocation.

Additionally, for future pandemics, we can expect that the same sorts of incentives would be in place. The relevant factors are not unique to the COVID pandemic but, rather, universal: countries can better secure their own supply of vaccines through bilateral procurements than dilute that supply via a cooperative scheme like COVAX.

Political considerations, then, are not a strong reason to prefer FPM over PAS. In other words, while political considerations may in theory give pragmatic weight to PAS over FPM, in practice they do not.

11.3 Flattening the Curve

Returning, then, to the more pressing issue of uncertainty, we should ask how FPM should be modified in order to account for this uncertainty. I propose an approach that applies need-based weights to a proportional, population-based baseline. This is designed to still prioritize countries that would benefit most, while hedging against the uncertainties inherent in estimates to determine which countries are actually in greatest need.

Under this proposal, we start from a proportional baseline, according to which each country's population is identified. This baseline, notably, has minimal degrees of uncertainty: while there may be some inaccuracy of total population counts of countries, these are likely to be small and in any case of much less variance than the cumulative uncertainties related to the FPM discussed above.

Independently, for each country, a score should be generated relating to the extent to which a country's population would benefit would be generated. Under the original FPM, this would be an estimation of the number of SEYLLs prevented by distributing a given quantity of vaccine to that country. If alternative metrics are preferred, such as simply the number of lives that could be saved, those could be used to generate a score instead.

The set of scores of all countries can be converted into a weighting function, with the lowest-scoring country set to 1, and each country's weighting set to a multiple of 1 directly proportionate to that country's score relative to the lowest-ranked country.

To illustrate this proposal, let us consider a simple scenario where country A and country B are the only potential recipients of a given supply of 100 vaccines. (See the summary at Table 11.1.) If country A would prevent 10 SEYLLs with a given supply of 100 vaccines (not a realistic number, but chosen for ease of illustration), and country B would prevent 30, country A's weight would be set to 1, and B's set to 3.

The country's population is then multiplied by the weighting number. If country A has 90 million people and country B has 10 million people, country A's weighted population would be 90 million (90 million × 1), and country B's weighted population would be 30 million (10 million × 3).

Finally, all countries in the scheme's weighted populations are added up, then each country assigned a percentage number generated by dividing that country's weighted population against the total weighted population of all countries in the scheme. This percentage is then used to determine what percentage of a given supply each country is given for a particular distributive tranche.

Supposing only country A and country B were part of the scheme: country A would receive about 75% of a given tranche (90 million is 75% of the total weighted population of 120 million), while country B would receive 25% (30 million is 18% of the total weighted population). In other words, out of a supply of 100 vaccines, country A would get 75 vaccines and country B 25.

Table 11.1

	Country A	Country B
SEYLLs prevented	10	30
Weight	1	3
Population	90 million	10 million
Weighted population (Weight × Population)	90 million	30 million
Fraction (Weighted Population/total Weighted Population)	.75 (90/120)	.25 (30/120)
Proposed allocation (doses)	75	25
FPM allocation (doses)	0	100
PAS allocation (doses)	90	10

Contrast with the alternative approaches: according to FPM, country B would get all 100 vaccines, since its people are in greater need. According to PAS, country A would get 90 vaccines, and country B would get 10 vaccines.

In order to account for the diminished marginal benefit of vaccines (given that vaccines are typically distributed to the most vulnerable parties first as a country receives more vaccines, the preventative effect of a given supply of vaccine is likely to go down as more of a population is vaccinated), this approach would have to be applied to small tranches of vaccines at one time. Subsequent tranches would modify the projected benefit of a given supply, accounting for the protective effects of previously allocated vaccines.

A weighted approach is not novel, and in fact a version of it has been used among other places by another Access to COVID Tools Accelerator pillar, in distributing diagnostic tests when very early on in the pandemic those were scarce ('Procurement Considerations for COVID-19 Diagnostics' 2021). It is undeniably complex, but its use in that diagnostic context should be indicative that despite this complexity it was acceptable to relevant stakeholders during the COVID-19 crisis.

This approach may seem objectionable because it will provide less expected benefit than FPM. In the illustration above, FPM would be expected to prevent 30 SEYLLs, whereas this modified approach would only prevent 15 (75 vaccines × 0.1 SEYLLs prevented/vaccine in country A + 25 vaccines × 0.3 SEYLLs prevented/vaccine in country B). By contrast, PAS would prevent 12.

In conditions of certainty, FPM would again be dominant. But because of the considerable uncertainty discussed above, it is prudent to hedge. Consider that, in conditions of absolute uncertainty where FPM had no predictive value, we would do well to default to a pure population approach, since there is almost no uncertainty of that metric. But even when we have some degree of confidence in FPM, there is a substantial risk that in real-world conditions PAS would do better than FPM. This is particularly so in light of potential LMIC under-reporting, which may systematically deflate FPM-based scores of those countries, perversely disadvantaging instead of prioritizing the worst-off countries. Hedging is also warranted in light of the rapidly shifting nature of global hotspots and lag between current data and when vaccines can be allocated. FPM prioritizing country B grappling a surge today instead of a country A that is perhaps stable may end up perversely costing numerous lives, if in the interim country B stabilizes and cases in country A surge.

But do we need to hedge this much, such that we are halving the number of SEYLLs expected to be prevented in the illustration, which may seem drastic? Perhaps not, and the above formula could be adjusted to give more weight to the SEYLL ranking and less weight to the population baseline. Another approach would be to estimate general levels of need, and weight countries according to a prioritarian principle where the utility gained from receiving vaccines of those in greater need would count more than those in lesser need (Nielsen 2022).

However, my proposal has the advantage of a certain degree of non-arbitrariness: weightings of populations are directly proportionate to the actual differences in how many SEYLLs are saved. A prioritarian model, by contrast, would require some amount of arbitrary determination of relative weights, compounded by the uncertainty in the data underlying estimates of need outlined above. It is also not straightforward to apply prioritarian principles to variable populations, and the preceding approach does not require controversial prioritarian modelling theories (Brown 2007).

Formal models to account for uncertainty in public health contexts could be deployed (Briggs et al. 2016; Metcalf et al. 2015), but even those would require subjective assessments of the degree of uncertainty and how this should appropriately translate into differential weighting. Additionally, the multiple sources of uncertainty outlined above cast doubt on the possibility of formally modelling uncertainty in this case. And there is furthermore a higher-order sense of uncertainty: we cannot be confident that we have identified all the relevant sources of uncertainty, and the degree to which we should hedge.

11.4 Conclusion

Allocation of scarce vaccines is not a mere theoretical exercise, but one that directly impacts the lives and livelihoods of millions around the world. All policy decisions are risky, but the degree and variety of sources of uncertainty concerning where vaccines would actually do the most good should give us pause in straightforwardly allocating according to need.

I have proposed an allocation framework that, in essence, is a combination of needs-based and proportional allocation schemes. In addition to helping hedge against uncertainty, this approach has the potential virtue of being a compromise position. While political considerations relating to incentivizing funding may not be applicable, the COVAX allocation model is one that has already been accepted by numerous stakeholders around the world. In terms of actually achieving a policy aim of getting more vaccines to those who need them, a proposal that meets groups halfway and does not require them to completely throw out their existing allocation frameworks may be more appealing (Emanuel, Luna, et al. 2021). So, even if the above is mistaken, and uncertainty is no reason to prefer my account over the original FPM, it may have further pragmatic value as being comparatively less revisionary with respect to COVAX's approach.

For future pandemics, it is less clear to what extent proportional allocation will be seen as an appropriate baseline for allocation of scarce vaccines or other interventions. Current discussions on pandemic preparedness are focused on procedural questions including governance and funding, but there has not to date been much attention from major potential stakeholders on working out an allocation scheme in advance. This, though, is a further degree of uncertainty that perhaps can be accounted for in planning: we don't have any idea how easy it will be to measure comparative need in a future pandemic, but at least we know that populations will be straightforward to measure.

One upshot from the preceding discussion is that substantial resources should be spent in reducing the different levels of uncertainty and thereby improving the extent to which distribution can appropriately meet global needs. This would mean gathering robust international data related to all levels of vaccine distribution, from accurately measuring need to estimating distribution impact, tracking variants, and so forth. Such efforts would overlap with broader disease surveillance efforts, and relevance to global allocation provides further reasons to support resource-strapped LMICs in gathering such data.

Still, in the face of unresolved uncertainty, retaining proportion of population as a baseline for allocation, with a commitment to weight or modify that baseline depending on degree of need around the world, may be the most pragmatic approach to thinking about allocation schemes for future pandemics.

Acknowledgments

I would like to thank Sreenivasan Subramanian, Dominic Wilkinson, Alex Voorhoeve, and other attendees of the 2021 Uehiro-Carnegie-Oxford workshop at which this chapter was presented for their helpful and challenging comments, as well as the very useful comments from an anonymous reviewer. I would also like to thank the other authors of "An ethical framework for global vaccine allocation" (*Science* 369(6509) (2020): 1309–12); this chapter builds on ideas developed and extensively discussed as part of that collaborative project, but of course any mistakes or shortcomings are solely my own.

Bibliography

Baraniuk, C. (2021). 'Covid-19: How effective are vaccines against the delta variant?', *BMJ*, n1960, DOI: 10.1136/bmj.n1960.

Bariyo, N., and Steinhauser, G. (2021). 'Covid-19 Vaccine Gap Between Rich and Poor Nations Keeps Widening', *The Wall Street Journal*, Sept. 5, 2021.

Beaton, E., Gadomski, M., Manson, D., and Tan, K.-C. (2021). 'Crisis Nationalism: To What Degree Is National Partiality Justifiable during a Global Pandemic?', *Ethical Theory and Moral Practice*, 24/1: 285–300, DOI: 10.1007/s10677-021-10,160-0.

Briggs, A., Scarborough, P., and Smith, A. (2016). 'Modelling in Public Health', in Regmi, K., and Gee, I. (eds), *Public Health Intelligence* (Cham: Springer International Publishing, 2016): 67–90.

Brown, C. (2007). 'Prioritarianism for Variable Populations', *Philosophical Studies*, 134/3: 325–61, DOI: 10.1007/s11098-005-0897-5.

Brown, T. S., and Walensky, R. P. (2020). 'Serosurveillance and the COVID-19 Epidemic in the US: Undetected, Uncertain, and Out of Control', *JAMA*, 324/8: 749, DOI: 10.1001/jama.2020.14017

Chinazzi, M., Davis, J. T., Dean, N. E., Mu, K., Piontti, A. P., Xiong, X., Halloran, M. E., et al. (2020). 'Estimating the effect of cooperative versus uncooperative strategies of COVID-19 vaccine allocation: a modeling study'. Network Science Institute: Northwestern University, https://www.networkscienceinstitute.org/publications/estimating-the-effect-of-cooperative-versus-uncooperative-strategies-of-covid-19-vaccine-allocation-a-modeling-study (accessed Oct. 28, 2021).

Eaton, L. (2021). 'Covid-19: WHO warns against "vaccine nationalism" or face further virus mutations', *BMJ*, n292, DOI: 10.1136/bmj.n292.

Emanuel, E. J., Buchanan, A., Chan, S. Y., Fabre, C., Halliday, D., Leland, R. J., Luna, F., et al. (2021). 'On the Ethics of Vaccine Nationalism: The Case for the Fair Priority for Residents Framework', *Ethics and International Affairs*, 35/4: 543–62, DOI: 10.1017/S0892679421000514.

Emanuel, E. J., Luna, F., Schaefer, G. O., Tan, K.-C., and Wolff, J. (2021). 'Enhancing the WHO's Proposed Framework for Distributing COVID-19 Vaccines Among Countries', *American Journal of Public Health*, 111/3: 371–3, DOI: 10.2105/AJPH.2020.306098.

Emanuel, E. J., Persad, G., Kern, A., Buchanan, A., Fabre, C., Halliday, D., Heath, J., et al. (2020). 'An ethical framework for global vaccine allocation', *Science*, 369/6509: 1309–12, DOI: 10.1126/science.abe2803.

Emanuel, E. J., Persad, G., Upshur, R., Thome, B., Parker, M., Glickman, A., Zhang, C., et al. (2020). 'Fair Allocation of Scarce Medical Resources in the Time of Covid-19', *New England Journal of Medicine*, 382: 2049_55, DOI: 10.1056/NEJMsb2005114.

Ferguson, K., and Caplan, A. (2020). 'Love thy neighbour? Allocating vaccines in a world of competing obligations', *Journal of Medical Ethics*, 47/12, DOI: 10.1136/medethics-2020-106887.

Gonsalves, G., and Yamey, G. (2021). 'The covid-19 vaccine patent waiver: a crucial step towards a "people's vaccine"', *BMJ*, n1249, DOI: 10.1136/bmj.n1249.

Guarascio, F. (2021). 'Global vaccines project to revamp rules after Britain got more than Botswana'. *Reuters*, Sept. 27, 2021.

Harris, J. (2021). 'Combatting Covid-19. Or, "All Persons Are Equal but Some Persons Are More Equal than Others?"', *Cambridge Quarterly of Healthcare Ethics*, 30/3: 406–14, DOI: 10.1017/S096318012000095X.

Herzog, L. M., Norheim, O. F., Emanuel, E. J., and McCoy, M. S. (2021). 'Covax must go beyond proportional allocation of covid vaccines to ensure fair and equitable access', *BMJ*, m4853, DOI: 10.1136/bmj.m4853.

Ibrahim, N. K. (2020). 'Epidemiologic surveillance for controlling Covid-19 pandemic: types, challenges and implications', *Journal of Infection and Public Health*, 13/11: 1630–8, DOI: 10.1016/j.jiph.2020.07.019.

James, E. R. (2021). 'Disrupting vaccine logistics', *International Health*, 13/3: 211–4, DOI: 10.1093/inthealth/ihab010.

Jecker, N. S., Wightman, A. G., and Diekema, D. S. (2021). 'Vaccine ethics: an ethical framework for global distribution of COVID-19 vaccines', *Journal of Medical Ethics*, 47/5, DOI: 10.1136/medethics-2020-107036.

Kiang, M. V., Irizarry, R. A., Buckee, C. O., and Balsari, S. (2020). 'Every Body Counts: Measuring Mortality From the COVID-19 Pandemic', *Annals of Internal Medicine*, 173/12: 1004–7, DOI: 10.7326/M20-3100.

Kim, J. H., Hotez, P., Batista, C., Ergonul, O., Figueroa, J. P., Gilbert, S., Gursel, M., et al. (2021). 'Operation Warp Speed: implications for global vaccine security', *The Lancet Global Health*, 9/7: e1017–21, DOI: 10.1016/S2214-109X(21)00140-6.

Kupferschmidt, K. (2020). 'Global plan seeks to promote vaccine equity, spread risks', *Science*, 369/6503: 489–90, DOI: 10.1126/science.369.6503.489.

Mahler, D. G., Yonzan, N., Lankner, C., Aguilar, R. A. C., and Wu, H. (2021). 'Updated estimates of the impact of COVID-19 on global poverty: Turning the corner on the pandemic in 2021?'. *Data Blog,* World Bank, https://blogs.worldbank.org/opendata/updated-estimates-impact-covid-19-global-poverty-turning-corner-pandemic-2021 (accessed Oct. 28, 2021).

Mancini, D. P., Bruce-Lockhart, C., and Schipani, A. (2021). 'Covax falters as rich countries buy up Covid vaccines'. *Financial Times*, Oct. 23, 2021.

Metcalf, C. J. E., Edmunds, W. J., and Lessler, J. (2015). 'Six challenges in modelling for public health policy', *Epidemics*, 10: 93–6, DOI: 10.1016/j.epidem.2014.08.008.

Nielsen, L. (2022). 'Pandemic prioritarianism', *Journal of Medical Ethics*, 48/4: 236–9, DOI: 10.1136/medethics-2020-106910.

Pifarré i Arolas, H., Acosta, E., López-Casasnovas, G., Lo, A., Nicodemo, C., Riffe, T., and Myrskylä, M. (2021). 'Years of life lost to COVID-19 in 81 countries', *Scientific Reports*, 11/1: 3504, DOI: 10.1038/s41598-021-83,040-3.

'Procurement Considerations for COVID-19 Diagnostics' (2021). World Health Organization, https://www.who.int/docs/default-source/coronaviruse/procurement-considerations-for-covid-19-diagnostics.pdf (accessed July 27, 2021).

Puranik, A., Lenehan, P. J., Silvert, E., Niesen, M. J. M., Corchado-Garcia, J., O'Horo, J. C., Virk, A., et al. (2021). *Comparison of two highly-effective mRNA vaccines for COVID-19 during periods of Alpha and Delta variant prevalence* (preprint). Public and Global Health, http://medrxiv.org/lookup/doi/10.1101/2021.08.06.21261707 (accessed Oct. 29, 2021), DOI: 10.1101/2021.08.06.21261707.

Reeves, P. (2021). 'Brazil Senate recommends Bolsonaro be charged with crimes against humanity'. *NPR*, Oct.27, 2021.

Robishaw, J. D., Alter, S. M., Solano, J. J., Shih, R. D., DeMets, D. L., Maki, D. G., and Hennekens, C. H. (2021). 'Genomic surveillance to combat COVID-19: challenges and opportunities', *The Lancet Microbe*, 2/9: e481–4, DOI: 10.1016/S2666-5247(21)00121-X.

Samuel, S. (2020). 'Who should get the Covid-19 vaccine first? Ethicists are fiercely debating how to vaccinate billions of people'. *Vox*, updated Nov. 20, 2020.

Santos Rutschman, A., and Barnes-Weise, J. (2021). 'The COVID-19 Vaccine Patent Waiver: The Wrong Tool for the Right Goal', *SSRN Electronic Journal*, May 7, 2021, DOI: 10.2139/ssrn.3840486.

Sharma, S., Kawa, N., and Gomber, A. (2021). 'WHO's allocation framework for COVAX: is it fair?', *Journal of Medical Ethics*, DOI: 10.1136/medethics-2020-107152.

Usher, A. D. (2021a). 'A beautiful idea: how COVAX has fallen short', *The Lancet*, 397/10292: 2322–5, DOI: 10.1016/S0140-6736(21)01367-2.

Usher, A. D. (2021b). 'Vaccine shortages prompt changes to COVAX strategy', *The Lancet*, 398/10310: 1474, DOI: 10.1016/S0140-6736(21)02309-6.

van der Hout, E., and McGann, A. J. (2009). 'Liberal political equality implies proportional representation', *Social Choice and Welfare*, 33/4: 617, DOI: 10.1007/s00355-009-0382-8.

Wagner, C. E., Saad-Roy, C. M., Morris, S. E., Baker, R. E., Mina, M. J., Farrar, J., Holmes, E. C., et al. (2021). *Vaccine nationalism and the dynamics and control of SARS-CoV-2* (preprint). *Epidemiology*, http://medrxiv.org/lookup/doi/10.1101/2021.06.02.21258229 (accessed Oct. 28, 2021), DOI: 10.1101/2021.06.02.21258229.

World Health Organization (2020). 'Fair allocation mechanism for COVID-19 vaccines through the COVAX Facility', https://www.who.int/publications/m/item/fair-allocation-mechanism-for-covid-19-vaccines-through-the-covax-facility (accessed Oct. 29, 2021).

World Health Organization (2021). 'WHO Coronavirus (COVID-19) Dashboard—India', https://covid19.who.int/region/searo/country/in (accessed Oct. 29, 2021).

Wouters, O. J., Shadlen, K. C., Salcher-Konrad, M., Pollard, A. J., Larson, H. J., Teerawattananon, Y., and Jit, M. (2021). 'Challenges in ensuring global access to COVID-19 vaccines: production, affordability, allocation, and deployment', *The Lancet*, 397/10278: 1023–34, DOI: 10.1016/S0140-6736(21)00306-8.

12

Tragic Choices during the COVID-19 Pandemic

The Past and the Future

Kristina Orfali

12.1 The Two Main Approaches for Resource Allocation: Ethical (USA) versus Medical (Europe) Framework

In a time of shortage of skilled staff, protective gear, ICU beds, respirators, dialysis, drugs, and others, 'triage'—a French word used mostly in wartime—aims at favoring the most likely to survive over the less likely. This utilitarian perspective is a common feature of all triage guidelines. All state that patients should be cared for regardless of status, income, ethnicity, race, or social status. But there is also an ethical consensus that neither a lottery nor a first come, first saved rule is an acceptable option. The notion of triage is not new in medicine; it is socially accepted, for instance, in the case of organ transplantation. Yet, despite such medical consensus, the specific features of the COVID-19 pandemic—and notably the exceptional level of uncertainty—created a greater need for urgent actions in an unprecedented public health emergency.

Looking back at the early period of the pandemic, the handling of resource allocation in anticipation and during the pandemic generated vivid debates at all levels in the USA, while leading to surprisingly few in Europe despite the alarming news from Italy, the first Western country hit by the virus.

12.1.1 The USA: Anticipatory Guidelines, Ethical Debates, and Planning for Scarce Resource Allocation

12.1.1.1 Anticipatory Guidelines and Preparedness
In 2019, the Global Health Security Index had ranked the US as the best-prepared nation to deal with pandemics. There had been considerable discussion within the professional healthcare community about disaster planning since Hurricane Katrina, the influenza epidemic of 2009, the SARS syndrome, and H5N1 influenza. In 2009, the Institute of Medicine provided a first report to lay out planning

Kristina Orfali, *Tragic Choices during the COVID-19 Pandemic: The Past and the Future* In: *Pandemic Ethics: From COVID-19 to Disease X.* Edited by: Dominic Wilkinson and Julian Savulescu, Oxford University Press.
© Oxford University Press 2023. DOI: 10.1093/oso/9780192871688.003.0013

for so-called Crisis Standards of Care (CSC). In 2015, the New York State Task Force on Life and the Law, for example—established in 1985 to address bioethical questions of significance to citizens of the state—and the New York State Department of Health revised their 2007 ethical and clinical guidelines for allocating ventilators to adults, children, and infants during an influenza pandemic. The original guidelines were among the first of their kind to be released in the United States and were widely cited and emulated by other states. Many in bioethics have participated in such disaster and pandemic planning, including using the best evidence about contagiousness, illness predictions, and fatality rates, to develop plans for how to fairly allocate extremely scarce resources in case of these events.

Careful planning has required a multidisciplinary approach to ensure that all voices would be heard both in updating previous plans and discussing new guidelines. The authors of the 2015 ventilators allocation guidelines, for example, were members of the New York Task Force on Life and the Law, made up of leaders in the fields of ethics, philosophy, religion, nursing, medicine, and law. The Minnesota Department of Health (2019) enlisted the Minnesota COVID Ethics Collaborative (MCEC), a multidisciplinary group of ethicists and other professionals (including physicians), to create ethical guidance for how to approach ICU and ventilator rationing under CSC conditions. MCEC's effort built on Minnesota Department of Health (MDH) guidance created during the 2009 influenza pandemic (Vawter et al. 2010). Their guidelines drew on ethical frameworks aimed at balancing utility and fairness. Minnesota's ethical objectives informed in turn the state of Montana to repurpose their plan for use during the COVID-19 pandemic in the event that the state needed to invoke the CSC emergency. Before that, Montana had adopted and modified the Washington state plan for COVID-19 use. The latter was based on a thorough review of the literature, guidelines from leading healthcare societies, recommendations of the National Academy of Medicine and the Washington State Disaster Medical Advisory Committee (DMAC) created in 2015, and input from both local and state engagement communities' reports (Li-Vollmer et al. 2010).

The continuous process of reviewing other state plans, revising and updating guidelines, and inviting both experts and laypeople into the discussion provided a foundation for CSC nationwide when the COVID pandemic hit hard. Ethicists and other non-medical disciplines were already part of these discussions on scarce resource allocation, paving the way for unprecedented debates around the ethical challenges of any potential triage situation.

12.1.1.2 Ethical Consensus

There are numerous medical and ethical publications (Berlinger et al. 2020; Emanuel et al. 2020; Truog 2020) on guidance in a pandemic that were drafted or updated as the pandemic unfolded. There are over sixty such guidelines in the US, mostly drafted by multidisciplinary teams, manifesting a concern to support any emergency triage plan at any level—state, hospital, and professional societies' guidelines—with an explicit ethical framework (Hick et al. 2020). A crucial aspect is that state plans usually require a formal emergency proclamation by the governor to be activated.

These guidelines express a wide consensus on saving more lives, and secondarily more years of life. Many plans include exclusion criteria such as 'severe baseline cognitive impairment', 'severe trauma', 'heart failure', 'severe burns', etc. Patients not excluded are then triaged according to a scoring system—for example, the 'sequential organ failure assessment' (SOFA), with measurements from six of each organ systems with a higher score indicating worse function. On the basis of such a score, patients are categorized in four groups.[1] This SOFA score is repeated to inform continuation (or not) of care in case of shortage. Finally, patients who are denied a respirator or whose ventilator is withdrawn should all get comfort care and palliative support. All guidelines address this dramatic situation with more or less clarity. While some have questioned the appropriateness of SOFA, most plans have adopted it in the absence of an alternative, accurate, evidence-based scoring system for likelihood of survival.

Most triage guidelines in the US emphasize that the treating physician should not be the one to make any triage decision. Hospitals should have a triage committee with a triage officer who will make such decisions. The separation between the clinical role and the triaging role is intended to keep intact the fiduciary doctor–patient relation and avoid any conflict of commitments and moral distress.

12.1.1.3 Guidelines Variations

Despite many similarities across the different triage plans, there are variations and notable differences. Some plans favor long-term survival over short-term. The New York guidelines focus on a patient's short-term likelihood of surviving the acute episode: saving more lives is explicitly prioritized in this plan. Other plans tend to go beyond maximizing survival at discharge and attempt to maximize the number of life years saved. The principle of 'life cycle', which is intended to provide each person with the same opportunity to live through the various stages of life, gives priority to younger individuals over older ones. Despite being criticized by many as potentially discriminating against the elderly, it seems to be socially accepted (Harris 1985; Neuberger et al. 1998) in a situation of absolute scarcity. Yet some plans (for example, Montana) only consider this appropriate in the event that there are 'ties' in priority scores/categories between patients and

---

[1] These groups are defined as follows: 1) the prognosis is too poor to justify intensive care and ventilation (if there is a shortage); 2) the patient is too well to need any ventilation; 3) the patient is in an intermediate position, and ventilation could be withdrawn or withheld if 4) the patient with high priority is presented when the ICU is full.

not enough critical care resources for all patients with the lowest scores. Some plans (for example Tennessee, Colorado, and Minnesota) permit prioritization on the basis of anticipated or documented duration of need of a ventilator. Some allocation frameworks do not have any categorical exclusion criteria (Pittsburg), while others have different ones. Louisiana excludes patients with severe dementia; North Texas and Washington guidelines rule out PVS and persistent coma patients. Scoring systems can also be used differently. A pregnant woman will get different points if she is in Pennsylvania, Utah, or Maryland. While New York's plan does not give a priority to healthcare providers (HCPs), many other state plans (Montana, Pennsylvania) do. The justification is that the so called 'instrumental value' of healthcare workers would make them more deserving of a priority to access a ventilator.

12.1.1.4 Challenging Issues

One of the greatest concerns in the USA has been the potential discrimination introduced by any triage plan. How can one draft a plan that would not amplify existing health disparities and structural inequalities such as racism, ableism, or ageism, to quote but a few of these complex issues? Insofar as triaging reinforces socially endemic discriminatory attitudes and behaviors targeted at certain groups, safeguards ought to be established to mitigate their conflation. Several plans were discussed to avoid discrimination as much as possible, attempting to take into consideration health disparities such as diabetes or high blood pressure which affect survival.

Biases against conditions of *disability* were quickly raised. In part because of pandemic planning and publicly available documents, robust debate has been intense on bioethics listserves, in blog posts, and in guidelines created by disability rights groups. Some states have been sued if their exclusion criteria were alleged to be discriminatory. For instance, the Washington State Health Department initially suggested that triage teams should consider "transferring patients out of hospitals or to palliative care if their baseline functioning was marked by 'losses of reserve in energy, physical ability, cognition and general health'. The Alabama plan considered "people with severe or profound mental retardation" as well as "severe to moderate dementia" as unlikely candidates for ventilator support during a period of rationing. In Tennessee's plan, those with spinal muscular atrophy who require help with activities of daily living would be denied treatment in a pandemic.

Several disability associations filed a complaint with the US Department of Health and Human Services Office for Civil Rights (OCR) over the rationing plan in Washington state, fearing discrimination. Similarly, the Disability Rights Education and Defense Fund (DREDF) appealed to the governor of California to prevent and prohibit any rationing based on disability. On March 28, the OCR started to investigate disability discrimination complaints in triage plans (Kansas and Tennessee were also targeted). The first federal intervention to enforce civil rights in rationing protocols required Alabama to rescind guidelines excluding people with "intellectual disabilities or dementia" from ventilator access. It was also required not to use categorical cut-offs linked to age or specific disabilities. Many debates around disability have been extensively reported not only in the bioethical literature (Savin et al. 2020) but also in the media (Millum et al. 2020). Should disability be considered a co-morbidity? There are not only ethical issues but legal ones, as rationing protocols could violate federal civil rights law in the case of "discriminatory healthcare decisions". The American Disability Act of 1990 bluntly forbids excluding an "individual with a disability" from any service by a federally funded entity.

A disability perspective clearly emerged from these debates (Ne'eman 2020; Savin and Guidry-Grimes 2020), leading to changes such as avoiding categorical exclusions based on particular disability diagnoses (Colorado, Pennsylvania, and Massachusetts), and reconsidering several existing and new guidelines. National disability rights organizations worked with advocates, policymakers, and ethicists to produce an evaluation framework for state crisis standards of care plans.

12.1.1.5 Age?

Age remained an intensely debated issue, especially since the pandemic hits the elderly harder than the young. Despite intense debates, some citizen groups, having looked at draft protocols, expressed fears that even using predicted survival to determine who would get access to resources—the most common strategy—might be discriminatory.

There was a very clear recommendation from many ethicists, relayed by the media, to consider life years as a secondary criterion only, and even then with caution—to avoid undermining the principle of an equal worth of the elderly and the disabled. The Age Discrimination Act of 1975 prohibits "discrimination on the basis of age in programs or activities receiving federal financial assistance." The ban covers all activities of recipient institutions, such as hospitals.

In the media as well as at the level of policymakers, ethical issues around discrimination were discussed at length, including not only disability or age cutoffs but also health disparities linked to lower income, lack of medical insurance, and those with lower life expectancy. How should we adjust scores to achieve greater fairness? Should we consider the Area Deprivation Index when triaging? How can we avoid amplifying existing inequalities in planning for scarce resource allocation?

Tools like triage protocols alone cannot rectify the problem of systemic inequity and racism; however, purposeful efforts were taken to ensure that triage protocols did not perpetuate or exacerbate prevailing inequities. These vivid debates were reported not only in the bioethical literature or within the health-care milieu but in popular media. Already in March 2020, a *New York Times* article reviewed triage plans of eleven states (Baker and Fink 2020), and all over the US biases were denounced (Jarvie 2020; Schmitt 2020), leading to challenges to existing plans and requiring accommodation (White and Lo 2021) to guidelines as the pandemic unfolded, hitting disproportionately the most disadvantaged groups including the poor and the African American and Latino communities. In April 2020, 500 healthcare professionals addressed an open letter to the Crisis Standards of Care Advisory in Massachusetts to advise against co-morbidities scoring which would hit some ethnic groups disproportionately and worsen their situation (Commonwealth of Massachusetts (2020).

A utilitarian approach can hardly avoid issues of discrimination, which only amplify existing social, physical, and economic inequalities; so they were debated and reviewed as much as possible in the American context, in an attempt to correct these ethically unacceptable situations.

12.1.2 Europe: Medically Drafted Guidelines

Compared to the USA, in most European public health systems, mitigating inequity is perhaps viewed as less of a concern because there is less social inequity and a more generally equal access to healthcare. Yet ignoring this concern leads also to ignoring other inequities, such as the specific issues raised by disability for example. While publicly endorsing a rhetoric of dignity and equal worth of all human beings, many European countries have in fact opted for an implicit utilitarian approach with little public discussion on exclusion criteria and the real ethical issues around triage planning. In fact, despite warnings from Italian physicians who were overwhelmed, there was little preparedness and no real plan of action when the pandemic hit several European countries. As mentioned by a physician in Denmark, "Despite a well-functioning health care system, no plan of action was prepared for a situation like this and the initial phase was filled with a lot of uncertainties and communication deficits between the government, health boards, hospital boards and department administration" (Andino et al. 2020).

The overall underlying assumption in public healthcare systems in Europe is that rationing or limiting life-saving care to maintain public resources are necessary constraints of the public system. In most European countries, great trust in the healthcare system is paired with an astonishing weakness of any independent clinical ethics framework. While some countries updated existing Ebola, influenza, or SARS guidelines when COVID-19 hit, most relied on professional societies of intensivists (Meyfroidt et al. 2020) or anesthesiologists (SFAR 2020, SIAARTI 2020, etc.) to draft guidelines on how to prioritize scarce resources as the pandemic swept in. Physicians are perceived as the gatekeepers of the system, with extensive experience on how to manage scarce resources in the ER, and in organ transplant, critical care, etc. Writing in *The Guardian*, Dr Rachel Clarke

(2020) said, "In the UK, unlike in north America, the decision whether or not to write a DNR-CPR order rests with the clinician, not with the patient or their family. Doctors, not patients, sign the order—contrary to some of the rumors on social media." Doctors are the ones best equipped to predict survival, to initiate intubation, deciding who will benefit or not from critical care, who will be discharged and when. Most critical care physicians are familiar with SOFA scores or frailty scores, and in most European systems it is generally accepted that there is no need to question their clinical judgement. The French professional society of intensivists SLRF produced updated guidelines in April 2020, stating: "Healthcare professionals have the professional experience of critical care and proportionality and collegiality in decision-making as well as in limitation and withdrawal of care; of commitment and communication with families. These are the foundation of the ethical values from which we should not deviate." In other words, any triage would fall into the hands of physicians and a strictly medical perspective should prevail precisely because of their expertise. There is an emphasis on a need for a medical 'collegial' decision-making process in most guidelines (Belgium, Switzerland, France, Italy), and no separate triage committees are considered in the situation of scarcity.

There has also been a tendency to omit explicit discussion of potential discrimination in medical decision-making regarding disability. Some guidelines do not admit elderly patients with any cognitive impairment (Belgium, Spain); but most do not at all address the issue of disability per se. However, the British Medical Association (2020) did publish some anticipatory guidance, cautioning against potential discrimination regarding age and disability without discussing ways to avoid it. After an uproar, NICE (the National Institute for Health and Care Excellence) in the UK amended its frailty score, deemed inappropriate for some disabled population (NICE 2021).

Age cut-offs are often indirectly taken into account with a careful wording: "Age in itself is not to be applied as a criterion", yet "[i]n connection to COVID-19, age is a risk factor for mortality and must therefore be taken into account" (Swiss Academy of Medical Science 2020). Many guidelines (Spain, France, Germany) tend to avoid explicitly age-related exclusion but include it indirectly in their different evaluations. Italy, one of the first countries to be hit by the pandemic, was among the few to acknowledge that "age limit may ultimately be set". In Sweden, guidelines were published by the Socialstyrelsen (National Board of Health and Welfare) and criticized by physicians themselves for taking into account only future survival years and not quality of life, making de facto discrimination against older people and contradicting the principle of 'equal worth of all human beings' stated in the introduction of the guidelines. The Karolinska Institute in Stockholm drafted a clear hierarchy of priority; for instance, patients over 70 with two organ failures or over 60 with three organ failures were not to be admitted in any ICU (Röstlund et al. 2020). The detail of most guidelines were rarely made public and usually discussed within the medical community only, except in the UK and in Italy. In Italy (Orfali 2020) the frontline physicians, unprepared for the dramatic reality and the wrenching decisions to be made, voiced publicly (and even internationally) their terrible dilemmas, leading to the publication of guidelines by the Italian Professional Society of Critical Care (SIAARTI). An uproar followed (Sorbi 2020), and ethical issues around triage were vividly debated at all levels of society and in the healthcare milieu. In France, on the contrary, the details of guidelines were not publicly discussed and almost never reached the public. In Germany, due to the constitutional constraints of the Basic Law of the country forbidding any form of discrimination, the state could not provide any specific guidance. Yet German intensivists, despite the constitutional hindrance, recommended taking into account comorbidities in much the same way as their European colleagues (Von Klaudija 2020).

In most European countries (except perhaps the UK), and unlike what happened in the USA, ethical input has been considered more often in the form of an ad hoc psychological assistance ('debriefing', or 'cellules éthique de soutien' in France [Comité Consultatif National d'Ethique, 2020]) for medical teams and has had little bearing on the drafting of the guidelines per se. There has been no public debate or input from patients' associations, chronic care associations, etc. on drafting any of these guidelines. In fact, there has been an overall reluctance to discuss any of these issues, even as the death toll increased. In France, a group of well-known physicians and researchers (Toussaint et al. 2020) appealed through the media for authorities to cease "instilling fear" and for the media to "stop relaying communication without some detachment as it has become counterproductive; our citizens no longer trust the official discourse". In France *triage* issues were converted into the more acceptable term of "prioritization of care". Interestingly, one of the first theoretical publications in France on such a topic was made by military physicians (Leclerc et al. 2020) in a critical care journal.

The question that comes to mind, given the USA's greater preparedness and greater ethical and public involvement in debates around the allocation of scarce resources (particularly during the first COVID-19 wave), is the following: did the USA do better in facing wrenching situations of scarcity? Or was, after all, the more medicalized European approach ultimately more acceptable, as argued by some (McCullough 2020)?

At this point, it is still too early to evaluate exactly the magnitude of the triage which took place both formally and informally. Yet, through observational data, cross-referencing accounts, media reporting, reviews, and interviews, we can attempt to give a critical account of the harsh reality of triage during the early context of the pandemic in different countries with different healthcare systems, despite numerous claims that it never or rarely happened.

12.2 Outcomes

12.2.1 Western Europe: Covert Triage

12.2.1.1 Common Features

Excess mortality was everywhere, but at different times. We know that the worst excess mortality almost everywhere happened in nursing homes. We also know that shortage of equipment, masks, ICU beds and staff, and ventilators were often extreme and day-to-day management took place in a context not only of scarcity but also of uncertainty. In most places, elective surgery was postponed (a form of triage of non-COVID patients), together with rearrangement of space allocation to increase critical care beds and redeploying of staff; new safety protocols were implemented. All this has been extensively documented early in the pandemic. However, despite media reports (Schmitt 2020; Jarvie 2020), blogs, and public outcry, less is known about any effective triage taking place. To our knowledge there is a dearth of empirical data and studies on that specific issue.

12.2.1.2 Formal/Informal Triage

What do we know? At the peak of the pandemic, in some hospitals in Italy, age cut-offs for ventilation went down from 80 to 75 (or even less) (Rosenbaum 2020). In Bergamo, the media reported these words from an intensivist: "We have to make choices…and decide quickly.… There is no written rule, we have to pay a great attention to the patients with cardio-pulmonary pathologies because they won't tolerate much…and won't survive a critical episode." Asked if the doctor would "let go", he responds, "it is a terrible sentence but alas true given the situation.… I have seen nurses with 30 years' experience cry.… You don't know what is going on in the hospital, that is why I have decided to talk to you [the journalist]" (Immarisio 2020). As the pandemic exploded, hospitals were pushed to the brink, forcing physicians and hospitals to make harrowing choices. Italy was the only country to acknowledge early on and openly that such tragic choices were being made. Interestingly, other European countries didn't listen as much as the Americans to these warnings and the corresponding dramatic accounts of triage.

In fact, in many European countries most of the triage took place *before* any hospital admission. People were often just not transferred to the hospital, but rather kept in their homes or nursing institutions. Even younger dialysis patients on transplant lists could be denied ICU care as they were considered as having a co-morbidity. Elderly sick patients were readily triaged as COVID patients and thus not being transferred at all (Röstlund et al. 2020). In France, there was huge media attention to the transfer of critically ill patients from one part of the country to another in trains to ease some overwhelmed hospitals in specific parts of the country. Much less mentioned was the fact that informal yet systematic triage was taking place at the level of the first responders. The French EMS (emergency medical service) SAMU (Urgent Medical Aid Service) was using a specific scoring system ('Aggir') evaluating patient's autonomy and level of dependency before allowing any transfer. On March 19, the Regional Health Agency (ARS) of Ile-de-France issued several guidelines to healthcare providers, recommending that they "take particularly into account for COVID patients the [criteria] of age". It was reported that on March 21, 19% of patients in the ICU of the most important hospital network in Ile de France (APHP) were older than 75. Fifteen days later they numbered only 7%; for those 80 years old or more, it went from 9% to 2% (Barré et al. 2022). In one of the first cluster which infected many in the hardest hit part of France (Mulhouse), a pastor reported: "Around me, 70 people had been tested positive and 31 died. My old friend Gerard who as the treasurer for our Church was 75, so he had no priority for a respirator..." (Blachère 2020).

There has been a more or less covert policy of triaging in many overstretched places. Depriving someone of care that is obviously non beneficial is a straightforward clinical judgment. But claiming (falsely) that this is the case, while the decision is in fact motivated by insufficient resources, is simply a concealed form of triaging. Reports in Sweden (Pancevski 2020) of too readily switching elderly COVID patients to palliative care, or in France of almost systematically declining to transfer them on the grounds that "elderly patients do not do well in the ICU", describe practices at odds with any current medical ethical standard. Too often, physicians have tended to convert an uncertain prognosis into a certain one, and to assess a treatment as "futile" and "outside the accepted practice", while in reality the treatment was only denied because of insufficient resources.

Though it is true that older patients in general receive a lower intensity treatment than their younger counterparts (Guidet et al. 2018; Sprung et al. 2019), there has been an implicit but real triage taking place almost systematically in several overwhelmed sites (Canard 2020). The unofficial covert triage policy has most often taken place at the EMS level by avoiding the transfer of patients. As a result, between March 1 and April 13, 2020, deaths at home increased by 99% in Ile de France and by 108% in the Belfort territory (Insee). Triage issues also came up in Spain, particularly in Madrid, with hospitals hastily drafting their own protocols with little ethical guidance. In Brussels, hospitals were left to vet for themselves, resulting in a patchwork of different protocols in the same city; and it was reported that in some cases COVID patients from nursing homes were turned away even when the intensive care units were only half full (Stevis-Gridneff 2020). In the UK, in order to free acute hospital beds in anticipation of the first wave of the pandemic, NHS providers were instructed to urgently discharge all medically fit patients as soon as it was clinically safe to do so, and care home residents were not tested on their discharge from hospital.[2] The lack of

---

[2] Letter from Sir Simon Stevens, Chief Executive of NHS England, to NHS providers, March 17, 2020.

testing, lack of equipment (PPE masks), shortage of staff, and lack of enough space for isolation contributed to amplify the high death toll of elderly people. In the UK, the number of deaths of people receiving domiciliary care between 10 April and 19 June, 2020, was over 120% higher than the three-year average over the same period between 2017 and 2019, with 12.6% of the total involving a confirmed case of COVID-19. The UK was not alone in suffering significant loss of life in care homes, but the tragic scale of loss was among the worst in Europe and could have been mitigated.[3] Finally, the overall general weakness of ethics in most European countries has also contributed to the prevailing strictly clinical approach; in fact, the crisis situation in a way facilitated suspension of any ethical reflection.

12.2.2 The US: Informal Triage and Suboptimal Care

By the fall of 2020, with 4% of the world's population, the USA had suffered 20% of its mortality. Its excess mortality for the first half of 2020 was substantially above Europe's (Aeron et al. 2020). We know now that many minorities, such as African Americans and Latinos, have been dying in disproportionately high numbers in every region of the USA. In Michigan, black people accounted for roughly one-third of deaths in April 2020, despite representing only 14% of the population; in Louisiana, which is 33% black, some 70% of deaths have occurred among African Americans.[4] Racial and ethnic minorities are on average poorer and more likely to live in overcrowded homes, to work in highly exposed jobs, to have chronic diseases, and to be uninsured. Despite all preparedness and carefully drafted plans, COVID-19 further exposed the racial gap and the structural inequalities of the whole system. No plan can fix a broken system, but did the anticipatory plans provide at least some guidance regarding the clinical management of scarcity?

12.2.2.1 Lack of Formal CSC Declaration: Unclear Situation and Suboptimal Care

The weakness of any federal management and response to the pandemic led to states implementing their own guidelines and relying on their governors. In New York, after a disastrous start, such as forcing nursing homes to take back COVID-sick patients from hospitals, Governor Cuomo requested that all hospitals in the

---

[3] For example, up to January 31, 2021, France recorded 31,795 deaths in all long-term care facilities, while England and Wales recorded 34,979 deaths in care homes over the same period; up to February 8, 2021, Germany had recorded 17,602 deaths in all long-term care facilities, while England and Wales recorded 38,645 deaths in care homes over the same period. England and Wales data from ONS; EU/EEA data from the European Centre for Disease Prevention and Control.

[4] Columbia Review, Spring/Summer 2020: 21.

city double their ICU beds to avoid being overwhelmed. Yet Governor Cuomo adamantly refused to declare crisis standards of care (CSC) despite the dramatic situation. In late March 2020, Governor Cuomo replied "that there is no protocol" for allocating scarce resources when asked about guidelines at his daily COVID press conference, and whether the state would provide guidance to institutions regarding how to decide who would get ventilators if there were too few (Kaste and Hersher 2020). No triaging plan was ever used despite much preparedness. No triage committee was ever consulted. Cuomo focused on extending as much as possible beds, hospital space, and staff, and even requested studies on ventilator-sharing to avoid at all costs the ethical and political difficulties of a triaging plan. Though healthcare providers and facilities were given immunity for civil or criminal liability for 'providing COVID-19 care in good faith',[5] and though "acts, omissions or decisions resulting from resources or staffing shortages" were within the scope of the immunity, many healthcare providers felt unsure about the protection, especially given the heated discussions (involving the religious right) in Albany and the Governor's reluctance to formally enact any triage. There are potential legal ramifications of either withholding or withdrawing a ventilator from a patient who would ordinarily receive such aid in the absence of a public health emergency. Clinicians' concerns about liability must be addressed because even a small chance of a serious lawsuit could push physicians toward a less ethical and suboptimal first come, first served allocation system for ventilators, leading to a major loss of lives (Cohen et al. 2020). In fact, at the bedside, given the stringent laws regarding end of life in New York State, the only thing conceded by the lawyers of some hospitals was not to perform CPR on COVID patients at the end of their life, even if this was against a family's wishes. For hospitals where PPE is low and there is a likelihood that people will run many ressuscitation codes, it was considered prudent to limit the provision of CPR for reasons of clinical judgment as well as for resources stewardship reasons. CPR does expose health care providers (HCP) to significant COVID risk. Yet there seems to have been many variations across institutions in New York City alone regarding what was done.

Many states have debated and approved Crisis Standards of Care (CSC) guidelines for the pandemic, but few have carried them out statewide. There are three levels of standard of care: conventional, contingency, and crisis capacity.[6] CSCs were activated for example by the state department of health in Arizona in June 2020, but hospitals only activated the contingency level of these standards of care. So several hospitals did operate under "crisis" level—but did not perform active reallocation. The definition of crisis includes other factors that did happen: use of crisis documentation, housing two patients in a single room, ICU patients in non-ICU areas, upskilling workers, non-standard staffing ratios, and others. In

---

[5] Article 30-D of New York Public health law.   [6] AAMC, Dec.18, 2020.

Maryland (Gwon et al. 2020), a well-prepared state regarding disaster planning with its Catastrophic Health Emergencies Act which specifically empowers the Governor to order the rationing of scarce resources with certain due-process standards in place, the Governor never issued such an order. In fact, governors rarely enacted CSC and triage plans and only when vaccines were already available and triage seemed therefore socially more acceptable as most patients were the unvaccinated ones (in Alabama March 2021; Nevada July 2021; Alaska, Utah, and Idaho Sept. 2021, etc.).

The result of such avoidance (Gutmann Koch and Han 2020) in the early period did in fact lead to informal triage such as overcrowded public hospitals turning away sick patients and often the most vulnerable ones. Private ambulance chartering, for example, lead to a de facto prioritization of the wealthy over the poor (Du Pont et al. 2020). In New York, one of the most hard- hit cities, the situation resulted in suboptimal care as the overstretched beds did not necessarily come with enough manpower to care for patients. The lack of dialysis machines and staff led to patients being given fewer hours of dialysis; many patients on anesthesia machines were supervised by non-ICU staff. In one facility, the ICU nurse-to-patient ratios went from 1:1–2 to 1:6–7 due to shortage of staff (Toner et al. 2020). In fact, the care provided under such extreme levels of resource shortage which would fall within the scope of 'crisis standard of care' can impact the use of any resource that is in short supply, from staff (nurses, respiratory therapists, etc.) to equipment (dialysis machines, Ecmo, N95 masks, etc.) to space (critical care beds). Admittedly, the care provided under such circumstances is often suboptimal. Yet if the care is much lower that normal without any formal acknowledgment, no official enactment of any plan and clear criteria, it imposes an unfair burden on distraught medical teams who have to face these dramatic situations. The CSC process is supposed to be fully transparent and formally allowed by the state. That was not the case, at least in New York, for the clinicians because of the state's failure to implement, with or without revision, long-standing guidance documents intended for just such a pandemic (Powell and Chuang 2020). Inevitably, it took an emotional toll on the overworked, understaffed frontline HCP (Farell et al., 2022).

12.2.2.2 Excessive Emotional Toll on Frontline Healthcare Providers

Many ICU providers wondered if the enactment of CSC and a clear triage plan would have done better than the suboptimal care that they had to carry out in a situation of scarcity. Although precise evaluations are difficult to make, it is clear that the situation did impact the teams profoundly and led to extensive moral distress. Clinicians who were forced to carry out such suboptimal care could hardly inform families in the absence of any formal declaration and legal shield. In two sites of New York-Presbyterian, the predominant ethical challenges centered around end-of-life decision-making, setting goals of care, and medical futility, all complicated by resource allocation questions and the ambiguity of state law under crisis standard (Fins and Prager 2020). Deaths occurred in hospitals at an unprecedented scale; HCPs were infected; families were not allowed at the bedside. Despite stretching resources, one of the ethicists and physicians (Powell and Chuang 2020) in the hard-hit Bronx in New York recognized: "However, even with an unprecedented augmentation of resources, tough choices and triage decisions have been made every day during the pandemic." It is quite a paradox that all the extensive debates on ethical frameworks for allocating scarce resources and plans to avoid biases in New York State ended up with teams left on their own with little guidance to tackle the tragic issues brought by the pandemic. In fact, several institutions across the state had to draft their own protocols in the absence of any state guidance, adding to the lack of consistency in medical practice. New York is not, of course, the only place in which HCPs experienced tremendous moral distress and burnout; but as the first hard-hit place in the country, much as Italy for the West, it epitomizes one of the worst trauma contexts for frontline HCPs. Sadly, but not surprisingly, the new law regarding mental health infrastructure supporting physicians and other HCPs is the Lorna Breen Health Care Provider Protection Act, named after a physician who died by suicide in April 2020 following recovery from COVID and an intense stretch treating COVID-19 patients at the onset of the pandemic in Manhattan.

12.3 Lessons for the Future

Despite different contexts, there are common lessons that need to be drawn from reviewing what happened and addressing the future: political leadership, legal protection, consistency, accountability, transparency, and building trust. Many governments (the UK, Sweden, France, etc.), as well as several states in the US, have now mandated reports from their health officials regarding the management of the pandemic. It is not in the purview of this chapter to review all these reports, which are not always easily accessed or are still in draft. The triage issue is rarely explicitly dealt with in these reviews; however, we have attempted to identify the most salient features in available reports (AAPG 2021; Comptes rendus de la Commission d'Enquête du Sénat 2020; SOU 2022 etc.) regarding scarcity management and issues to be addressed in the future.

12.3.1 Strong Political Centralized Leadership Needed

In the USA context, extensive preparedness and ethical input regarding triage plans were jeopardized by the weakness of a central political leadership and a lack of formal declaration allowing health professionals to effectively enact triaging.

This in turn raised legal liability questions in the absence of official activation of crisis standards. There was also a reluctance to put any sensitive aspects of planning into writing, leading to confusion and ambiguity at the level of care. Ethical and clinical preparedness is insufficient without a political will to carry out guidelines. Stalled leadership leads to several negative consequences.

Many guidelines cite the ethical obligation of political authorities not only to produce such documents (rather than force beleaguered frontline providers to invent solutions during disasters, while enduring great risk and burnout) (Institute of Medicine 2009; Powell and Chuang 2020) but also to enact a protective formal declaration. Such a declaration needs to include specific guidance about its scope. Indeed, one of the principal lessons of Hurricane Katrina was that it is unjust to force frontline providers to tackle problems that should have been addressed in advance. Leaving triage decisions up to frontline clinicians because there is no formal acknowledgment of the reality of the situation is likely to result in decisions that adversely affect vulnerable populations and generate unfair moral distress and burden on HCPs. Studies have repeatedly shown that physicians have implicit biases (Maina et al. 2018) and that these biases are more likely to affect care when clinicians are under stress (Stepanikova 2012; Dyrbye et al. 2019). In the Johns Hopkins report (Toner et.al. 2020) on the experiences of critical care teams during the first wave in New York City, it became clear that there was a lack of education regarding what CSC really meant (particularly in the absence of an emergency declaration), and a lot of confusion regarding any triaging protocol. In preparing for the future, it might be important to anticipate that CSC plans must factor in that a formal declaration from the state may not be made in time and should include how to proceed without it.

One question remains: can the political leadership be immune to pressures and electoral calculations in a situation of scarcity? Europe was, as we now know, less prepared. The UK post-pandemic report suggested setting up an external agency: "I do not believe that we are anything like as well prepared for future problems as we could be if we were, as a nation, to have some external body that is not subject to the pressures that are on Whitehall's Ministers and civil servants, that has its funding somehow enshrined in law, and has the sole task of looking at what is not happening but might happen, and to which we could respond better if we were better prepared to do so..." (House of Commons 2021: 23). This could be an avenue to explore elsewhere; in France as well, given the multiplicity of agencies (Agences Régionales de Santé) and lack of coordination experienced during the first wave of the pandemic (Assemblée Nationale 2020:27).

A more centralized system can also optimize the management of resources. In France, it was possible to quickly transfer patients from the overstretched hospitals of the East and Ile de France to hospitals in other parts of the country with greater capacity. In Italy, healthcare itself is not centralized, so such transfers were less common. Later on, transfers between European countries took place to ease overwhelmed sites. In New York City, although a lot of collaboration took place between hospitals (particularly for those affiliated to health systems), there was a lack of coordination across the state. The state government did not enable or facilitate the transfer of patients to other parts of the state where capacity existed.

12.3.2 Consistency and Transparency

Even in the European context a more centralized system did not always come with more consistency. In Brussels, for example, a study of three hospitals with three different triage protocols showed that survival did in some cases depend on which hospital people went to. The allocation of resources was more heterogeneous than expected, even if age remained the most salient criteria in most places. "Protocols kept changing daily, that was hard" (resident, New York); "As caregivers and citizens, we had a hard time living with so many contradictory and daily changing recommendations which were not in fact driven by scientific knowledge" (Dr. S. Crozier, Paris). In New York, critical care directors spoke to the lack of consistency between plans made at the local hospital level and at the health system level. They also stated that plans were often too theoretical and not operational enough. There was room for improvement in getting more input from clinicians. Contrary to many existing resource allocation frameworks in the USA, the critical care teams in New York City argued that a triage committee would be cumbersome and too slow in a real-life context (Toner et al. 2020). They advocated a more European model of bedside decision involving the treating physician and other physicians to make the best decision for the immediate patient in the context of the status of resources if there was adequate situational awareness and education of the clinician about CSC policy. Organizational leaders and government officials need to support physicians and other clinicians by recognizing their expertise not just during but before planning for public health crises, and protecting them from harm.

Though it is almost impossible to develop a clinical scoring system without bias, there needs to be clarity and consistency (Orfali 2021b) on the protocols in place at all levels when triage decisions have to be made. Any triage plan has also to be communicated clearly to families and the public in a situation of resource scarcity. There has to be "an ethical consensus to safeguard the societal cohesion which today we are starting to question" (Hirsch 2020). Though there has been an avalanche of publications regarding triaging plans worldwide, we still do not know what guidelines, if any, were really in use at the bedside at the peak of the pandemic. Empirical research has to be done to understand the failures or success of managing these tragic situations for future pandemic planning. For example, is insulating 'clinical judgement' from any social consideration after all the best option, as mostly defended by European clinicians? Evaluating the application of the different protocols can help shed light on what could be the least bad option in a scarcity situation such as experienced in the first wave.

12.3.3   Support for HCP: from Moral Distress to Moral Injury

HCPs were exposed to COVID-19 on a dramatic scale. In the UK alone, during the first peak of the pandemic between March and May 2020, the Office for National Statistics recorded 760 deaths of people working in care—nearly twice the average during the same period from 2014 to 2019. In addition to facing the high risk of infection, many HCPs and especially the younger ones were troubled by the unprecedented number of deaths they were experiencing, particularly in the most hard-hit places. When the pandemic ravaged different countries, starting with Italy, frontline physicians in Lombardy were begging "not to be alone facing difficult choices".[7] The emotional toll of the pandemic on HCPs is now well recognized worldwide, with a wealth of studies on post-traumatic stress syndrome and moral distress. Yet, given the dramatic shortage of resources during the first wave, the absence of family support for inpatients, particularly at the end of life, the high risk and fear of infection, and the uncertainty around an unknown disease, many frontline HCPs have been forced to make tragic decisions or to suffer the consequences of unbearable situations over which they had no power. This specific part of the frontline HCP's dramatic experience—the so-called 'moral injury' (MI)—they have experienced in unexpected high-stake situations has been less studied. MI (Koenig and Al Zaben 2021) is a common syndrome described among veterans and military personal. It is defined as a "deep sense of transgression including feelings of shame, grief, meaninglessness, and remorse from having violated core moral beliefs" (Brock and Lettini 2012); and also as "a betrayal of what's right".

Was it possible to alleviate the pain and trauma, particularly regarding tragic choices? The Hopkins Report (Toner et al., 2020) suggests that there was no time really to process the stress during the wave but reported that, in one place, the inclusion of a trauma psychologist afterwards helped to normalize the psychological stress. In several European countries, psychologists are routinely part of the ICU team and can help with coping skills. In the US, clinical ethicists have often played a similar role and lately support for mental health of HCPs has finally been taken into account at the federal level. In any case, there needs to be an additional support mechanism in place to address moral distress and support HCPs through forced choices both during the crisis and afterwards.

---

[7]   *La Repubblica*, March 2020.

Another important feature is the *legal shield* needed for HCPs, as they have to confront shortages and scarcity, altering the standard of care. Adhering to crisis standards of care in the USA may expose healthcare providers and entities to considerable costs and burdens, including the risk of both civil and criminal liability. Liability shields may be necessary when, due to the circumstances of the emergency, a state faces scarce resources and activates its crisis standards of care. There needs, however, to be a specific ethical oversight in such circumstances.

12.3.4 The Role of Experts

Many political leaders announced their adherence to a science-led policy and publicly identified (and praised) the experts on whom they relied (Cairney and Wellstead 2020). The public often trusted the experts more than their leaders. Yet there were no universally informed experts for COVID-19 decisions. That has been obvious in many instances. In the early days many experts downplayed the severity of the virus. SAGE (the Scientific Advisory Group for Emergencies) in the UK, stated, for example, on March 3, 2020, "that there is currently no evidence that cancelling large events would be effective", which led to stalling lockdown decisions until March 23 (SAGE 2020). Had they done so a week earlier, the death toll would have been reduced by at least by half according to Niall Fergusson.[8] The most astonishing aspect has been the incredible reluctance of experts to recognize the need for mask wearing early on—one of the most obvious and simple means to reduce transmission. Despite the example of Italy suggesting to citizens that they protect themselves, even with a cloth due to mask shortage, it was not until early June that SAGE advised the UK government to announce the need to wear masks. In France, the head of the scientific advisory body for the pandemic, Professor J–F. Delfraissy, when asked why he had not recommended mask wearing, responded, "because there was a shortage of them". Similarly, while A. Fauci, along with several other US health leaders, initially advised people not to wear masks, he later said that he was concerned that there wouldn't be enough protective equipment for healthcare workers. In Sweden, an outlier regarding COVID-19 management, the whole country relied exclusively (Pierre 2020) on the state epidemiologist Anders Tegnell and his vision of 'herd immunity' with the least restrictive measures possible, avoiding any draconian policies in pandemic times. Subsequent analysis indicates that Swedish mortality would have more than halved had they adopted the Danish or even the UK policies (Mishra et al. 2021). The role of experts has been ambivalent in terms of advising governments and even the public during the pandemic due to resource

---

[8] *The Economist*, June 20, 2020, p. 24.

scarcity, uncertainty around the disease, and a misguided political desire to reassure the public. Paradoxically, experts themselves have too often provided recommendations born out of political expediency rather than science. Unclear or misleading information increases public suspicion towards the authorities.

These few examples show that expertise and politics are often too intertwined, and we should advocate stronger independence for experts in health agencies from politics. Additionally, procedures to report political meddling in health agencies should also be addressed (Stephenson 2022), as demonstrated in the recent GAO report in the USA (Scientific Integrity 2022). There might be a lesson to be learned here: avoid having experts being used for purposes out of their realm. By claiming to follow science and the experts, governments tend to avoid accountability.

In a situation of uncertainty, reliance on data-based evidence is problematic, but real-time data sharing at an international level should be paramount. Experts claim authority that most non-scientists cannot independently evaluate. By international collaboration and immediate systematic peer reviewing of what was going on at the most local levels of communities and through networks, experts are also under peer scrutiny, which could make their advice more 'objective'. Sweden, for example, relied heavily on one scientific approach only, with the result indicated above.

12.3.5 Accountability, Transparency, and Ethics

There cannot be any social closure, confidence in authorities and governments, or preparation for future pandemics without a clear and honest inquiry and review in each country of what really happened. Sociologist Lee Clarke (1999: 8) observes: "crises, disasters and scandals result in public disquiet and in loss of confidence in the body of politics. Confidence can be effectively restored only by thoroughly investigating and establishing the truth and exposing the facts to public scrutiny". Accountability has the essential function of restoring, maintaining, and building trust. Early on, there have been many calls for a public inquiry into different national responses to COVID-19: in the UK (McKee, Martin, et al. 2020; Calvert and Arbuthnott 2021), in Spain from physicians (García-Basteiro et al. 2020), and so on. Several governments (UK, France, and Sweden for example) and states in the USA have had to start investigating their own response to the COVID pandemic and reviewing dysfunctions through parliamentary commissions or others to improve future pandemic management (AAPG 2021; Comptes rendus de la Commission d'Enquête du Sénat 2020; Hall 2020). There has to be at this point rapid feedback to allow for better future governance (Boin et al. 2020). There is a need for a systematic evaluation of decision-making. I focus mostly here on the issue of allocation of scarce resources, a difficult topic for governments to explicitly acknowledge and most often driven by litigation (Jacquin et al.2020), the media, and public pressure.

In France, the prevailing norm seems to still be secrecy regarding the reality of triaging despite increasing examples of litigation from distraught families and some media accounts. Yet, in one of the auditions of the Senate investigating the French response to the pandemic, the coordinator for Ethics at the APHP, Dr. S. Crozier (2020), clearly acknowledged it: "I want to specify that the prioritization of patients during the crisis did take place. It would be wrong and dishonest to deny it. In reality, the true ethical question is: on what criteria did we make these choices? How can we justify them? We should analyze now the past experiences and eventually the lost opportunities for some people." She added: "Why didn't we admit the lack of means? Was it more dangerous to tell the truth? Why did we hide the situation? What would have been the consequence of revealing the situation of scarcity?"[9]

In France, families have created associations such as "Coronavictimes" after one of their members had been turned down by SAMU (the French EMS) and left to die at home or in nursing homes. But even the different commissions investigating the management of the pandemic, while acknowledging that there was de facto triage due to shortage situations, will hardly recognize that there were written official recommendations to do so. In the UK, recently, the government was held liable for the death of nursing home residents because asymptomatic COVID-19 persons were returned to these homes,infecting frail elderly people. More than 20,000 residents, elderly or disabled, died between March and June 2020 in these homes.

Ethical input (Dunham et al. 2020) and transparency at all levels, not only in anticipation but during crisis, can help make difficult choices more acceptable (Fischkoff et al. 2020). In the UK, the ongoing ethical debates pointed to the need to make explicit political decisions which the government wanted to avoid. The noninvolvement of ethics during the crisis in France (Hirsch 2022), such as the refusal of the authorities to include lay citizens despite calls from the head of the Scientific Board for COVID-19, Professor Delfraissy, will now impact public opinion, when litigations and investigations reveal what really happened. Ethics should not be reduced to mere psychological support or to some humanistic sugarcoating; it must be integrated within larger frameworks of planning for future situations of scarcity. Because there are multiple ethically permissible approaches to allocating scarce life-sustaining resources (see Dominic Wilkinson's Chapter 10 in this volume), and because the public will bear the consequences of these decisions, the knowledge of public perspectives and moral points of reference on these issues is critical. Policymakers should involve communities (Daugherty et al. 2018) to identify values and principles that should guide any rationing. The

---

[9] Commission d'Enquête du Sénat, Sept.2020.

whole process should be transparent, efficient, and accountable in the eyes of public (Orfali 2021a).

12.3.6 Trust

An important reason for trust being generally seen as a critical factor in managing a pandemic is probably the extensive research showing that trust is an important condition for a society to function well (Fukuyama 1995; Yamagishi 2011). Trust in science, first, and secondly trust in government were consistently found to have positive and significant effects during the pandemic (Reiersen et al. 2022). Trust increases the public's tolerance of uncertainty and reduces the perception of unanticipated complexity of possible events. It is, of course, difficult for any government to obtain public support for any form of triage, but interestingly while the dialysis utilitarian triage in the early days led to a public outcry, the penicillin shortage of 1943 for civilians in the US was accepted because it was based on absolutely egalitarian access in a time of war. A triage panel in each hospital decided such allocation.

However, trust is a fairly stable variant and, in a time of crisis, it is difficult to suddenly build up trust *ex nihilo*. It must be developed before the crisis. Shared moral values are asserted in a normal context and will impact what is acceptable or not in a given society, including in the abnormal context of a disaster. In fact, trust means that there is a confident expectation that all people involved will act competently and dutifully. Pre-existing trust in Scandinavian countries led to a greater acceptance of different choices: Denmark versus Sweden with its risky course of action at the time. In Sweden the controversial response to the pandemic did lead to criticism within the country, and support for the policy decreased with the knowledge of the heavy death toll among the elderly population (Anderson et al. 2021). However, it did not really erode the prevailing trust in the authorities (SOU 2022:102).

12.4 Conclusion

The more a given society is structurally unequal, the more there is a lack of trust in the authorities and little expectation of justice. Therefore, there has to be a clear and explicit mechanism to ethically justify and legitimate any process that could aggravate these inequalities. The reverse is also true for countries with less inequality and greater access to healthcare; there is an implicit assumption that the state or the authorities will provide the least harmful triage process. Yet at this point there is a clear need for more information and understanding of the pandemic to get the complete story of what really happened and a need for serious empirical work rather than limited and scattered information on how physicians or others allocated and performed bedside rationing.

On an optimistic note: will this pandemic lead to 'emancipatory catastrophism' (Beck 2015), creating new systems, more justice, and 'cosmopolitan' respect for others? Never before has the world experienced such a crisis at the same time. Never before has there been so much scientific collaboration and interconnectivity across the world. In fact, according to a new report (Wellcome Global Monitor 2020), trust in science and in each country's scientists has increased 9% since 2018; unsurprisingly, doctors and nurses also get a high score. Some countries have denied or lied about the reality of the pandemic; many have advocated nationalization of supply chains, but most countries have attempted to share information and have had to expose their dramatic situation. In Beck's view, disasters and potentially catastrophic risks generate new normative horizons, specifically the emergence of 'global justice frames' (Beck 2015). He applied his view to climate and environmental risk; however, it seems that the pandemic, 'a global risk', has brought a unique 'process of metamorphosis of the world' no longer embedded in traditional boundaries but a "change in the frame of reference of change". Let's hope this is the future that will apply to Pandemic X.

Bibliography

AAPG (All Party Parliamentary Group) (2021), *The Long COVID Report*, March 2022; *The Public Inquiry Report* (October 2021), https://www.appgcoronavirus.uk/

Aeron, J., and Muelbauer, J. (2020), 'Mortality Rate from COVID-19 Is Substantially Worse Than Europe's', *VoxEU*, 29/09.

Andersson, O., Campos-Mercad, P., Wengstrom, E. (2021), 'Attityder och beteende under COVID pandemin', *Ekonomiskdebatt*, 6(49): 1–18.

Andino, J.J., Dupree, J., Jensen, C., et al. (2020), 'COVID and CopMich, comparing and contrasting COVID-19 experiences in the USA and in Scandinavia, Nature Reviews', *Urology*, 17: 493–8.

Assemblée Nationale (2020), 'Mission d'information sur l'impact, la gestion et les conséquences dans toutes ses dimensions de l'épidémie de Coronavirus-COVID-19 en France', *Rapport N° 3053*, https://www2.assemblee-nationale.fr/15/missions-d-information/missions-d-information-de-la-conference-des-presidents/impact-gestion-et-consequences-dans-toutes-ses-dimensions-de-l-epidemie-de-coronavirus-COVID-19/(block)/76900/(instance_leg)/15/(init)/0-15.

Baker, M., and Fink, S. (2020), 'At the top of the COVID -19 curve: how do hospitals decide who gets treatment', *New York Times*, March 31, 2020.

Barré, I., and Liffran, H. (2022), 'COVID: un hôpital à corps et a tri', *Canard Enchaîné*, January 12, 2022.

Beck, U. (2015), 'Emancipatory catastrophism: What does it mean to climate change and risk society?' *Current Sociology*, 63(1): 75–88.

Berlinger, N., Wynia, M., Powell, T., et al. (2020), 'Ethical Framework for Health Care Institutions and Guidelines for Institutional Ethics Services Responding to the Novel Coronavirus Pandemic', *The Hastings Center*, March 16, 2020.

Blachère, E., (2020), 'Coronavirus: le rassemblement évangélique de *Mulhouse* accusé à tort. Nos révélations', *Paris-Match*, May 20, 2020.

Boin, A., McConnel,l A., and Hart, P. (2020), *Governing the Pandemic: The Politics of Navigating a Mega-Crisis* (London:Palgrave MacMillan, 2020).

British Medical Association (2020), 'COVID-19- Ethical Issues. A Guidance note', https//www.bma.org.uk.

Brock, R.N., and Lettini, G. (2012), *Soul repair: Recovering from moral injury after war* (Boston, MA: Beacon Press, 2012).

Cairney, P., and Wellstead, A. (2020), 'COVID-19: effective policy-making depends on trust in experts, politicians and the public', *Policy Design and Practice* 4/1: 1–14.

Calvert J., and Arbuthnott, G., (2021), *Failures of State: The Inside Story of Britain's Battle with Coronavirus* (London:HarperCollins, 2021).

Canard, J. (2020), 'Le suffocant bulletin de santé des EHPAD', *Canard Enchaine*, April 15, 2020.

Clarke, L. (1999), *Mission improbable: Using fantasy documents to tame disaster (Chicago:* University of Chicago Press, 1999).

Clarke R. (2020), "Do not resuscitate orders" have caused panic in the UK. Here is the truth', *The Guardian*, April 8, 2020.

Cohen, G. I., Crespo, A., White, D. B. (2020), 'Potential Legal Liability for Withdrawing or Withholding Ventilators During COVID-19. Assessing the Risks and Identifying Needed Reforms', *Jama*, 323/19: 1901–2.

Comité Consultatif National d'Éthique (2020), 'COVID-19: Contribution du CCNE: Enjeux éthiques face à une pandémie' (13 March) 4, 9, https://www.ccne-ethique.fr/.

Commonwealth of Massachusetts (2020), 'Crisis Standards of Care: Planning Guidance for the COVID-19 Pandemic', 04/7, https://d279m997dpfwgl.cloudfront.net/wp/2020/04/CSC_April-7_2020.pdf.

Comptes rendus de la Commission d'Enquête du Sénat. (2020), 'Evaluation des Politiques Publiques face aux Pandémies', October 14, 2020, http://www.senat.fr/commission/enquete/gestion_de_la_crise_sanitaire.html

Crozier, S. (2020), 'Audition, Table Ronde', in *Comptes rendus de la Commission d'Enquête du Sénat.*

Daugherty, B., E. Lee, Howard S. Gwon, Monica Schoch-Spana, Alan C. Regenberg, Chrissie Juliano, Ruth R. Faden, and Eric S. Toner. (2018), 'Scarce Resource Allocation During Disasters A Mixed-Method Community Engagement Study', *Chest* 153 (1): 187–95.

Dunham, A., Rieder, T., and Hymbryd, C. (2020), 'A bioethical perspective for navigating moral dilemmas amidst the COVID-19 pandemic', *Journal of the American Academy of Orthopedic Surgeons*, 28(11): 471–6.

Du Ponta, D., and Baren, J. (2020), 'Ambulance Charters during the COVID-19 Pandemic and Equitable Access to Scarce Resources', *AJOB*, 20(10): 7–9.

Dyrbye, L., et al. (2019), 'A cross-sectional study exploring the relationship between burnout, absenteeism, and job performance among American nurses', *BMC Nursing* 18: 57.

Emanuel, E.J., Govind, P., Ross, U., et al. (2020), 'Fair Allocation of Scarce Medical Resources in the Time of COVID-19', *New England Journal of Medicine*: 382: 2049–55.

Farrell, C. M., Hayward, B. J. (2022), 'Ethical Dilemmas, Moral Distress, and the Risk of Moral Injury: Experiences of Residents and Fellows During the COVID-19 Pandemic in the United States', *Academic Medicine*, 97(3S): S55–S60.

Fins, J. J., and Prager, K. (2020), 'The COVID-19 Crisis and Clinical Ethics in New York City', *Journal of Clinical Ethics*, 31(3): 228–32.

Fischkoff, K., Neuberg, G., Dastidar, J., Williams, E.P., Prager, K., and Dugdale, L. (2020), 'Clinical Ethics Consultations During the COVID-19 Pandemic at a New York City Medical Center', *Journal of Clinical Ethics*, 31(3): 212–18.

Fukuyama, F. (1995), *Trust. The Social Virtues and the Creation of Prosperity* (New York, NY: Free Press, 1995).

García-Basteiro, A., Alvarez-Dardet, C., Arenas, C., et al. (2020), 'The need for an independent evaluation of the COVID-19 response in Spain', *The Lancet*, 396(10250): 529–30.

Global Health and Security Index (2019), www.ghsindex.org/wp-content/uploads/2020/04/2019-Global-Health-Security-Index.pdf.

Guidet B., Vallet H., Boddaert J., et al. (2018), 'Caring for the critically ill patients over 80: a narrative review', *Annals of Intensive Care*, 8, Article no. 114.

Gutmann Koch, V., and Han, S. A. (2020), 'COVID in NYC: What New York Did, and Should Have Done', *American Journal of Bioethics*, 20:7, 153–5.

Gwon, H., Haeri, M., Hoffmann, D. E., et al. (2020), 'Maryland's Experience With the COVID-19 Surge: What Worked, What Didn't, What Next?' *American Journal of Bioethics*, 20(7): 150–2.

Hall, B. (2020), 'Sweden Launches Inquiry into Coronavirus Handling', *Financial Times*, 30 June, 2020.

Harris J. (1985), *The Value of Life*. London: Routledge and Kegan Paul.

Hick, J. L, Hanfling, D., Wynia, M. K., and Pavia, A. T. (2020), 'Duty to Plan: Health Care, Crisis Standards of Care, and Novel Coronavirus SARS-CoV-S', Discussion Paper, National Academy of Medicine. March 5, 2020.

Hirsch, E. (2020), 'Audition, Table Ronde', in *Comptes rendus de la Commission d'Enquête du Senat*, October 14, 2020, http://www.senat.fr/commission/enquete/gestion_de_la_crise_sanitaire.html

House of Commons (2021), *Coronavirus: lessons learned to date, 6th Report of the Health and Social Care Committee and Science and Technology Committee of Session 2021–2022*, Sept. 21, 2021, https://committees.parliament.uk/publications/7496/documents/78687/default/.

Immarisio, M. (2020), 'Coronavirus, il medico di Bergamo: 'Negli ospedali siamo come in guerra. A tutti dico: state a casa', Interview of Christian Salaroli in *Corriere della Sera*, March 9, 2020.

Institute of Medicine (2009), *Guidance for establishing crisis of standards of care for use in disaster situations: a letter report*, Washington DC, National Academies Press, 2009.

Jacquin, J. B., et al. (2020), 'L'exécutif face à la menace de suites judiciaires', *Le Monde*, March 25. 2020.

Jarvie, J., (2020), 'Ethical Dilemmas in the Age of Coronavirus: whose Lives should we Save?' *Los Angeles Times*, March 19, 2020.

Kaste, M., and Herscher, R. (2020), 'Ventilator shortage looms as state ponders rule for rationing', *National Public Radio*, 04/03.

Koenig, H. G., and Al Zaben, F. (2021), 'Moral Injury: An Increasingly Recognized and Widespread Syndrome', *Journal of Religion & Health*, 60(5): 2989–3011, doi: 10.1007/s10943-021-01328-0.

Leclerc, T., Donat, N, Donat, A., Pasquier, P. Libert, N., Schaeffer, E., et al. (2020), 'Prioritization of ICU treatments for critically ill patients in a COVID-19 pandemic with scarce resources', *Anaesthesia Critical Care & Pain Medicine*, 39(3): 333–9.

Li-Vollmer, M. (2010), 'Health Care decisions in Disasters : Engaging the Public on Medical Prioritization during a Severe Influenza Pandemic'. *Journal of Participatory Medicine*, 2, Dec. 14, 2010.

McCullough, L. (2020), 'In Response to COVID-19 Pandemic Physicians Already Know What to Do', *The American Journal of Bioethics*, 20(7): 9–12.

McKee, M., Gill, M., and Wollaston, S. (2020), 'Public inquiry into UK's response to COVID-19', Editorial, *BMJ*, 369: m2052.

Maina, I. W., Belton, T. D., Ginzberg, S., Singh, A., and Johnson, T. J. (2018), 'A decade of studying implicit racial/ethnic bias in healthcare providers using the implicit association test', *Social Science & Medicine*, 199: 219–29.

Meyfroidt, G., Vlieghe, E., Biston, P., et al. (2020), 'Ethical principles concerning proportionality of critical care during the COVID-19 pandemic', Advice by the Belgian Society of Intensive Care medicine (SIZ), March 18, 2020.

Millum J., and Persad G. (2020), 'Guest Commentary: Fair Triage Guidelines Not Business as Usual, Will Save More Patients with Disabilities', *Denver Post*, April 7, 2020.

Minnesota Department of Health (2019), 'Patient Care Strategies for Scarce Resource Situations', Updated April 2019. https//www.health.state.mn.us/communities/ep/surge/crisis/standards/pdf.

Mishra, S., Scott, J. A., Laydon, J. D., et al. (2021), 'Comparing the responses of the UK, Sweden and Denmark to COVID-19 using counterfactual modelling', *Scientific Reports*,11: 16342.

Ne'eman, A. (2020), 'I will not apologize for my needs', *New York Times*, March 23, 2020.

Neuberger J, D. Adams, P. MacMaster, A. Maidment, M. Speed. (1998), Assessing priorities for allocation of donor liver grafts: survey of public and clinicians. *Bmj*; 317:172-5.

NewYork Public Health Law §3082 (2020), https://law.justia.com/codes/new-york/2020/pbh/article-30-d/3082/.

NICE (2021), 'Covid-19 rapid guidelines: managing COVID-19, NG 191', National Institute for Health and Care Excellence, London, www.nice.org.uk/guidance/ng191.

Orfali, K. (2020), 'What triage issues reveal: ethics in COVID-19 pandemic in Italy and France', *Journal of Bioethical Inquiry*, 9:1–5.

Orfali, K. (2021a), 'Getting to the Truth: Ethics, Trust, and Triage in the United States versus Europe during the COVID-19 Pandemic', *The Hastings Center Report*, January 2021.

Orfali, K. (2021b), 'Triage criteria: medically, ethically or socially defined?', *The American Journal of Bioethics*, 21(11): 77–79.

Pancevski B. (2020), 'Coronavirus Is Taking a High Toll on Sweden's Elderly. Families Blame the Government', *Wall Street Journal*, 18 June, 2020.

Pierre, J. (2020), 'Nudges against pandemics: Sweden's COVID-19 containment strategy in perspective'. *Policy and Society*, 39(3): 478–93.

Powell, T., and Chuang, E. (2020), 'COVID in NYC: What We Could Do Better', *The American Journal of Bioethics*, 20(7): 62–6.

Reiersen, J., Roll, K., Williams, J. D., and Carlsson, M. (2022), 'Trust: A Double-Edged Sword in Combating the COVID-19 Pandemic?' *Frontiers in Communication*, 7:822302.

Rosenbaum, L. (2020), 'Facing COVID-19 in Italy: Ethics, Logistics, and Therapeutics on the Epidemic's Front Line', *New England Journal of Medicine*, May 14, 2020.

Röstlund L., and Gustafson A. (2020a), 'Dokument visar vilka som inte får intensivvård', *Dagens Nyheter*, 10 April, 2020.

Röstlund L., and Gustafson A. (2020b), 'Läkare: Vi tvingas till hårda prioriteringar', *Dagens Nyheter*, 24 April, 2020.

SAGE (2020), Scientific Advisory Group for Emergencies meetings (UK), https://www.gov.uk/government/collections/sage-meetings-march-2020

Savin, K., and Guidry-Grimes, L. (2020), 'Confronting Disability Discrimination during the Pandemic', Bioethics Forum Essay, *Hastings Report*, April 2, 2020.

Scientific Integrity (2022), 'HHS Agencies Need to Develop Procedures and Train Staff on Reporting and Addressing Political Interference', US Accountability Office, Gao-22-1041613, April 20, 2022.

Schmitt, Harald (2020), 'The way we ration ventilators is biased', *New York Times*, April 15, 2020.

SFAR (2020), Société Française d'Anesthésie- Réanimation, 'Priorisation des traitements de réanimation pour les patients en état critique en situation d'épidémie de COVID-19 avec capacités limitées', April 3th, 2020.

SIAARTI (2020), Italian College of Anesthesia, Anelgesia, Resuscitation, and Intensive Care, 'Clinical ethics recommendations for the allocation of intensive care treatments, in exceptional, resource-limited circumstances', March 16, 2020.

Sorbi, M. (2020), 'Terapie intensive, il documento choc: liste dei meritoveli per essere curati', *Il Giornale.It*, March 8, 2020.

SOU. 2022:10 2. *Sverige under pandemin, Statens Offentliga Utredningar.*

Sprung, C. L., et al. (2019), 'Changes in End-of-Life Practices in European Intensive Care Units from 1999 to 2016', *Journal of the American Medical Association*, 322(17): 1692–1704.

Stepanikova, I. (2012), 'Racial-Ethnic Biases, Time Pressure and Medical Decisions', *Journal of Health & Social Behavior,* 53(3): 329–43.

Stephenson, J. (2022), 'Report Says US Health Agencies Need Better Processes to Address Political Interference', *JAMA Health Forum,* 3(4): e221534.

Stevis-Gridneff, M., et al., (2020), 'When COVID-19 Hit, Many Elderly Were Left to Die', *New York Times,* August 8, 2020.

Swiss Academy of Medical Science (2020), 'COVID-19 pandemic: triage for intensive-care treatment under resource scarcity, Guidance on the application of Section 9.3 of the SAMS Guidelines, Intensive-care interventions', March 20, 2020.

Toner, C., Mukherjee, V., Hanfling, D., et al. (2020), *Crisis Standard of Care: Lessons from New York City Hospitals COVID-19 Experience. A Meeting Report.* Johns Hopkins Center for Health Security, Nov. 2020.

Toussaint, J. F., et al., (2020), 'COVID-19 : 'nous ne voulons plus être gouvernés par la peur'. La Tribune des chercheurs et des médecins. *Le Parisien*, September 10, 2020.

Truog, C., Mitchell, C., and Daley, G. (2020), 'The toughest triage- Allocating ventilators in a pandemic', *NEJM*, 382(21): 1973–5.

Vawter, D. E., Garrett, J. E., Gervais, K. G., et al. (2010), 'For the Good of Us All: Ethically Rationing Health Resources in Minnesota in a Severe Influenza Pandemic', St. Paul, MN, Minnesota Department of Health.

Von Klaudija A. (2020), 'COVID-19 Ethik Abbildung Endfassung, 03-25', https://www.bda.de/docman/alle-dokumente-fuer-suchindex/oeffentlich/aktuelles-1/2027-COVID-19-ethik-abbildung-endfassung-2020-03-25/file.html.

Wellcome Global Monitor (2020), COVID-19, Report, Nov.29, 2021, https://wellcome.org/reports/wellcome-global-monitor-covid-19/2020.

White, D. B., and Lo, B. (2020), 'A Framework for Rationing Ventilators and Critical Care Beds During the COVID-19 Pandemic', *JAMA* 323(18): 1773–4.

Yamagishi, T. (2011), *Trust. The Evolutionary Game of Mind and Society* (London: Springer, 2011).

PART IV

PANDEMIC EQUALITY AND INEQUALITY

13

Ethical Hotspots in Infectious Disease Surveillance for Global Health Security

Social Justice and Pandemic Preparedness

Michael Parker

At the time of writing, the world remains in the grip of the COVID-19 pandemic. Approximately 14.9 million people have died and every country in the world has been affected directly or indirectly (WHO 2022a). This, together with recent experiences of Ebola and Zika, has led to calls for the development and implementation of international strategies for pandemic preparedness, response, and prevention. An Independent Panel established by the Director-General of WHO has called for

> ...a fundamental transformation designed to ensure commitment at the highest level to a new system that is co-ordinated, connected, fast-moving, accountable, just, and equitable – in other words, a complete pandemic preparedness and response system on which citizens can rely to keep them safe and healthy.
>
> (WHO Independent Panel 2021: 4)

World leaders have proposed a 'new international treaty for pandemic preparedness and response', arguing that,

> Today, we hold the...hope that as we fight to overcome the COVID-19 pandemic together, we can build a more robust international health architecture that will protect future generations. There will be other pandemics and other major health emergencies. No single government or multilateral agency can address this threat alone. The question is not if, but when. Together, we must be better prepared to predict, prevent, detect, assess and effectively respond to pandemics in a highly coordinated fashion. The COVID-19 pandemic has been a stark and painful reminder that nobody is safe until everyone is safe.
>
> (Bainimarama et al. 2021)

These calls have been supported by leading public health scientists (Khor and Heymann 2021; Duff et al. 2021), and philanthropists (Gates 2022). Such calls are,

Michael Parker, *Ethical Hotspots in Infectious Disease Surveillance for Global Health Security: Social Justice and Pandemic Preparedness* In: *Pandemic Ethics: From COVID-19 to Disease X.* Edited by: Dominic Wilkinson and Julian Savulescu, Oxford University Press. © Oxford University Press 2023. DOI: 10.1093/oso/9780192871688.003.0014

of course, not new (Fidler 1996). However, at the time of writing, the WHO is indeed coordinating work on a new pandemic treaty (WHO 2022b).

13.1 Requirements for Effective Pandemic Preparedness

The factors implicated in the emergence of new infectious diseases with pandemic potential are increasingly well understood. Most new pathogens are zoonotic, having their origins in shifts from transmission between animals—wildlife and livestock—to transmission among humans (G20 Independent Panel 2021). Relatively recent examples of infectious diseases with zoonotic origins include three new coronaviruses, a number of new and highly pathogenic influenza viruses, Zika, and Ebola (Carroll et al. 2021). The emergence of these pathogens and their transformation into human infectious diseases with pandemic potential are increasingly being driven by intensified land use, environmental degradation, and urbanization, and are further enhanced by significant economic and social inequalities, climate change, and increased global connectedness (Carroll et al 2021).

Taken together, this suggests five possible courses of action which together might be required for an effective model of pandemic preparedness. The first might be thought of as *preventative*. This would include actions of various kinds aimed at creating the conditions in which zoonotic transmission is less likely to happen. This would include policies to encourage moves away from (the harmful aspects of) current farming and land use practices, and interventions to halt and reverse processes of environmental degradation. A second cluster of actions might be thought of as *containment, mitigation*, and *suppression*, an approach called for most recently by the WHO Independent Panel (WHO Independent Panel 2021). This would include surveillance-informed interventions aimed at elimination. A third requirement is going to be *health system strengthening and resilience* to ensure that health services are sufficiently robust to cope with the additional pressures of an epidemic/pandemic (G20 Independent Panel 2021). A fourth would be the building and maintaining of sustainable infrastructure, scientific resources, and economic arrangements for *rapid production and equitable distribution of diagnostics, therapeutics, and vaccines*. The fifth would be the development of regulations and agreed practices to protect the effectiveness of existing drugs through *coordinated action to address antimicrobial resistance (AMR)*.

This list is not intended to be comprehensive or particularly fine-grained. Its purpose is to map out in broad terms the range and scale of interventions likely to be needed as part of any effective global approach to pandemic preparedness. All of these interventions are interconnected and interdependent. For example, increasing success in *prevention* would make efforts in *containment, mitigation, and suppression* more effective, as would the development of more *resilient health systems*, and *coordinated action to address AMR*.

13.1.1 The Central Role of Surveillance

The majority of the remainder of this chapter will focus on the role of infectious disease surveillance in informing containment, mitigation, and suppression. Calls for more effective infectious disease surveillance and intelligence have been particularly prominent in the light of the COVID-19 pandemic and Zika and Ebola prior to this, and a central role has been claimed for surveillance in recent high-level calls for action on pandemic preparedness. For example, the WHO Independent Panel urges

> …WHO to establish a new global system for surveillance, based on full transparency by all parties, using state-of-the-art digital tools to connect information centres around the world and including animal and environmental health surveillance, with appropriate protections of people's rights.
>
> (WHO Independent Panel 2021: 53)

As did an independent panel established by the G20:

> We must prioritize installing a global genomic and epidemiological surveillance program within the next five years to prevent and detect cross-species spillovers and to rapidly share data.   (G20 Independent Panel 2021: 32)

These calls echo those made by many leading scientists in the area:

> Key to these efforts is building a surveillance system that spans wildlife, livestock, and human populations. Such a system would use known geographical 'hotspots' for early detection of any viral transfer into human and livestock populations, and pre-emptively disrupt further transmission of the virus locally.
>
> (Carroll et al 2021: 2)

In addition to its prominence in post-COVID calls for pandemic preparedness, a second reason for my focus on surveillance in this chapter is that programmes of infectious disease surveillance—particularly when combined with measures for containment, mitigation, and suppression—raise problems of social justice in a particularly acute way. This suggests that an exploration of the moral and political significance of requirements for effective surveillance may offer an interesting and productive starting point for thinking about questions of justice in pandemic preparedness more broadly. It also has the potential to offer a perspective from which to reflect upon the implications of different conceptualizations of 'global health security'.

13.1.2 What Does Surveillance Entail for Those who Are Surveilled?

Given the scientific consensus that almost all pandemics have their origins in wildlife and that their transmission to humans 'involve[s] dynamic interactions between wildlife, livestock and people, within rapidly changing environments' (Daszak et al. 2007), an effective surveillance system will need to be capable of spanning wildlife, livestock, and human populations (Carroll et al. 2021). A particularly important focus will be the 'biosecurity of the wild-life domestic animal interface' (Zinstag et al. 2020). A central feature of any such system would be routine viral surveillance of humans and animals to enable early detection of spillover from wildlife into livestock and humans. This involves collecting and analysing data about viruses in wildlife, livestock, and humans in ways that are sufficiently intensive and rapid to be capable of identifying such spillover in real time to anticipate and interrupt high-consequence epidemics and pandemics (Carroll et al. 2021:3).

An important component of this early warning system is going to be the sequencing of pathogen genomes and the identification and analysis of transmission networks. The value of this was illustrated in Ebola, where

[a] recent analysis of 1,610 Ebola virus genomes – approximately 5% of all cases – reconstructs the movement of the virus across West Africa and reveals drivers of its spread.   (Gardy and Loman 2017: 12)

Such approaches were also used effectively in response to Zika (Worobey 2017) and in COVID-19 (Viana et al. 2022). The achievement of this kind of analysis, particularly in the context of outbreaks, depends in turn upon fast, affordable sequencing of pathogen genomes directly from collected samples with portable sequencing platforms (Gardy and Loman 2017). To be effective, at scale and in remote locations, this in turn is going to depend upon better techniques for recovering and analysing viral genetic material from low-quality samples (Worobey 2017).

When it comes to human health, viral surveillance will need to be supplemented by the routine analysis of other forms of health-related information. This will include the collection and real-time sharing of information from routine medical sources such as clinical reports, notifiable diseases reporting systems, laboratory reports, pathology results, diseases registries, and death records (Morse 2007). It will also need to be supplemented by other forms of health-related data sometimes referred to as 'syndromic'. These include pharmacy records, ambulance calls information, data on absences from work, and emergency department records (Morse 2007):

> Most modern surveillance systems use human, animal, environmental and other data to carry out disease-specific surveillance, in which a single disease is monitored through one or more data streams, such as positive laboratory test results or reportable communicable disease notifications....Syndromic surveillance systems might leverage unique data streams such as school or employee absenteeism, grocery store or pharmacy purchases of specific items or calls to a nursing hotline as signal of illness in a population. Increasingly, digital streams are being used as an input to these systems [including] the automated analysis of trending words or phrases on social media sites...such as Twitter.
>
> (Gardy and Loman 2017: 14)

Beyond animal and human health, an effective surveillance system will also need to be capable of monitoring and analysing environmental degradation, infrastructure developments such as major road programmes, increases in farming activity, and changes to smallholder livestock practices and live animal markets (Zinstag et al. 2020). Much of this will involve the use of drones and satellite imagery. Patterns of human movement can also be identified and analysed using mobile phone data or the 'patterns of city lights at night' (Gardy and Loman 2017: 15). This is important because it is possible that by using such sources of information, including, 'monitoring sewage, social media, mobility data, or crowdsourced reports, we can identify threats much faster than the traditional microbiology surveillance system did' (Davies et al. 2021).

Any successful surveillance strategy with these highly complex, diverse, and contextual sources of data is going to need to find ways to combine national, regional, and global data in a way that is fast, accurate, and globally coordinated and connected. This will involve the development of sophisticated digital tools, novel methods of analysis including the application of machine learning and artificial intelligence, and cutting-edge informatics resources (WHO Independent Panel 2021). It will also require the development of secure and effective forms of data storage and capacity building to ensure that there are skills, institutions, and experience locally to successfully engage with the data including training and the provision of necessary IT support and resources. The effectiveness of global coordination and cooperation in the context of a great many different data formats and sources depends crucially upon the agreement and implementation of shared international data standards. The data systems will need to be interoperable and compatible. An important component of this is going to be the development and sharing of 'standardised case definitions for influenza-like illnesses and severe acute respiratory influenza' (Carroll et al 2021: 3). Meaningful scientific work across multiple diverse settings depends crucially upon shared disease definitions and practices of classification. There is a need for worldwide coordination of data standards and systems, and for the appropriate training and retraining of clinicians and health officials (Morse 2007).

The technical and data harmonization requirements are daunting. However, even well-curated data are not useful unless they are shared. Perhaps most importantly of all, therefore, it will be crucial to achieve high-level international agreement about the *importance* of sharing data. It is vital that those who direct health information systems relating to wildlife, livestock, and humans are committed to sharing knowledge, information, and diagnoses (Morse 2007). There needs to be real-time sharing of samples and of data, including data on new pathogens and genomic sequences (Haseltine 2021; G20 Independent Panel 2021). Enhanced molecular diagnosis and surveillance capacity are only going to be effective if they are coupled with agreed and supported open-data principles and platforms, and data-sharing frameworks (Gardy and Loman 2017). And this in turn depends upon the establishment of governance systems capable of achieving the well-founded trust and confidence of publics and of governments and scientists in very different parts of the world.

13.1.3 A Global Focus on the Local: Where Will Surveillance Actually Happen?

Despite the rhetoric, the reality is that global infectious disease surveillance is unlikely to be truly global. An effective pandemic preparedness surveillance system will be one in which particular attention is paid to known geographical 'hotspots' for any viral transfer from wildlife into human and livestock populations and to pre-emptive disruption of any further transmission of the virus locally (Carroll et al. 2021: 2). As described above, the factors creating the greatest risk of spillover from wildlife to livestock and ultimately into humans are well known (Allen 2017). They include recent demographic changes and environmental degradation, increasing farming activity, and high wildlife diversity (particularly among mammals) (Jones et al. 2008). The evidence suggests that the focus of surveillance activities will need to be on locations fitting this description in Africa, Latin America, and Asia (Jones et al. 2008: 992).

The establishment of an effective infectious disease surveillance system will turn hotspots within these regions and the populations living and working within them into some of the most highly surveilled, mapped, and intervened-upon people and communities in the world in the interests of the health of the global population. Data sharing and the analysis of data may well be a global endeavour. However, the vast majority of the data will come from these regions. Those who are the objects of surveillance for pandemic prevention will almost exclusively be those living and working in places with the characteristics listed above. That is, they will mostly be poor and living on the margins. What does this mean for people living and working in these regions?

13.2 Global Justice and Infectious Disease Surveillance

Broadly speaking, justice questions relating to pandemics might be said to arise in two quite different ways. There are questions arising in the context of pandemic response. These include considerations of the equitable distribution of vaccines, the impacts of non-pharmaceutical interventions such as 'lockdowns' on already disadvantaged groups and individuals, the need to decide how to prioritize between prevention of health risks and the impact of school closures on life chances of children, and so on. These kinds of questions have become very familiar during the current COVID-19 pandemic. The discussion above, however, suggests another domain in which important and urgent questions of justice arise. Partly driven by technological and scientific developments and partly by post-COVID calls for action, it is increasingly clear that important questions in social justice, and in ethics more broadly, also arise with respect to the impacts of pandemic preparedness and prevention in the periods between pandemics. Infectious disease surveillance is a particularly important example.

The achievement of a world free of, or effectively protected from, emerging infectious diseases with pandemic potential would be good for everyone. As we have all seen and to differing degrees learnt from experience during COVID-19, such diseases have the potential for devastating impact on well-being, and particularly on those who are already disadvantaged and do not have access to effective health systems. So too do the measures—such as lockdowns—introduced to address their spread. The emergence of infectious diseases is a profound threat to all and is particularly so to those who are already disadvantaged. Against this backdrop, the need for establishment of an effective system of infectious disease surveillance is of great urgency and moral importance.

13.2.1 Pandemic Preparedness as a Collective Action Problem

The mapping out above of the requirements for effective pandemic preparedness, and in particular those for effective emerging infectious disease surveillance, has highlighted the scale and complexity of this hugely important task. Solutions need to be found, but the demands of achieving these are not going to be easy to meet, even for well-meaning people and states. The securing of a world free of, or effectively protected from, infectious diseases with pandemic potential cannot be achieved by individuals and/or single states (Bainimarama et al. 2021). This is not only because of the complexity and scale of the problem but also because, although its achievement would be good for everyone, those actors whose actions are essential to its success have other competing interests. It is a situation in which all—individuals, institutions, nations—would be better off through collaboration but where competing values, commitments, and interests make such collaboration unlikely.

At the level of the state, a truly effective global health surveillance system will require countries to relinquish some aspects of national sovereignty. There may be legitimate worries about the possibility that information sharing will present risks to national security. Information about infectious disease risk may affect tourism and other aspects of the national economy, as might imposed changes in farming practices. Sharing information may have the potential to affect public and international perception of the competence of the government. And in some cases, it may be judged contrary to the national interest for marginal regions and the situation of those who live there to be visible at all. Tensions are also likely to arise for individuals, families, and communities. Changes in farming practices, control on uses of antibiotics, regulation of animal markets, and controls on land use, for example, may all have the potential to undermine the livelihoods of those who are already living in poverty (OUCRU 2016). The collection, sharing, and analysing of this data and its use in the design, targeting and implementation of strategies for containment, mitigation, and suppression may well all have negative impacts on farmers, communities, and families living in hotspots.

Its potential as a tool for avoiding or controlling the emergence of infectious diseases with epidemic or pandemic potential means that there is good prima facie reason for countries and citizens to collaborate to achieve effective surveillance. This is, however, a problem the solution to which cannot be found in appeal to the interests of individual states, communities, and farmers. It is a complex and very demanding cluster of collective action problems.

13.2.2 Infectious Disease Surveillance as a Global Public Good

What kinds of obligations might the value of surveillance be said to generate for individuals, states, and international bodies? One way of grounding reasons to participate in interventions of this and similar kinds is to understand them as global public goods (Kaul et al. 1999). The concept of the global public good aims to solve collective action problems of this kind by explaining why coordinated action is required (to those who would otherwise think in market terms, focus on the moral obligations of individuals, or be motivated by narrower, more local concerns). It is a useful reminder that the value of many important goods cannot be understood or realized individually, or even in terms of the interests of individual states. A global public good is defined by Kaul, Grunberg, and Stern as one that is non-rivalrous in consumption, non-exclusionary, and of global importance. The sustainable achievement of a world free (or at least well protected) from the emergence of infectious diseases with epidemic or pandemic potential clearly meets all of the requirements of a global public good. It is non-rivalrous in consumption because the fact that one person benefits from a world free of or protected from such diseases does not mean that others cannot. It is non-exclusionary because, wherever they are in the world, people cannot easily be excluded from the benefits of a world free from such diseases. Finally, a world free of or well protected from diseases with pandemic potential is undoubtedly of profound global importance (Khor and Heymann 2021: e357).

Does the fact that a world free of or effectively protected from infectious diseases with pandemic potential meets the requirements of a global public good mean that an effective system of infectious disease surveillance also meets them? Infectious disease surveillance cannot by itself do all the work of effective pandemic preparedness or prevention. It needs to be combined with resilient health systems, preventative actions—e.g. reducing/reversing environmental degradation—rapid production and distribution of vaccines, diagnostics, and therapeutics, and so on. Surveillance is nonetheless an essential requirement for the achievement of a profoundly important global public good.

13.3 Surveillance and Social Justice

The concept of a global public good is a useful way of highlighting the fact that pandemic preparedness and response are best thought of as morally significant public health goals unachievable through the actions of individuals or single states. What is doing the ethical work here is not the mere fact that surveillance requires collective action but that its achievement has important implications for well-being. The establishment of an effective and sustainable surveillance system is a necessary condition for successful pandemic preparedness and for the achievement of conditions necessary for flourishing lives. A world free of infectious diseases with pandemic potential is one in which it is more likely that basic needs will be met. The key role of surveillance in promoting and protecting the well-being of the most disadvantaged provides good reason to collaborate and also generates important obligations for all, including those living in emerging infectious disease hotspots. Surveillance, even if combined with effective containment, mitigation, and suppression, will clearly not *guarantee* flourishing lives. However, it is clear that without these measures flourishing lives will be harder to sustain. This provides the basis of a strong obligation on states and individuals to participate in pandemic preparedness.

The moral importance of effective efforts at pandemic preparedness and prevention cannot be overstated. States, international organizations, institutions, and individuals with the opportunity to make a difference all have important obligations to contribute to its achievement. But what is owed to those who live and work on the infectious disease surveillance front line and whose contribution is likely to be central? This is an important moral question because the burdens on those living in infectious disease hotspots are likely to be significant. Although calls for action on infectious disease surveillance have tended to focus on the roles of states and international bodies, the reality is that its successful achievement will require action—and sacrifices—primarily from people living in these regions. Importantly, those who are going to be the focus of surveillance and asked to do most in the cause of global health security are often people who are already significantly disadvantaged. This is an important consideration because, whereas most people both now and in the future stand to gain from the achievement of a world free from infectious diseases with pandemic potential, it is possible that the combination of surveillance, containment, mitigation, and suppression would result in those who are on the front line being made significantly worse off.

Many of the most effective interventions to disrupt transmission from wildlife to livestock and humans are going to disproportionately impact small-scale farmers, many of whom are already living on the edge of poverty and inevitably have pressing concerns other than freedom from emerging infectious diseases. What is it going to be like to live in a pandemic preparedness hotspot? What will containment, mitigation, and suppression mean for those who are subject to them? It is likely that this will involve significant restrictions on liberty and requirements to adapt to interventions such as changes to farming practices and land use, combined with various forms of control, regulation, and oversight that have the potential for real hardship. It is also important to note that many of these populations will already be subject to other pre-existing forms of structural injustice. In addition to the possibility of it leading to interventions with a range of harmful effects, an effective global health surveillance system will also require individuals and communities, often living in authoritarian states, to give up significant amounts of privacy. As outlined above, surveillance will include not only the collection of a wide range of health information, including genomic sequences, phylogenetic mapping of pathogens with the potential to identify transmission pairs and broader patterns of transmission, statistics about hospital admissions, pharmacy records, and absences from work, but also the collection and analysis of information such as social media, mobile phone mobility data, analyses of sewage, and observation by drones. It will involve not only the collection and global sharing of information about farming practices and animal markets but also satellite imagery analysis of land use, environmental degradation, and infrastructure change.

Taken together, then, the demands of surveillance and associated interventions necessary for effective pandemic preparedness are likely to impose a significant burden upon some of the most disadvantaged people in the world. The fact that the benefits of a surveillance system are obtained through the contribution of people, many of whom are living on or near the threshold below which lives are seriously compromised, suggests significant obligations are owed to them. But what is the nature and scope of these obligations, and by whom are they owed?

Once source of such obligation is the fact that, as illustrated above, some who are living in infectious disease hotspots and are currently able through farming or other roles to provide for themselves and their families may as a direct consequence of pandemic preparedness programmes no longer be able to do so. In such cases, it is the actions of others, albeit in the interests of global health security, that will have reduced the quality of their lives. Those who live and work in infectious disease hotspots can only reasonably be expected to participate in surveillance if this does not involve putting themselves or their families at significant risk of serious harm. This suggests both the success and the moral justifiability of a global infectious diseases surveillance system is going to depend upon effective protections and support for these populations whose disadvantage is caused to at least some degree by pandemic preparedness. Importantly, however, obligations generated by the foreseeable consequences of coordinated action for pandemic preparedness and prevention are likely in such settings to be part of a larger picture of broader and pre-existing obligations of social justice owed by those in high-income countries to those who are significantly worse off (Powers and Faden 2006). This suggests that obligations to those living in infectious disease hotspots are grounded not only in responsibilities associated with the impact of surveillance but also in broader grounds of social justice.

How might such obligations be met? Any legitimate approach to resolving these important questions of social justice needs to be grounded in genuine co-production and engagement with and leadership by the communities and individuals who live in hotspots and who are going to be subject to surveillance and the interventions informed by it (Fricker 2007). It is possible to imagine different ways in which such obligations might be met, all of which will involve significant efforts to improve the living conditions of those living in hotspots, guarantees of non-discrimination, and economic support to enable changes such as those of farming practice. One possible component might be an international and national commitment to the creation of sustainable and resilient health systems, which would have the advantage of both improving well-being and contributing to global health security.

A further quite different kind of obligation, one of reciprocity, might also reasonably be said to be owed to those who live in infectious disease hotspots. The fact that surveillance and other activities of containment, mitigation, and suppression, all of which come at a significant cost e.g. to privacy, are to be endured by those who are disadvantaged in the interests an often wealthier global population might be said to create important obligations of reciprocity. This suggests that obligations to those living or working in infectious disease hotspots might reasonably be thought to go beyond those owed to them solely on the grounds of social justice or arising out of the fact that those who instigated pandemic preparedness have made them significantly worse off. It might be argued that over and above this those who are asked or required to live under conditions of surveillance are owed significant additional obligations of reciprocity.

13.4 Three Tests of Ethical Commitment

In this final section, I briefly introduce three additional ways in which difficult questions of justice are likely to arise in the context of infectious disease surveillance for global health security. Each of these presents difficult questions regarding what is owed to those who live in infectious disease hotspots.

13.4.1 Acceptable Sources of Surveillance Data

The sincerity of international commitments to the well-bring of those living in infectious disease hotspots will be tested early. Effective global systems of infectious disease surveillance will involve some uncomfortable ethical trade-offs. To what extent will it, for example, be ethical to accept important surveillance data from authoritarian regimes, or from countries where information has not been gathered according to internationally acceptable ethical standards? More weakly, should information be accepted from countries that are not meeting their obligations to those who live and work in infectious disease hotspots? How should the international community respond to intelligence that successful interventions to prevent the emergence of infectious diseases with pandemic potential are being imposed by countries without due regard to the well-being of those who are subject to them? Practical politics is likely to require that countries committed to global infectious disease surveillance will need to work closely with countries failing to meet their obligations to those in hotspots to solve these problems of social justice over time—providing assistance and possible incentives. What should they do if no progress is made? Should they (we) ultimately be willing to accept a less than perfect surveillance system in the interests of global justice, or should they (we) accept less than perfect global justice in the interests of effective pandemic prevention?

13.4.2 Data and Duties of Care

One of the key components of surveillance in infectious disease hotspots is going to be the sequencing of pathogen genomes in both humans and non-human animals and the identification and analysis of transmission networks (Gardy and Loman 2017). Such approaches have already been used in the context of identification of new variants in COVID-19 (Viana 2022). Phylogenetic analysis is a rapidly developing method of identifying patterns of transmission and the linking of individuals to 'transmission events'. The identification of new infectious diseases and novel variants, and the mapping and analysis of transmission events and networks in the context of ongoing, population-level infectious disease surveillance, raise a number of new ethical questions (Johnson and Parker 2020). Some of these relate to the nature and scope of responsibilities of public health systems, or other bodies undertaking genomic surveillance, to those who provide the samples for analysis. One example of an issue requiring attention concerns the fact that an approach to sequencing for novel infections is going to have the potential to identify a range of other currently known infections. What should be done with this information? Does its generation create responsibilities of care in those who are undertaking the surveillance? Does its possibility lead to an obligation to provide effective health services? A second set of ethical questions is going to relate to the potential for information about transmission chains and events, and increasingly accurate analyses of the direction of transmission, to be used in ways that are harmful.

13.4.3 Prioritization Decisions between the Needs of Those in the Future and Those in the Present

Finally, just how much resource should be put into pandemic preparedness and surveillance? In the immediate aftermath and enduring impact of COVID-19, there is likely to be national and international pressure on funders, governments, and public health authorities to place a great deal of weight on and resources into efforts to protect future generations from the emergence and spread of new infectious diseases with pandemic potential (Gates, 2022). But just how much resource should be targeted at pandemic preparedness and prevention is a complex and complicated question. As was seen in the midst of the COVID-19 pandemic, reducing mortality and morbidity is often in tension with other important values and commitments. Given other important and urgent priorities in the present and immediate future—underfunded health systems and persistent inequalities which mean that many people do not currently meet any reasonable threshold for a good life—it seems unlikely that a convincing case could be made for pandemic preparedness to be the overriding priority. There are likely to be limits to public support for investment in these kinds of future-oriented measures. How should the interests of people in the future to be free of pandemics be judged against the needs of people in the present? It is vital that these difficult questions are addressed as a matter of urgency.

13.5 Conclusion: Infectious Disease Hotspots Are also Ethical Hotspots

World leaders have recently argued that

> The COVID-19 pandemic has been a stark and painful reminder that nobody is safe until everyone is safe.... (Bainimarama et al. 2021)

This is not in fact true. It is possible that the vast majority of the world's population could achieve 'safety' by means of the observation and surveillance of, and use of interventions upon, those in hotspots without meeting their obligations to them. This is, itself, a rather 'stark and painful reminder' of the potential for pandemic preparedness and response to greatly increase and intensify existing global health and other inequalities (Olatunbosun-Alakija 2021). It is not inevitable, however. In this chapter, I have described the various ways in which the development and implementation of an effective system of surveillance capable of offering protection from emerging infectious diseases with pandemic potential—a vitally important global public good—is a highly complex task requiring new and demanding forms of international collaboration and coordination, and is also an initiative many of the most important costs of which will be borne by those who live in emerging infectious disease hotspots in Africa, Latin America, and South East Asia. Many of those affected will be poor and living in marginalized communities that are going to be on the front line of surveillance and of interventions to address emerging infectious diseases with epidemic and pandemic potential. The practices of infectious disease surveillance mean that these populations will become some of the most highly observed, monitored, and intervened-upon in the world. And many of the proposed interventions to address, and protect the wider world from, emerging infectious diseases have the potential for significant negative impact upon their well-being in ways that could, if unchecked, push them below any meaningful threshold of acceptable well-being. I have argued that significant obligations are owed to those who live in these regions and are at such risk. I have also suggested that, in addition to obligations of social justice, obligations of reciprocity may exist.

These are, however, imperfectly specified obligations, and little has been said thus far about those who are their bearers. This is one reason why recent calls for an international treaty for pandemic preparedness and response are potentially of great importance (Bainimarama et al. 2021). For the negotiation of such a treaty provides a possible mechanism for setting out, even if only in broad terms, what is owed to those who live in infectious disease hotspots by states, international organizations, and other actors. For this to be achieved, any such treaty needs to engage with the social justice considerations and questions of reciprocity identified above. At a minimum, it has to include a clear commitment to ensuring that those who live in emerging infectious disease hotspots are the recipients of interventions that ensure their lives meet the requirements of threshold well-being (Powers and Faden 2006). Many farming practices and other behaviours are driven by poverty. Meeting obligations to such communities may also be an important part of what it takes to achieve the global public good of a world free from, or effectively protected from, the emergence of infectious diseases with pandemic potential. A key part of successful infectious disease management in ways that are respectful and supportive of local communities is likely to require the development through co-production of creative sustainable ways of changing farming practices and reducing environmental degradation in ways that protect existing communities.

A treaty cannot, of course, by itself address these problems of global health justice. Surveillance, and the governance of it, need to be understood as part of a bigger cluster of problems in global health justice, a key part of which is going to be the development of mechanisms to ensure health system strengthening and the existence of robust health systems and equitable access in all countries, particularly in the regions under discussion here. They also need to be understood against a background of broader concerns about global health injustice (Olatunbosun-Alakija 2021). This is going to call for careful consideration about the appropriate balance of responsibilities at different levels. For example, whilst emphasizing the importance of coordinated international action, it is also going to be important to avoid suggesting that the needs of those in hotspots are solely the responsibility of global actors. This may have the potential to encourage states to come to view their own responsibilities to these populations as thereby lessened.

A final thought. The issues outlined and discussed in this chapter support and illustrate the importance of a number of recent calls for a refocusing of bioethics research and scholarship towards a greater engagement with questions of global justice and equity, and global public health (Kahn et al. 2020; O'Neill 2016; Nuffield Council on Bioethics 2020). It has also shown that achieving this is likely to require bioethicists to develop new methods and theoretical perspectives capable of engaging meaningfully with large, complex problems without oversimplifying them. An important implication of the argument in this chapter is that an infectious disease ethics capable of engaging with the questions of responsibility etc. will need to be able to respond to three dimensions. The first of these is scale. The ethics of surveillance is a complex multilevel problem ranging all the way from difficult decisions in the clinic, through national-level public health policy, up to and including the making of international global health policy. These levels of analysis and types of ethical problem have tended to be viewed separately in bioethics. Is this a clinical ethics problem, a research ethics problem, a public health ethics problem, or a political philosophy problem? An ethics adequate to the task set out here needs to be coherent and convincing across multiple levels of analysis. It needs to be scalable (Parker 2015). Secondly, in addition to these levels of analysis, in normative terms, there is the question of how to make sense of the complexity and contextual meaning of the various interconnected moral worlds and moral problems which together constitute the different aspects of global health security. How empirically does one go about making sense of the nature of the ethical problem and the problem of moral responsibility as they arise for different actors and across radically different contexts? How does one speak meaningfully about the nature and scope of responsibility in this kind of complex relational whole? The answer cannot be that it is impossible. A third dimension requiring further attention is the development of an understanding of the moral aspects of the relationships in infectious disease surveillance between infectious disease hotspots and what might perhaps be conceptualized as 'ethical hotspots'.

Acknowledgements

My work on infectious disease ethics and on global health bioethics more broadly, and that of the Ethox Centre and the Global Health Bioethics Network, are supported by Wellcome Trust grants (096527), (221719), and (203132). The trust and confidence research theme of the Oxford Pandemic Sciences Institute is supported by the Moh Family Foundation.

Bibliography

Allen, T., Murray, K. A., Zambrana-Torrelio, C., et al. (2017), 'Global hotspots and correlates of emerging zoonotic diseases', *Nature Communications* 8/1124, doi- 10.1038/s41467-017-00923-8.

Bainimarama, V., et al (2021), 'COVID-19 shows why united action is needed for more robust international health architecture', *WHO News,* https://www.who.int/news-room/commentaries/detail/op-ed---covid-19-shows-why-united-action-is-needed-for-more-robust-international-health-architecture.

Carroll, D., Morzaria, S., Briand, S., et al. (2021), 'Preventing the next pandemic: the power of a global viral surveillance network', *British Medical Journal* 372:n485, doi - 10.1136/bmj.n485.

Daszak, P., Plowright, R. K., Epstein, J. H., et al. (2007), 'The emergence of Nipah and Hendra virus: Pathogen dynamics across a wildlife-livestock-human continuum', in S. K. Collinge, and C. Ray (eds.), *Disease Ecology: Community Structure and Pathogen Dynamics* (New York: Oxford University Press, 2007), https://doi.org/10.1093/acprof:oso/9780198567080.003.0013

Davies, S. C., Farrar, J., and O'Neill, J., (2021), 'An ounce of pandemic prevention', *Project Syndicate,* https://www.project-syndicate.org/commentary/pandemic-prevention-digital-public-health-monitoring-by-sally-c-davies-et-al-2021-03?barrier=accesspay.

Duff, J. H., Liu, A., Saavedra, J., et al. (2021), 'A global public health convention for the 21st Century', *Lancet Public Health* 6: e428–33.

Fidler, D. P. (1996), 'Globalization, international law, and emerging infectious diseases', *Emerging Infectious Diseases* 2/2: 77–84.

Fricker, M., (2007), *Epistemic injustice: power and the ethics of knowing* (Oxford: Oxford University Press, 2007).

G20 Independent Panel (2021), 'A global deal for our pandemic age', Report of the G20 High Level Independent Panel on Financing the Global Commons for Pandemic Preparedness and Response, https://pandemic-financing.org/report/foreword/.

Gardy, J. L., Loman, N. J. (2017), 'Towards a genomics-informed, real time, global pathogen surveillance system', *Nature Reviews Genetics* 19: 9–20, doi- 10.1038/nrg.2017.88.

Gates, B. (2022), *How to prevent the next pandemic* (London: Allen Lane, 2022).

Haseltine, W. A. (2021), 'How to end the pandemic', *Project Syndicate*, 29 July 2021, https://www.project-syndicate.org/commentary/how-to-end-the-pandemic-by-william-a-haseltine-2021-07.

Johnson, S. B., Parker, M. (2020), 'Ethical challenges in pathogen sequencing: a systematic scoping review', *Wellcome Open Research* 5: 119, https://doi.org/10.12688/wellcomeopenres.15806.1)

Jones, K. E., Patel, N. G., Levy, M.A., et al. (2008), 'Global trends in emerging infectious diseases', *Nature* 451: 990-3, doi- 10.1038/nature06536.

Kahn, J. P., Mastroianni, A. C., and Venkatapuram, S. (2020), 'Bioethics in a post-Covid world: time for future-facing global health ethics', in Brands, H., Gavin, F. J. (eds.), *Covid-19 and World Order: The Future of Conflict, Competition, and Cooperation* (Baltimore, Johns Hopkins University Press, 2020), 114–32.

Kaul, I., Grunberg, M., and Stern, M. (1999), 'Defining Global Public Goods', in Kaul, I., Grunberg, M., and Stern, M., (eds.), *Global Public Goods: International Cooperation in the 21st Century* (Oxford: Oxford University Press, 1999), 2–19.

Khor, K. S., and Heymann, D. (2021), 'Pandemic Preparedness in the 21st century: which way forward?', *Lancet* 6: e428.

Morse, S. S. (2007), 'Global infectious disease surveillance and health intelligence', *Health Affairs* (Millwood) 26: 1069–77, doi- 10.1377/hlthaff.26.4.1069.

Nuffield Council on Bioethics (2020), 'Research in global health emergencies: ethical issues', published by Nuffield Council on Bioethics, https://www.nuffieldbioethics.org/publications/research-in-global-health-emergencies.

Olatunbosum-Alakija, A. (2021), 'Unless we address the inequity in global health, then the world will not be prepared for the next pandemic', *British Medical Journal* 375: n2848, doi: 10.1136/bmj.n2848.

O'Neill, O. (2016), *Justice across boundaries: whose obligations?* (Cambridge: Cambridge University Press, 2016).

OUCRU (2016), 'Project report: Health in the backyard, Vietnam', https://mesh.tghn.org/articles/case-study-health-backyard-vietnam/.

Parker, M. (2015), 'Scaling ethics up and down: moral craft in clinical genetics and in global health research', *Journal of Medical Ethics* 41: 134–7, doi:10.1136/medethics-2014-102,303.

Powers, M., and Faden, R. (2006), *Social justice: the moral foundations of public health and health policy* (Oxford: Oxford University Press, 2006).

Viana, R., Moyo, S., Amoako, D. G., et al. (2022), 'Rapid epidemic expansion of the SARS-CoV-2 Omicron variant in southern Africa'. *Nature* 603: 679–86.

WHO (2022a), '14.9 million excess deaths were associated with the COVID-19 pandemic in 2020 and 2021', WHO News Release, 5 May 2022, https://www.who.int/news/item/05-05-2022-14.9-million-excess-deaths-were-associated-with-the-covid-19-pandemic-in-2020-and-2021.

WHO (2022b), 'WHO Director General's opening remarks at the public hearing regarding a new international instrument on pandemic preparedness and response, 12 April 2022', https://www.who.int/director-general/speeches/detail/who-director-general-s-opening-remarks-at-the-public-hearing-regarding-a-new-international-instrument-on-pandemic-preparedness-and-response---12-april-2022.

WHO Independent Panel (2021), 'COVID-19 Make it the last pandemic', Independent Panel for pandemic preparedness and response, https://theindependentpanel.org/wp-content/uploads/2021/05/COVID-19-Make-it-the-Last-Pandemic_final.pdf.

Worobey M. (2017), 'Molecular mapping of Zika spread', *Nature* 546: 355–7.

Zinsstag, J., Utzinger, J., Probst-Hensch, N., et al. (2020), 'Towards integrated surveillance-response systems for the prevention of future pandemics', in Infectious Diseases of Poverty 9: 140, doi – 10.1186/s40249-0200-00757-5.

14

COVID-19: An Unequal and Disequalizing Pandemic

S. Subramanian

14.1 Introduction

The simple thesis of this chapter is that the COVID-19 pandemic is one that has afflicted the poor and the non-poor undiscriminatingly.[1] Given the propensity of the world to privilege the interests of the relatively affluent over those of the relatively impoverished, this has meant that both the policy response to the pandemic and the pre-existing distribution of resources in favour of the rich have worked to the disproportionate disadvantage of the poor—making for a pandemic which, between and within countries, has been both intrinsically unequal and consequentially disequalizing.

The implementation of draconian lockdowns, it is argued, is one important manifestation of such a state of affairs and the orientation underlying it. It is an orientation that is compatible with a 'politics of visibility' and an accompanying 'politics of invisiblization'. By a 'politics of visibility' is meant a poor country's disposition to be *seen* to be combating the pandemic rather than actually addressing it substantively, one instrument for which is the imposition of stringent lockdown—a response that attracts both international and intranational attention as an essentially spectacular policy measure. This has been discussed in the context of India, at some length, in Ray and Subramanian (2020c), and, even more explicitly, in the terms of 'spectacle and social murder' by Nilsen (2021).

The orientation in question is compatible, too—given a poor country's long prior history of inequity in both social practice and state policy—with unpreparedness as much as unwillingness for attending to the needs of the vulnerable in a time of crisis, in some sudden departure from the norms of attitude and behaviour that have presided over 'normal times'. This paves the way for neglecting the predicament of the poor and the marginalized, both on the ground and in

[1] Parts of this paper draw heavily on earlier published work in which the author was involved, specifically Ray and Subramanian (2020a, b, c; 2021). Large parts of the last-mentioned article have been directly reproduced from the original source, permission for which, from the Editor of *Frontline* and my co-author Debraj Ray, is gratefully acknowledged. I would also like to record my debt to Debraj, from whom I have learnt so much. The usual caveat applies.

S. Subramanian, *COVID-19: An Unequal and Disequalizing Pandemic* In: *Pandemic Ethics: From COVID-19 to Disease X*. Edited by: Dominic Wilkinson and Julian Savulescu, Oxford University Press. © Oxford University Press 2023.
DOI: 10.1093/oso/9780192871688.003.0015

the record and public revelation of statistical data. This is what is signalled by the term 'politics of invisiblization'.

The themes mentioned above are discussed with reference to the coronavirus experience in India (until September 2021). This chapter is organized as follows. It begins with the thesis that the coronavirus disease is an intrinsically 'unequal' one, compared to other communicable diseases, and one which advanced-country interests dictate will be globally arrested by mechanisms such as drastic lockdowns, without any apparent regard for the differential impact which such mechanisms will have on rich and poor countries. This is followed by a brief account of the two 'waves' of the disease which India has been exposed to, in 2020 and 2021, respectively, and the policy responses to these. We then have a quick review of the implications of the pandemic for certain demographic and economic outcomes, with specific reference to mortality, growth, poverty and inequality, hunger, education, unemployment, and access to vaccine. In the concluding section we have some observations on what might be learnt from India's experience of the coronavirus disease. These prescriptions for a future Pandemic X lay an emphasis on long-term orientation rather than short-term responses to a crisis.

14.2 COVID-19: An 'Unequal' Disease?

14.2.1 Communicable Diseases, Rich Countries, and Poor Countries

According to the World Health Organization (WHO 2020), the top ten causes of global mortality can be classified into three major categories: communicable, non-communicable (chronic), and injuries. The total death count for 2019 is estimated at 55.4 million. Our concern here is with the category of communicable diseases. WHO (2020) provides information on the ten leading causes of death for each of four country groupings based on the World Bank's categorization by economic standing (as reflected in per capita gross national income): low income countries; lower-middle income countries; upper-middle income countries; and high income countries.

We find, from the WHO information just alluded to, that there are four communicable diseases such that each of these figures among the top ten causes of death in at least one of the four country groupings. These are neo-natal conditions (NNCs), lower respiratory infections (LRIs), diarrhoeal diseases (DDs), and tuberculosis (TB), which together we shall call the four communicable diseases (or 4C diseases, for short). We reduce the World Bank's four-fold classification of countries into a binary one, consisting of one group we call the set of (relatively) poor countries (obtained by combining the low and lower-middle income countries into a single category), and a second group we call the set of (relatively) rich countries (obtained by merging the higher-middle and high income countries).

Using WHO (2020) and other data, Table 14.1 constructs a picture of the global distribution of deaths due to the 4C diseases in 2019, and the global distribution of deaths due to COVID-19 in 2020, across poor and rich countries.[2] Among other things, Table 14.1 shows that in 2019 the 4C diseases together accounted for 7.9 million of the global count of 55.4 million deaths, which makes for a substantial share of 14.3 per cent. However, the global distribution of deaths by these causes is highly asymmetrical across the categories of rich and poor countries: the former accounted for just 26.3 per cent of all 4C disease deaths. The contrast is particularly well marked in the case of diarrhoeal diseases (with a rich countries' share of 7.3 per cent), and less evident in the case of lower respiratory infections (with a rich countries' share of 40.4 per cent, still considerably lower than the halfway mark).

Where COVID-19 is concerned, two features are worth remarking. First, the 2020 COVID-19 global mortality figure is actually *less* than the corresponding figures for neonatal conditions and lower respiratory infections, while tuberculosis, with the lowest aggregate mortality count of 1.51 million, nevertheless registers a magnitude which is a substantial 83 per cent of the magnitude of COVID-19 mortality. Second, and as we have seen, the rich countries accounted for just 26.3 per cent of mortality from the 4C diseases in 2019, while, by contrast, they account for all of one-half of global COVID-19 mortality in 2020. That is to say, COVID-19 is by no means the single most deadly communicable disease in the world, but it is the only one which, in terms of aggregate mortality, is as significant for the rich countries as it is for the poor countries. Or, in summary, aggregate COVID-19 mortality is *absolutely* less quantitatively important than for some other communicable diseases (while other such diseases are not far behind), but it is *relatively* important for the rich countries—both in relation to the rich–poor distribution of COVID-19 deaths, and in relation to the significance of respective shares in mortality by disease.

These elementary observations are reinforced by the numbers in the last three columns of Table 14.1, where we switch the focus on absolute numbers of deaths to deaths per capita. Presumably, the lethality of a disease, as measured by the risk of dying from it, is best conveyed by the number of deaths per million population from the disease. The last three columns of Table 14.1 indicate that the risk of dying from any of the 4C diseases is, by a variable but large order of magnitude, higher for poor as compared to rich countries, whereas the risks for COVID-19 are not much different between poor and rich countries.

---

[2] Our country group estimates of mortality are rough estimates: the WHO data on the 4C diseases which we have accessed are presented on line charts without precise accompanying numbers, which we have arrived at by measuring lengths with a foot rule against a normalized scale.

Table 14.1 The global distribution of five major communicable diseases between poor and rich countries: 2019 and 2020

Disease	Deaths in Millions: Rich Countries	Deaths in Millions: Poor Countries	Deaths in Millions: All Countries	Share of Rich Countries' Mortality in Global Mortality (per cent)	Deaths/Million: Rich Countries	Deaths/Million: Poor Countries	Ratio of Poor Countries' to Rich Countries' Per Capita Mortality
Diarrhoeal Diseases (2019)	0.11	1.40	1.51	7.29	26.9	390.9	14.53
Tuberculosis (2019)	0.36	1.04	1.40	25.71	88.0	290.4	3.30
Neonatal Conditions (2019)	0.56	1.84	2.40	2.33	136.9	513.7	3.75
Lower Respiratory Infections (2019)	1.05	1.55	2.60	40.39	256.6	432.7	1.69
Total for the 4C Diseases (2019)	2.08	5.83	7.91	26.30	508.3	1627.7	3.20
COVID-19 (2020)	0.91	0.90	1.81	50.27	218.9	247.2	1.13

Notes and sources: Mortality figures for the 4C diseases are from WHO (2020). Mortality figures for COVID-19 are from country-specific data at https://ourworldindata. org/grapher/total-covid-cases-deaths-per-million?time=2019-12-31.latest, and are valid as of December 30 or 31. 2020. The data have been aggregated separately for the categories of 'rich' and 'poor' countries (employing the World Bank's country groupings into Low Income, Lower-Middle Income [combined here into 'Poor'], Upper-Middle Income and High Income [combined here into 'Rich'] countries). Additionally, country and world population figures from 2019 are from World Bank)(https://data.worldbank.org/indicator/SP.POP.TOTL), global population figure for 2020 is from Population Reference Bureau, July 10, 2020 (https://www.prb.org/2020-world-population-data-sheet/#:~:text=The per cent20world per cent20population per cent20projected,as per cent20in per cent20the per cent20United per cent20States). Country population shares in 2020 have been assumed to be the same as in 2019. The share of 'poor' countries' population in global population is nearly 47 per cent.

No doubt these findings require qualification. One has to allow for the strong likelihood that COVID-19 mortality in poor countries has been underestimated, and in rich countries overestimated, with the net outcome in favour of overall actual mortality exceeding reported mortality. (This, however, is subject to the observation that under-registration of deaths for all diseases is not uncommon in poorer countries.) Further, it is likely that lockdown itself, especially in the richer countries, has contributed to lowering COVID mortality. (But then, mortality-reducing interventions, both preventative and curative, must also be taken into account for the other communicable diseases.) In the end, I have gone by the global statistics put out by international agencies like WHO, and in the belief that, while qualifying factors might alter the precise numbers reported, they would perhaps not reverse the broad tendencies observed.

The differential implications of communicable diseases for the rich and the poor are also, obviously, mediated by *how* these communicable diseases are typically communicated. In the case of lower respiratory infections, the principal mode of transmission is through person-to-person contact. This is, of course, true for COVID-19 as well. This is also why, as Table 14.1 reveals, lower respiratory infections and COVID-19 are relatively more salient than the other three communicable diseases in the rich countries. TB flourishes in poor, rather than rich, populations (see Figueroa-Munoz and Ramon-Pardo 2008: 733). Again, in the case of diarrhoeal diseases, WHO (2017) indicates that 'Infection is spread through contaminated food or drinking-water, or from person-to-person as a result of poor hygiene'. In the matter of neonatal infections, observing good hygiene practices during childbirth and the post-partum period acquires considerable importance (Mannava et al. 2019). Countries like India still have a substantial incidence of births delivered at home, and fare poorly when it comes to access to clean drinking water and toilets. Briefly, communicable diseases like COVID-19 would be of greater significance for rich countries than ones like diarrhoeal diseases, neonatal conditions, or tuberculosis—exactly as, *within* each country, rich populations would be relatively more concerned about COVID-19, which by its nature is nowhere near as class-conscious as the other communicable diseases we have mentioned.

Thus, both across and within countries, a pandemic like COVID-19 assumes a global dimension not so much from considerations of a common fate shared by rich and poor alike as from the consideration that the poor are now a source of transmission threat to the rich. It becomes imperative, then, that a communicable disease like COVID-19 be stopped in its tracks, in a way that other equally or more lethal diseases have not merited similar urgency of attention. It should therefore come as no surprise that control and mitigation measures such as lockdown should be an accompanying feature of the global sway exercised by COVID-19. We turn now to this issue.

14.2.2 Lockdown

By lockdown we have in mind a collection of stringent and generalized measures of mitigation and control involving stay-at-home requirements, closure of educational institutions and business enterprises, and embargoes on large meetings. In this understanding, lockdown does not include other non-pharmaceutical measures such as testing, tracing, and quarantining (within limits against intrusive surveillance imposed by the right to privacy), mask wearing, maintaining physical distance, and observing hygienic practices such as hand- and face-washing. The time purchased by the lockdown is supposed to be used for priming the health infrastructure, preparing for the acquisition of personal protective equipment, raising capacity for testing-tracing-isolating, and generally preventing an overload on the public health system until a vaccine or other prophylactic/curative pharmaceutical treatment of the disease is discovered. This, in principle, is how a lockdown is expected to work. The underlying logic is that lockdown will assist in 'flattening the curve' of infections, and therefore deaths; defer and reduce peak mortality; and reduce overall mortality in relation to what would have obtained in the absence of lockdown.

It is worth underlining that the preceding account relates only to the epidemiological implications of lockdown for COVID-19-related benefits. But lockdown, as is becoming increasingly clear (even if this should not have been hard to predict at the outset) has a whole host of other costs, including the possibility of lives lost for reasons of non-availability or infeasibility of treatment for non-COVID morbidities; the rigours of mass migration of informal-sector workers from urban workplaces to rural homes (as happened in India); starvation and other undernutrition-related conditions caused by loss of livelihoods and incomes on account of lockdown; suicide, caused by the psychological oppression of enforced long-duration stay-at-home measures; and domestic violence.[3] In fact, Ray and Subramanian (2020a) signalled these issues at a relatively early stage of the pandemic (28 March 2020): '...the general economy-wide costs and the household-specific burdens of a comprehensive lockdown are enormous. A spiralling macroeconomic downturn is an obvious consequence, but what we have in mind is the protracted stress on household incomes, employment, and nutrition, *ultimately measured in human lives and not in rupees*' [emphasis in original].[4]

To preclude all misunderstanding, what is being advanced is not some blanket anti-lockdown sentiment. The fact of the matter is quite far from this, as the following clarification, in Ray and Subramanian (2020b: 539–40), should indicate:

---

[3] We do not deal here with the question of a reasonable alternative to stringent and comprehensive lockdowns: the question has been dealt with elsewhere (for example, in Ray, Subramanian, and Vandewalle 2020, and, indeed, in the Great Barrington Declaration mentioned below).

[4] Such a perspective on overridingly stringent measures of disease control is also clearly reflected in the so-called Great Barrington Declaration (Kulldorf et al. 2020).

... in our opinion, the first-best (or 'unconstrained') approach to tackling the viral epidemic is a fully implemented lockdown which is also accompanied by a comprehensive package of welfare measures designed to compensate for the negative impact on human lives of such a lockdown. We believe that this is a clear enough articulation of an ethical position that one might, in principle, adopt... But this position-in-principle inevitably also provokes the pragmatic question: what if the State is unable to implement the first-best option just outlined—for reasons that could range from financial constraints to lack of expertise to ignorance to incompetence? [Emphasis in original.]

It is lockdown without its compensating features that is contentious. It is for this reason that, in the end, stringent lockdowns in poorer countries are a different proposition from what they are in richer countries, though such lockdowns in the poorer countries might benefit the richer countries through control of cross-border incursions by the virus. Overall, therefore, it is fair to assert that the geopolitics of COVID-19 has been one in which it is the interests of the global North that have been prioritized, and, within countries, those of the relatively affluent constituency of citizens who make opinion and influence policy. The case of India, dealt with in what follows, is a case in point.

14.3 The Pandemic and the Policy Response to it

14.3.1 Introduction

As of November 2022, there have been two major waves of the pandemic in India. At the time of writing (November 23, 2022), the cumulative number of confirmed COVID-19 cases is 44.67 million, and the cumulative number of confirmed deaths is 530,601.[5] These are the official figures, which, as we shall see later, are probably severe undercounts of the true figures. A bald summary picture of the trajectory of the pandemic, in terms of daily cases and daily deaths, would suggest that the first wave of daily cases peaked around the middle of September 2020, and the second wave around the middle of May 2021, and that the first wave took longer to peak than the second. The second wave has been of a massively larger order, in terms of both cases and deaths, than the first wave: the peak daily count of cases in the second wave, at 391,008, was 4.2 times the corresponding figure of 93,180 for the first wave; and the peak daily count of mortalities in the second wave, at 4190, was 3.6 times the corresponding figure of 1165 for the first wave.

---

[5] These figures are from the Our World in Data website (https://ourworldindata.org/coronavirus/country/india), and sourced from the Johns Hopkins University COVID database.

The principal policy response to the first wave was a stringent lockdown, which for obvious reasons must be expected to have impacted particularly harshly on the poor. The response, of any sort, to the second wave was hard to discern, which again would have impacted disproportionately on the poor simply because resource constraints were more binding on the poor than on the rich in accessing such ameliorative health intervention as was available.

14.3.2 The First Wave

This section will be a very quick précis of ground already covered in elaborate detail in Ray and Subramanian (2020b). The predominant policy response of the government to the first wave of the pandemic was the imposition of a stringent lockdown. In the month leading to the somewhat abrupt imposition of lockdown in the last week of March, the government was busy with at least three events: President Trump's visit to India on February 24–25; communal riots in Delhi for at least three days from February 23, believed to have been instigated by Hindus against Muslims, which left fifty-three people dead, of whom more than 60 per cent were Muslims; and the resignation of the Congress government, which lost its majority in the state of Madhya Pradesh in the third week of March (March 16) and the installation in its place of a BJP government (on March 23). On March 22, a fourteen-hour-long 'Janata [People's] Curfew' was abruptly announced, and this was followed, on March 24, by the declaration of a complete lockdown for a period of three weeks, till April 14, which was extended till May 3, with allowance for relaxation for selected businesses and activities. The lockdown was renewed on May 1, and again on May 17, when it was extended to May 31. Subsequently, the lockdown was relaxed over six phases, from the beginning of June till the end of November 2020.[6]

The object of a lockdown is presumably to employ the interim respite afforded by it to prime the health infrastructure, provide relief measures to those particularly hard hit by it, and to undertake testing, tracing, and quarantining on a large scale. None of these objectives seems to have received the state's undivided attention. In the matter of testing, India compares unfavourably even with countries that are not part of the 'advanced' league; according to data from Worldometer,[7] as of September 22, 2021, the numbers of tests (in thousands) per million population for some selected countries were roughly as follows: India 400; Colombia 459; Peru 524; Argentina 531; Malaysia 885; and Chile 1103.

---

[6] For a timeline of the lockdown, see the Wikipedia entry 'COVID-19 lockdown in India': https://en.wikipedia.org/wiki/COVID-19_lockdown_in_India.

[7] https://www.worldometers.info/coronavirus/#countries.

In the matter of the provision of relief, it is noteworthy that several commentators came up in remarkably quick time with proposals for clearly specified and doable measures of meaningful response to the emergency caused by the corona crisis. Here is a considerably incomplete list of papers carrying recommendations for policy intervention: Iyer and Krishnamurthy (2020); Narayanan (2020); Khera (2020); Borah et al (2020); Ghosh (2020); a response, with 635 signatories,[8] to a relief measure announced by the Finance Minister; Sen, Rajan, and Banerjee (2020); and Sinha (2020). The huge gap between recommendation and response in the matter of relief measures actually deployed on the ground has been extensively dealt with in Ray and Subramanian (2020b), and will not be repeated here. A quick clue to the quantum of assistance provided can be gathered from the financial outlays available, or created, for addressing the pandemic. Two fiscal stimuli were announced, one on March 27, and the other on May 12, 2020, the latter of which was advertised as accounting for 10 per cent of GDP. Ray and Subramanian (2020b: 563) provide an elaborate assessment of these financial packages, and their summary is all we have space for here:

> At a stretch, we could count under 'fiscal stimulus' *all* of the Plan 1 allocation of Rs. 1.7 tr, reduced, let us say, to Rs.1.3 tr to account for elements of double-counting…, the provisions for tax relief (Rs. 0.78 tr), the PM's announcement for the health sector (Rs. 0.15 tr), the provident fund payments of Rs. 0.025 tr, the Rs. 0.035 tr provision for foodgrain to migrant workers without ration cards, and the entire new expenditure of Rs. 0.4 tr on NREGA, to arrive a bit south of Rs. 2 tr, which is around 1 per cent of India's GDP. (In fact, Barclay's estimate of the actual fiscal impact of the package, at Rs. 1.5 tr, is even more pessimistic, and only 0.75 per cent of GDP;….) The rest of the items appear to be loans and liquidity injections from the Reserve Bank and from nationalized banks, or reductions in provident fund contributions and taxes deducted or collected at source. For a country already so flush with liquidity that banks are very reluctant to on-lend…, this sort of strategy appears to be somewhat unthinking, to put it mildly. Alternatively, it is a strategy conceived with only some economic agents—principally business enterprises and tax assessees—in mind. This is a very gently reproving evaluation when compared with one journalistic assessment (Jha 2020), which suggests that 'Modi's "Stimulus Package" is a Gigantic Confidence Trick Played on the People of India'.

---

[8] 'Concerned citizens' response to the COVID 19 relief package announced by the finance minister', *Caravan Magazine*, March 27, 2020, https://caravanmagazine.in/noticeboard/citizens-response-to-covid-relief-package-nirmala-sitharaman.

14.3.3 The Second Wave

If the policy response elicited by the pandemic's first wave was almost entirely constituted by the single instrument of lockdown, the latter was conspicuously absent, in a swing of the pendulum in the other direction, as a response from the central government to the second wave. Indeed, there was little in the way of *any* discernible policy response to the second wave. If anything, it seems to have been preceded by wholesale complacence about the possibility of any such occurrence. This is clearly reflected in a statement made by the country's Prime Minister on February 16, 2021 (coinciding roughly with the beginning of the second wave): 'At the beginning of this pandemic, the whole world was worried about India's situation. But today India's fight against corona is inspiring the entire world…'[9] Even more remarkable is the quiet confidence in this declaration by the Union Health Minister, made on March 6, 2021, in the course of a speech addressed to the Delhi Medical Association's 62nd Annual Delhi State Medical Conference: 'We are in the end-game of the COVID-19 pandemic in India…'[10] Most remarkable of all is the suggestion that the central government was not unaware of the impending wave: according to a Reuters report of early May 2021 (Ghoshal and Das 2021),

> A forum of scientific advisers set up by the government warned Indian officials in early March of a new and more contagious variant of the coronavirus taking hold in the country, five scientists who are part of the forum told Reuters. Despite the warning, four of the scientists said the federal government did not seek to impose major restrictions to stop the spread of the virus. Millions of largely unmasked people attended religious festivals and political rallies that were held by Prime Minister Narendra Modi, leaders of the ruling Bharatiya Janata Party and opposition politicians. The warning about the new variant in early March was issued by the Indian SARS-CoV-2 Genetics Consortium, or INSACOG.

The 'religious festivals and political rallies' alluded to in the Reuters report are by far the most egregious precursor to/accompaniment of the second wave. The Kumbh Mela is a Hindu religious festival held once every twelve years in the state of Uttar Pradesh, and attracts congregations of pilgrims running into the millions: when there was every case for calling off the festival in the cause of avoiding

---

[9] This is from a valedictory address on the occasion of the platinum jubilee celebration of the Heartfulness Institute of Shri Ram Chandra Mission, reported in *The Hindu* of February 16, 2021: https://www.thehindu.com/news/national/indias-fight-against-covid-19-is-inspiring-the-world-pm-modi/article33852627.ece.

[10] Reported in *The Times of India*, March 7, 2021: https://timesofindia.indiatimes.com/india/we-are-in-the-endgame-of-covid-19-pandemic-in-india-harsh-vardhan/articleshow/81378288.cms.

a superspreader event, it was nevertheless held, and proceeded from April 1 to April 17, when it was eventually called off (Kamal 2021). The second major superspreader event relates to the campaigns for elections to the State Legislatures of West Bengal and Tamil Nadu. These states witnessed large election rallies in the time leading up to the West Bengal election that ended on April 29 and the Tamil Nadu election that ended on April 6. The situation was particularly serious in West Bengal, where the elections were held over *eight phases*, in the period covering March 27 to April 29.

The second wave—believed to be the outcome of a virulent Delta variant of the virus called B.1.617.2—was, as mentioned earlier, far more widespread, lethal, and swift in its unfolding than the first wave. There is little to suggest that the central government was prepared for the wave, and the states of the Indian Union, many of which resorted to lockdowns of varying durations, were largely left to their own devices to deal with the crisis. It would be no exaggeration to suggest that what prevailed in the absence of anything like considered state policy was an anarchy of tragic proportions. It is by now well recognized that the period from February to July 2021, and especially the first half of this period, was one that witnessed a completely overwhelmed healthcare system in which patients were frequently turned away at hospital gates; there were severe shortages of hospital beds and ventilators; and, above all, there was a fatal gap between the demand for and supply of oxygen cylinders for COVID patients struggling to breathe. The problem was one of both absolute shortage of oxygen and poor logistics for the distribution of what was available. While the production of liquid oxygen was about 7000 MT per day (*India Today* 2021), the demand for it had risen to 8400 MT per day by April 25 and to 11,000 MT by May 1, before gradually declining (Thadhani 2021). Added to this were inadequate transport tankers and logistical inflexibilities in the delivery of oxygen according to need. Inevitably, a black market for oxygen emerged: reports suggest that in April oxygen cylinders were selling at four to five times the normal price in Patna, Bihar (Rumi 2021), seven times the normal price in Noida near Delhi (Salaria 2021), and nine times the normal price in Lucknow, Uttar Pradesh (France 24 2021). In the face of all of this, the Union Minister of State for Health and Family Welfare, responding to a query from an Opposition leader in the Upper House of Parliament in July, blandly stated that states did not specifically report any deaths due to oxygen shortage during the second wave (Scroll Staff, 2021)! (This is presumably part of the federal politics of disavowal by the central government of responsibility for 'state subjects' such as health.)

Excess mortality during the second wave found tragic reflection in the phenomenon of overwhelmed crematoria, the running out of wood for funeral pyres, and bodies dumped in rivers failing access to normal modes of disposal. A BBC report (Pandey 2021) says:

India's holiest river, the Ganges, has been swollen with bodies in recent days. Hundreds of corpses have been found floating in the river or buried in the sand of its banks…The bodies on the river banks, taken together with funeral pyres burning round-the-clock and cremation grounds running out of space, tell the story of a death toll unseen and unacknowledged in official data.

In the matter of vaccination, while this was initially prioritized for the 45+ age group, from May 1 the central government determined that vaccination would be open to all above the age of 18. Further, it determined that responsibility for finding the funds to vaccinate the 18–45 age group would lie with the states of the Indian Union—a remarkable decision that goes against the grain of the near-universal principle that vaccination of a country's citizens is a federal government's responsibility. Following a *suo motu* intervention in the matter by the Supreme Court, the union government's policy was revised. But even under this revised policy, which stipulated the prices at which a set of identified private suppliers could sell their vaccine on the open market, it turned out that private citizens would end up bearing a large part of the aggregate vaccine bill (the relevant calculations are available in Subramanian 2021a): with such a pricing policy, the major casualties must be expected to be poor citizens who will be rationed out of the market by the vaccine prices. In any event, these considerations are of somewhat academic interest only, for they are premised on the assumption of availability of production capacity and steady supplies of vaccine—an assumption of heroic proportions given the actual record of vaccination to date, which is: 67 per cent of persons with a complete initial protocol, and 5 per cent of those only partially vaccinated, as of November 23, 2022.[11]

Where has all this left India?

14.4 Policy and the Pandemic: Some Fallouts

14.4.1 Introduction

Space constraints dictate no more than a rapid reader on some of the fallouts of the pandemic and the manner in which it has been addressed by state policy. We consider specific outcomes in the dimensions of mortality, economic growth, money-metric poverty, livelihoods, hunger, education, and disadvantage peculiar to citizens of particular demographics. The burden of the pandemic's consequences, it is suggested, has been disproportionately borne by the socio-economically weaker sections of the population, for reasons of restricted

---

[11] https://ourworldindata.org/covid-vaccinations.

withholding capacity in a time of crisis, of restricted state assistance in tiding over the crisis, and of settled attitudes of discrimination against members of specific religions and castes.

14.4.2 The Reach of Infections and Mortality

Given the limitations and unreliability of official data, (Zimmermann et al. 2021; Vasudevan et al. 2021), various attempts have been made to assess the probable true magnitude of COVID-related mortality in India. Employing estimates of the infection fatality rate and the scale of countrywide infection from official sero-surveys, Banaji (2021) estimates that actual mortality could be between five and eight times the level of reported mortality. Mortality figures have also been sought to be reckoned by estimating 'all-cause excess mortality' attributable directly or indirectly to the pandemic: this would entail, broadly, employing Civil Registration System (CRS) data from the Census, to compare mortality over the COVID-19 period with mortality over a corresponding proximate period in a non-COVID regime. Leffler et al. (2021), employing the 'excess deaths' approach, suggest that the factor by which excess mortality exceeds reported mortality for a set of seventeen states could range between 2.8 and 4.1. Employing data from the CRS, from around 200,000 public hospitals and smaller facilities, and a nationally representative telephonic survey, Deshmukh et al. (2021) arrive at an excess mortality figure which is between 6.8 and 8.6 times the reported mortality.

14.4.3 Economic Growth

The effect of the pandemic on economic growth must be seen in *cumulative* terms, as coming on top of two earlier disastrous policy interventions—those of the cash-absorbing demonetization move of 2016 and the hasty introduction and shoddy implementation of the Goods and Services Tax. The first affected the poor and those in the informal sector, and the second, additionally, small enterprises. The collective effect on growth is evident from Reserve Bank of India statistics on Gross Domestic Product (GDP)[12]: from 2019/20 to 2020/21, GDP has *declined* by 7.25 per cent, from Rs.145,693 billion to Rs.135,127 billion.

---

[12] Reserve Bank of India (2021), *Handbook of Statistics on Indian Economy*, https://www.rbi.org.in/scripts/AnnualPublications.aspx?head=Handbook per cent20of per cent20Statistics per cent20on per cent20Indian per cent20Economy. GDP figures in the text are from Table 4 of the *Handbook*, 'Components of Gross Domestic Product', https://rbidocs.rbi.org.in/rdocs/Publications/PDFs/04T874 2F20432F549289B10AE9828C12FEC.PDF.

14.4.4 Money-Metric Poverty

There have been at least two efforts at reckoning the additional numbers of people that might have slipped into poverty over the period of the first wave of the pandemic—one by the Pew Research Center (Kochhar 2021) in the US, and the other by the Azim Premji University (Azim Premji University 2021) in India; and both these studies have been reviewed by the present author (Subramanian 2021b). The two studies come up with vastly differing estimates, employing, as they do, different data sets relating to income distributions, mean incomes, and poverty lines; and a good deal of the difference seems to be because of variations in the poverty line employed. The more convincing of the two estimates, as argued in Subramanian (2021b), is the one due to the Azim Premji University, which reckons that over the post-lockdown period March–October 2020 of the first wave of the pandemic, in relation to the pre-lockdown period July 2019–February 2020, an additional *230 million people* may have been precipitated into poverty.

14.4.5 Livelihoods

The Periodic Labour Force Surveys (PLFSs) brought out by the Ministry of Statistics and Programme Implementation are an important source of data on employment, unemployment, and earnings. In an analysis of the PLFSs of 2017–18, 2018–19, and 2019–20, Anand and Thampi (2021)[13] note, among other things, that real earning declined by 7.6 per cent in April–June 2020 compared to the same quarter in 2019 for wage/salaried workers; daily wages declined by 5.5 per cent for casual labourers; and earnings declined by 26.4 per cent for the self-employed. Bhardwaj and Deshpande (2021) provide further evidence of distress in the massive increase in the issue of new job cards, of the order of 17.5 million, under the Mahatma Gandhi National Rural Employment Guarantee Act (MGNREGA) public works programme; the spurt in the numbers of younger people in the 18–30 age group seeking employment; and the failure of employment supply to match employment demand, with just 4.1 per cent of all registered families finding the promised one-hundred days of employment on the programme.

Survey data on the immediate effect of the lockdown in 2020 indicate massive losses in livelihoods. Azim Premji University (2021) cites the findings of three survey-based studies—the Azim Premji, Dahlberg, and Action Aid surveys—on

---

[13] Another important analysis of recent rounds of the PLFS is the paper by Deshpande and Singh (2021).

the proportion of people who lost their employment in the lockdown months of 2020: the figures, for the three respective surveys, are 66 per cent, 72 per cent, and 75 per cent. The APU study also suggests that the Scheduled Caste community was the one most likely to have both suffered unemployment and recovered employment during and after the lockdown, for reasons of engagement in jobs of relatively greater informality and flexibility; this is also true for workers from poorer households in general. The differential impact of the pandemic on persons of relatively disadvantaged caste and religious affiliation is brought out in the following figures. While 43 per cent of Muslims in the category of permanent salaried workers had to transit to self-employment and 15 per cent to daily wage work, the corresponding numbers for Hindus were lower, at 34 per cent and 9 per cent respectively; and while 18 per cent of Scheduled Caste/Scheduled Tribe workers among permanent salaried workers had to transit to daily wage work, this was the case for 'only' 3 per cent of workers in the general category.

The impact of the pandemic and the attendant lockdown on unemployment is perhaps most clearly reflected in the time series of monthly unemployment rates generated by the surveys of the Centre for Monitoring Indian Economy (CMIE). Table 14.2 presents these data (based on assessment of employment status on the date of the survey) for the last three years. The simple average of monthly unemployment rates is highest, at 10.4 per cent, in 2020, which was the year of a national lockdown. The spikes in unemployment rates, when the pandemic raged most fiercely, can be seen in the months of April, May, and June of 2020, and the months of May and June of 2021.

14.4.6 Hunger

According to a survey carried out by the Azim Premji University (2021), only 10 per cent of all households reported that their food intake had not been affected by the pandemic; 30 per cent reported a diminution in food intake and complete recovery post lockdown; 40 per cent reported partial recovery; and 20 per cent no recovery. The same study also reports a Hunger Watch Survey conducted by the Right to Food Campaign in September and October of 2020, which found that two-thirds of the households surveyed had suffered a reduction in food intake which persisted even five months after the lockdown. These statistics must be seen in the light of a 2020 Global Hunger Index score for India of 27.2, which places it in the 'serious' category of hunger, and awards India a lowly rank of 94th out of 107 countries. A particularly harsh aspect of the lockdown has been the prolonged closure of educational institutions, in which the worst sufferers were schoolchildren with no access to the Midday Meals Scheme over the period of the closure.

Table 14.2 Monthly unemployment rates (per cent) for India: 2019, 2020, and 2021

	J	F	M	A	M	J	J	A	S	O	N	D	Simple Average
2019	6.9	7.2	6.7	7.3	7.0	7.9	7.3	8.2	7.1	8.1	7.2	7.6	7.4
2020	7.2	7.8	8.8	23.5	21.7	10.8	7.4	8.3	6.7	7.0	6.5	9.1	10.4
2021	6.5	6.9	6.5	8.0	11.8	9.2	7.0	8.3					7.2

Source: From Centre for Monitoring Indian Economy: 'CMIE-Unemployment Rate in India', https://unemploymentinindia.cmie.com/kommon/bin/sr.php?kall=wsttimeseries&index_code=050050000000&dtype=total.

14.4.7 Education

Following the pandemic, schools in India remained closed for nearly seventeen months, and have witnessed tentative and gradual reopening only from August and September of 2021. This has been a drastic setback to learning and the creation of human capital in a society already seriously deficient in both resources. A major source of information on the impact of the pandemic on rural school education is the 2020 Annual Status of Education Report (ASER 2021). (ASER is an autonomous unit engaged in survey, research, and evaluation, and it operates within the framework of the government organization Pratham.) The 2020 Report points to both considerable absolute deprivation in education and relative disparity in the distribution of that deprivation. A major casualty of school closure has been enrolment. ASER's survey findings indicate that the proportion of all children not enrolled in school has risen from 4 per cent in 2018 to 5.5 per cent in 2020.

The Survey highlights, among other things, both educational deprivation as a major casualty of the pandemic-cum-lockdown and its disequalizing effects in terms of differentiation according to the nature of schools (government/private), access to smartphones, and level of parental education (which can also stand in for level of parental income). To this must be added the urban–rural divide. The ASER Report is based on an entirely rural survey. More recently (September 2021), the People's Archive of Rural India (PARI, 2021) has come up with a survey of both rural and urban areas, and some of its key findings are as follows. The urban (rural) proportion of sample children who (a) are 'studying online regularly' is 24 per cent (8 per cent); (b) are 'not studying at all nowadays' is 19 per cent (37 per cent); (c) did 'not meet their teacher(s) in the last 30 days' is 51 per cent (58 per cent); (d) did 'not have a test or exam in the last 3 months' is 52 per cent (48 per cent); and (e) are 'unable to read more than a few words' is 42 per cent (48 per cent). Further comment is surely superfluous.

14.4.8 Casualties of Caste, Religion, and Gender

The Scheduled Castes and Tribes, religious minorities (specifically Muslims), and women have traditionally been disadvantaged in the distribution of society's benefits and burdens. Instances of such group-related inequalities have already been encountered in the subsection dealing with 'livelihoods' (14.4.5). These are accentuations of well-defined existing tendencies of social stratification. But there have, in addition, been certain specific and distinctive forms of disequalizing and discriminatory outcomes caused by the pandemic, and these have fallen with severity upon persons of particular caste and religious affiliation, and women.

A particularly odious aspect of occupational specialization by caste is that relating to the virtual reservation of manual scavenging, and, more generally, menial sanitation work for members of the Scheduled Castes (SCs). Members of these castes have also been co-opted to the exhausting job of presiding over the disposal of bodies in overflowing crematoria. The sudden and incremental burdens imposed on sanitation workers by the pandemic, in terms of mortality, inadequate protection against risk of infection, and lack of transparency on welfare provisions and compensation packages, are available in the accounts of Rajput (2021), Ravichandran (2020), and Bhatnagar (2021), among others.

The marginalization of the Muslim community, and the attribution of various 'antinational' sentiments and activities to its members, have become an increasingly prominent feature of India's political landscape today. A particularly ugly crystallization of this trend is to be found in the so-called Tablighi Jamaat incident, involving allegations against a Muslim religious congregation in Nizamuddin, Old Delhi, of a deliberate attempt to spread the coronavirus disease (see Singh and Bhandari 2021 for a comprehensive account). While all of this is bizarre on its own, it acquires a particularly outlandish aspect when set against the subsequent event of the Kumbh Mela discussed in Section 3.3 of this chapter.

A specifically gender-related adverse fallout of lockdown has been the phenomenon of intimate-partner violence: the link between the two phenomena has been explored by, among others, Ravindran and Shah (2020) and Gulati (2020).

14.5 Concluding Observations

A pandemic of the proportions of COVID-19 must be expected to leave behind a trail of devastation in its wake. It is not our intention to lay all of the unhappy outcomes of the disease at the door of state policy. Having said this, it is also undeniable that the more severe effects of the pandemic could have been vastly more successfully mitigated by policy than has been the case. In particular, public policy mediated by the deployment of a blunt instrument such as lockdown, in combination with a mix of unpreparedness, incompetence, and insensitivity, has accentuated the havoc wrought by the disease. This is particularly the case with a pandemic that is inherently unequal (in the Orwellian sense of all pandemics being equal, but some more equal than others) and, like other 'natural' disasters, is also disequalizing in its differential impact on the already vulnerable sections of society (the poor, the labouring classes, and those burdened by the disadvantage of caste and religious affiliation).

There are at least three aspects of public policy, or rather its failure, that are rendered salient by India's experience of the coronavirus disease. The first has to do with the manner in which state policy has both vindicated and betrayed Amartya Sen's (1981) theory of 'entitlement failure', which he advanced in the context of an analysis of famine: namely, that the first object of state policy should be to anticipate and alleviate the distress of those members of society who are known to be particularly disadvantaged in terms of endowment and entitlement— typically, those who are poor, those who depend on their labour power for their livelihood, and those who bear the social burdens of stigma and discrimination. In the present case, these claims and interests have not only been disregarded but have arguably been sacrificed for the claims and interests of those with more robust endowments and entitlements.

Second, and this is a manifestation of the orientation just discussed, state policy has been distinguished by what Ray and Subramanian (2020c) have called a 'politics of visibility', accompanied by a 'politics of invisiblization'. The first is reflected in the implementation of a draconian policy of lockdown which has the advertisement value of attracting international kudos for ostensibly effective leadership, and the second is reflected in the glossing over of lives that are marginal in the perspective of an elitist society, as much as in suppression of statistics on the reach of infection and the magnitude of mortality from the pandemic.

Third, the utter unpreparedness of the state for a crisis points to a long prior history of obtuse social policy marked by the failure to take budgetary allocations for nutrition, health, and education with any measure of seriousness: good habits are not acquired overnight. The case of the state of Kerala is just the opposite, and explains why it—unlike much of the rest of the country—was so well prepared for the pandemic. Everything about India's pandemic experience points to the absolute paramountcy, especially in a country with as much poverty and informality as India, of having a system of socialized health, education, and distribution of food. In stark contrast, the presently discernible orientations of privatization of state responsibilities, and the sacrifice of the public sector to the interests of crony capitalism, bode ill for crises of the COVID-19 type in future.

Taking everything into account, the state's 'management' of the pandemic in India is reflected sharply in the alliance of the state's interests with the interests—both nationally and globally—of those who are relatively advantaged in the scheme of things. One is speaking here of extreme myopia and extreme self-centeredness. This is the case on such a large and obvious scale that it is actually somewhat embarrassing to draw attention to the 'lessons' that might be drawn from the country's experience or the implications for ethical thought and action for a future pandemic X which that experience might entail. What is assailed by a review of India's coronavirus record is, at basis, an understanding of human motivation and desirable human ambition that has been privileged by the mainstream economic idea of 'self-interest'. That idea, in its extreme and devastatingly exclusionary form, is at the heart of the issue.

Bibliography

Anand, I., and A. Thampi (2021), 'Growing Distress and a Falling Unemployment Rate', *The India Forum*, September 17, 2021, https://www.theindiaforum.in/article/rising-distress-and-falling-unemployment-rate-what-going?utm_source=website&utm_medium=organic&utm_campaign=category&utm_content=Economy.

ASER (2021), *Annual Status of Education Report (Rural) 2020 Wave 1*, February 2021, http://img.asercentre.org/docs/ASER per cent202021/ASER per cent202020 per cent20wave per cent201 per cent20- per cent20v2/aser2020wave1report_feb1.pdf.

Azim Premji University (2021), *State of Working India 2021: One year of COVID-19*, Centre for Sustainable Employment, Azim Premji University, https://cse.azimpremjiuniversity.edu.in/wp-content/uploads/2021/05/State_of_Working_India_2021-One_year_of_COVID-19.pdf.

Banaji, M. (2021), 'Estimating COVID-19 Fatalities in India', in *The India Forum*, May 10, 2021: https://www.theindiaforum.in/article/estimating-covid-19-fatalities-india

Bhardwaj, A., and A. Deshpande (2021), 'High Demand for MGNREGA is a Ringing Fire Alarm', *The Wire.in*, September 17, 2021, https://thewire.in/labour/high-demand-for-mgnrega-is-a-ringing-fire-alarm.

Bhatnagar, G. V. (2021), 'Across Waves of COVID-19 in India, Sanitation Workers Remain Most Ignored', *The Wire.in*, May 31, 2021, https://thewire.in/rights/across-waves-of-covid-19-in-india-sanitation-workers-remain-most-ignored.

Borah, A., S. Das, A. Dasgupta, A. Deshpande, K. Mahajan, B. Ramaswami, A. Saha, and A. Sharma (2020), 'Coronavirus Pandemic: The Policies We Need to Be Ready for the Long Haul' and 'Coronavirus Pandemic: How to Mitigate the Lockdown Impact on Vulnerable Populations', *The Wire*, March 30 and April 1, 2020, https://thewire.in/government/coronavirus-long-haul-comprehensive-relief-policy-framework and https://thewire.in/political-economy/coronavirus-pandemic-how-to-mitigate-the-lockdown-impact-on-vulnerable-populations.

Deshmukh, Y., W. Suraweera, C. Tumbe, A. Bhowmick, S. Sharma, P. Novasad, S. H. Fu, L. Newcombe, H. Gelband, P. Brown, and P. Jha (2021), 'Excess Mortality in India from June 2020 to July 2021 during the COVID Pandemic: Death

Registration, Health Facility Deaths, and Survey Data', medRxiv preprint, https://doi.org/10.1101/2021.07.20.21260872, https://www.medrxiv.org/content/10.1101/2021.07.20.21260872v1.full.pdf.

Deshpande, A., and J. Singh (2021), 'Dropping Out, Being Pushed out or Can't Get In? Decoding Declining Labour Force Participation of Indian Women', Ashoka University Discussion Paper 65, July 2021, https://dp.ashoka.edu.in/ash/wpaper/paper65.pdf.

Figueroa-Munoz, J. I., and P. Ramon-Pardo (2008), 'Tuberculosis control in vulnerable groups', *Bulletin of the World Health Organization*, 86(9): 733–5, https://www.ncbi.nlm.nih.gov/pmc/articles/PMC2649499/pdf/06-038737.pdf.

France 24 (2021), 'India's COVID-19 Shortages Spur Black Market for Drugs, Oxygen', April 22, 2021, https://www.france24.com/en/live-news/20210422-india-s-covid-19-shortages-spur-black-market-for-drugs-oxygen.

Ghosh, P. (2020), 'We need a Marshall Plan to Fight COVID-19', *Ideas for India*, April 8, 2020, https://www.ideasforindia.in/topics/macroeconomics/we-need-a-marshall-plan-to-fight-covid-19.html.

Ghoshal, D., and K. N. Das (2021), 'Scientists say India government ignored warnings amid coronavirus surge', Reuters, May 1, 2021, https://www.reuters.com/world/asia-pacific/exclusive-scientists-say-india-government-ignored-warnings-amid-coronavirus-2021-05-01/.

Gulati, N. (2020), 'COVID-19: Lockdown and Domestic Abuse', *Ideas for India*, April 19, 2020, https://www.ideasforindia.in/topics/social-identity/covid-19-lockdown-and-domestic-abuse.html.

India Today (2021), 'Explained: Why India is Facing a Shortage During 2nd COVID Wave', April 22, 2021, https://www.indiatoday.in/coronavirus-outbreak/story/explained-why-india-is-facing-oxygen-shortage-during-2nd-covid-wave-1793435-2021-04-21.

Iyer, Y., and M. Krishnamurthy (2020), 'COVID-19: An emergency economic manifesto', *Hindustan Times*, March 25, 2020, https://www.hindustantimes.com/analysis/covid-19-an-emergency-economic-manifesto/story-8GFWu7HWJJqPHIpYCsHL5M.html.

Jha, P. S. (2020), 'Modi's "Stimulus Package" is a gigantic confidence trick played on the people of India', *TheWire.in*, https://thewire.in/politicaleconomy/modis-stimulus-package-is-a-gigantic-confidence-trick-played-on-the-people-of-india.

Kamal, H. M. (2021), 'Kumbh Mela and election rallies: How two super spreader events have contributed to India's massive second wave of COVID-19 cases', *Firstpost*, April 22, 2021, https://www.firstpost.com/india/kumbh-mela-and-election-rallies-how-two-super-spreader-events-have-contributed-to-indias-massive-second-wave-of-covid-19-cases-9539551.html.

Khera, R. (2020), 'COVID-19: What can be done immediately to help vulnerable population' *Ideas for India*, March 25, 2020, https://www.ideasforindia.in/topics/poverty-inequality/covid-19-what-can-be-done-immediately-to-help-vulnerable-population.html

Kochhar, R. (2021), 'In the pandemic, India's middle class shrinks and poverty spreads while China sees smaller changes', Pew Research Centre, March 18, 2021, https://www.pewresearch.org/fact-tank/2021/03/18/in-the-pandemic-indias-middle-class-shrinks-and-poverty-spreads-while-china-sees-smaller-changes/.

Kulldorf, M., S. Gupta, and J. Bhattacharya (2020), 'Great Barrington Declaration', https://gbdeclaration.org/

Leffler, C. T., J. D. Lykins, and V. E. Young (2021), 'Preliminary Analysis of Excess Mortality in India During the COVID-19 Pandemic (updated August 4, 2021)', in medRxiv preprint, doi: https://doi.org/10.1101/2021.08.04.21261604, https://www.medrxiv.org/content/10.1101/2021.08.04.21261604v1.full.pdf.

Mannava, P., J. C. S. Murray, R. Kim, and H. L. Sobel (2019), 'Status of Water, Sanitation and Hygiene Services for Childbirth and Newborn Care in Seven Countries in East Asia and the Pacific', *Journal of Global Health*, 9(2): 1–10, https://www.ncbi.nlm.nih.gov/pmc/articles/PMC6925970/pdf/jogh-09–020430.pdf.

Narayanan, S. (2020), 'Food and Agriculture During a Pandemic: Managing the Consequences', *Ideas for India*, March 27, 2020, https://www.ideasforindia.in/topics/agriculture/food-and-agriculture-during-a-pandemic-managing-the-consequences.html.

Nilsen, A. G. (2021), 'Spectacle and Social Murder in Pandemic India', *Boston Review*, March 23, 2021, https://bostonreview.net/articles/alf-gunvald-nilsen-spectacle-and-social-murder-pandemic-india/.

Pandey, G. (2021), 'COVID-19: India's Holiest River is Swollen with Bodies', *BBC News, Delhi*, May 19, 2021, https://www.bbc.com/news/world-asia-india-57154564.

PARI (2021), *Locked Out: Emergency Report on School Education*, September 2021, https://ruralindiaonline.org/en/library/resource/locked-out-emergency-report-on-school-education/.

Rajput, A. (2021), 'Delhi: Half of COVID dead under municipal corporations are safai karmacharis', *Indian Express*, May 28, 2021, https://indianexpress.com/article/cities/delhi/delhi-half-of-covid-dead-under-municipal-corporations-are-safai-karamcharis-7333365/.

Ravichandran, N. (2020), 'Sanitation Workers Holding the Fort against COVID-19 Have No Protective Equipment', *The Wire.in*, March 30, 2020, https://thewire.in/rights/sanitation-workers-covid-19-working-conditions.

Ravindran, S., and M. Shah (2020), 'COVID-19:"Shadow Pandemic" and Violence Against Women', *Ideas for India*, September 17, 2020, https://www.ideasforindia.in/topics/social-identity/covid-19-shadow-pandemic-and-violence-against-women.html.

Ray, D., and S. Subramanian (2020a), 'Is There a Reasonable Alternative to a Comprehensive Lockdown?', *Ideas for India*, https://www.ideasforindia.in/topics/macroeconomics/is-there-a-reasonable-alternative-to-a-comprehensive-lockdown.html.

Ray, D., and S. Subramanian (2020b), 'India's Lockdown: An Interim Report', *Indian Economic Review*, 55: 531–79, https://doi.org/10.1007/s41775-020-00094-2.

Ray, D., and S. Subramanian (2020c), 'India's Response to COVID-19 is a Humanitarian Disaster', *The Boston Review*, July 16, 2020, https://www.bostonreview.net/articles/debraj-ray-s-subramanian-indias-unconscionable-response-covid-19/.

Ray, D., and S. Subramanian (2021), 'COVID And Other Diseases: An Animal Farm Perspective', *Frontline*, February 26, 2021.

Ray, D., S. Subramanian, and L. Vandewalle (2020), 'India's Lockdown', *Center for Economic Policy Research Policy Insight No. 102*, April 2020, https://cepr.org/publications/policy-insight-102-indias-lockdown.

Rumi, F. (2021), 'Oxygen Cylinders and Remdesivir being sold on black market', *The Times of India*, April 22, 2021, https://timesofindia.indiatimes.com/city/patna/oxygen-cylinders-remdesivir-being-sold-on-black-market/articleshow/82185040.cms

Salaria, S. (2021), 'Making hay in the black market: Remdesivir sold at Rs.40.000, oxygen cylinder at Rs.35,000', *The Times of India*, April 22, 2021. https://timesofindia.indiatimes.com/city/noida/making-hay-in-the-black-market-remdesivir-sold-at-rs-40000-oxygen-cylinder-at-rs-35000/articleshow/82187715.cms

Scroll Staff (2021), 'No deaths due to lack of oxygen reported by states during second COVID wave, claims Centre', *The Scroll.in*, July 21, 2021, https://scroll.in/latest/1000671/no-deaths-due-to-lack-of-oxygen-reported-by-states-during-second-covid-wave-claims-centre.

Sen, A. (1981), *Poverty and Famines: An Essay on Entitlement and Deprivation*, (Oxford: Clarendon Press, 1981).

Sen, A., R. Rajan, and A. Banerjee, 'Huge numbers may be pushed into dire poverty or starvation...we need to secure them', *The Indian Express*, April 17, 2020, https://indianexpress.com/article/opinion/coronavirus-india-lockdown-economy-amartya-sen-raghuram-rajan-abhijit-banerjee-6364521/.

Singh, R. S., and H. Bhandari (2021), 'Tablighi Jamaat: Much Ado About One Thing', *The Hindu*, March 22, 2021, https://www.thehindu.com/news/cities/Delhi/tablighi-jamaat-much-ado-about-one-thing/article34126409.ece.

Sinha, D. (2020), 'Food for All During Lockdown: State Governments Must Universalise PDS', in *The Wire*, April 20, 2020, https://thewire.in/rights/covid-19-lockdown-food-supply-pds

Subramanian, S. (2021a), 'A Slow Learner's Difficulty with the New Vaccine Policy', *The India Forum*, June 9, 2021, https://www.theindiaforum.in/letters/slow-learner-s-difficulty-new-vaccine-policy.

Subramanian, S. (2021b), 'Pandemic-induced Poverty in India after the First Wave of COVID-19: An Elaboration of Two Earlier Estimates', Issue Brief No.12, The Hindu Centre for Politics and Public Policy, August 19, 2021, https://www.thehinducentre.com/publications/issue-brief/article35974299.ece.

Thadhani, A. (2021), 'Preventing a Repeat of the COVID-19 Second-Wave Oxygen Crisis in India', *Observer Research Foundation*, June 25, 2021, https://www.orfonline.org/research/preventing-a-repeat-of-the-covid-19-second-wave-oxygen-crisis-in-india/

Vasudevan, V., A. Gnasekaran, B. Bansal, C. lahariya, G. G. Parameswaran, and J. Zon (2021), 'Assessment of COVID-19 Data Reporting in 100+ Websites and Apps in India', OSF Preprints, DOI: 10.31219/osf.io/wa3gn.

WHO (2017), 'Diarrhoeal Disease', May 2, 2017, https://www.who.int/news-room/fact-sheets/detail/diarrhoeal-disease#:~:text=Infection per cent20is per cent20spread per cent20through per cent20contaminated,soap per cent20can per cent20reduce per cent20disease per cent20risk.

WHO (2020), 'The Top 10 Causes of Death', December 2, 2020, https://www.who.int/news-room/fact-sheets/detail/the-top-10-causes-of-death#:~:text=The per cent20top per cent20global per cent20causes per cent20of,birth per cent20asphyxia per cent20and per cent20birth per cent20trauma per cent2C.

Zimmermann, L. V., BS, Maxwell Salvatore, MS, Giridhara R. Babu, PhD, MPH, and Bhramar Mukherjee, PhD (2021), 'Estimating COVID-19-Related Mortality in India: An Epidemiological Challenge With Insufficient Data', *American Journal of Public Health*, July 2021, https://ajph.aphapublications.org/doi/pdf/10.2105/AJPH.2021.306419.

15

Pandemic and Structural Comorbidity

Lasting Social Injustices in Brazil

Maria Clara Dias and Fabio A. G. Oliveira

15.1 Introduction

This article intends to point to the COVID-19 epidemic as an accelerator of social inequalities and the structural vulnerability situation experienced by specific segments of the Brazilian population, particularly, and by countries in the Global South, in general. To this end, we intend to present the effects of the pandemic on certain groups. Also, we aim to link the intensification of these groups' vulnerabilities to structural factors. Such factors are related to the colonial matrix (Quijano 2000; Lugones 2005, 2008; Dias 2020c and 2020d; Oliveira et al. 2020). In the Brazilian case, they get more potent due to the election of a president who explicitly reproduced and stimulated—in a paradigmatic and almost caricatural way—the prejudices imposed by the model of colonial capitalist exploitation. Thus, in this article we aim to demonstrate that a fundamental measure to be adopted in order to mitigate the effects of future pandemics is to immediately address the structural injustices that always make certain groups the most affected. This must be done through public policies adequate to the specific demands—vulnerabilities and functioning—of these groups.

As a theoretical reference, we will adopt the moral and justice perspective developed by Dias (2014; 2020a; 2020b), namely, the Functionings Approach (FA). It is a perspective that (1) aims to abandon current paradigms that violate basic functionings of individuals who remain at the margins of hegemonic epistemologies, and (2) claims a decolonial paradigm as a way to understand the colonial legacies that are still present in the structuring of social inequalities at global and local levels. FA's proposal is part of what has been called the decolonial turn in the literature produced by the Global South (Maldonado-Torres 2007; 2017). In this sense, this article is part of a broader movement carried out by intellectuals and scientists from the Global South to promote a critical review of the colonization process and the expansion of European capitalism over the countries of the Global South. Through interdisciplinary studies—philosophy, anthropology, political science, among others (Mignolo and Walsh 2018)—the aim is to recover original cultures, knowledge, and forms of social organization

Maria Clara Dias and Fabio A. G. Oliveira, *Pandemic and Structural Comorbidity: Lasting Social Injustices in Brazil*
In: *Pandemic Ethics: From COVID-19 to Disease X*. Edited by: Dominic Wilkinson and Julian Savulescu,
Oxford University Press. © Oxford University Press 2023. DOI: 10.1093/oso/9780192871688.003.0016

that have been silenced through the imposition of the so-called colonial thinking matrix (Restrepo 2018). These studies show how the subjugation of native peoples created racial (Quijano, 2000) and sex/gender (Arisi and Fernandes, 2017; Lugones 2007; 2008; 2010) categories as a way of naturalizing and, consequently, justifying the imposition of hierarchical relations and domination between colonizers and colonized. Criticism of the categories created then becomes part of the resistance to the model still in force today, which invisibilizes other ways of being and relating in the world, at the margins of the system of capitalist exploitation and its forged conception of progress and development (Costa 2016).

15.2 COVID-19 in Brazil: Background and Pandemic

Brazil has experienced an intensification of sociocultural conservatism and neoliberal policies between 2018 and 2022. It is marked, among other things, by the worsening of violence against the LGBTI+ population and women, the advance of deforestation in the Amazon, the flexibility of the demarcation of indigenous lands, the impoverishment of families involved in family farming, and the dismantling of social policies and Brazil's Unified Health System (SUS), which, since the end of the 1980s, has been an international reference in disease prevention, primarily through the implementation of mass vaccination programmes. In this context, the country was surprised by the COVID-19 pandemic. We reached the half a million deaths mark in just over a year, ranking among the ten countries with the highest death rate from COVID.

In January 2019, Jair Messias Bolsonaro assumed the republic's presidency in Brazil. He self-declares as a far-right conservative, opposed to LGBTI+[1] and indigenous rights[2], committed to the expansionist agenda of agribusiness[3], i.e. the advance of deforestation of the Amazon, politically permissive and a supporter of the removal of land from the indigenous population[4], besides the implementation of a rather pernicious version of economic neoliberalism. Bolsonaro not only discredited the real risk of infection and death from the COVID-19 virus but actively interfered in the governors' attempt to seek protection for the population of their

[1] There are numerous records that prove our statement, from interviews to public speeches at official events or in live streaming organized on the president's own social media. Here we list some of them: a) https://www.youtube.com/watch?v=3pautVX23lY; b) https://www.youtube.com/watch?v=prB3BS2wWCE; c) https://www.youtube.com/watch?v=NY8YH-nMlrQ (accessed 1 Apr. 2021).
[2] See https://www.theguardian.com/world/2020/jan/24/jair-bolsonaro-racist-comment-sparks-outrage-indigenous-groups (accessed 21 May 2022).
[3] See https://www.youtube.com/watch?v=lcXJNGhUQy8.
[4] See https://www.brasildefato.com.br/2021/03/25/lack-of-land-demarcation-hinders-indigenous-access-to-public-policies-vaccine (accessed 21 May 2022).

states.[5] He delayed the purchase and production of vaccines and strongly criticized the wearing of masks and social isolation. All this combined with public appearances without masks or any other health precautions.[6]

At the beginning of the pandemic, Bolsonaro declared that only the elderly and people with some kind of disability would die, which, in his perception, made the disease no more than "an insignificant flu", in no way alarming.[7] The pandemic appeared to be in line with his governmental policy, removing from the scene those who were no longer actively contributing to the country's economy. Brazil reached, within a little more than a year, the mark of half a million deaths.

To which groups do the majority of the deceased belong? Although a current discourse expressed that we were all in the same boat,[8] in a short time the profile of the victims showed that we definitely were not—and never have been. On the contrary, considering a colonial heritage based on asymmetrical power relations, government policies or medical councils have gradually reinforced the structural vices of Brazilian society. In line with this, the medical protocols adopted, imported from the Global North, prioritized the distribution of emergency resources to individuals with fewer "comorbidities".

The Brazilian Intensive Care Medicine Association (AMIB) was the first to release a document with recommendations. The protocol proposes adopting a scoring system to classify individuals, whereby the lower the score, the higher the priority. Evaluation includes using the Sequential Organ Failure Assessment (SOFA), the identification of severe comorbidity with an expectation of survival of less than one year, and the Eastern Cooperative Oncology Group (ECOG) tool. As a tie-breaker, the lowest SOFA score should be considered. The adoption of a clinical evaluation by the screening team is also suggested.

The SOFA score implies the evaluation of six fundamental systems: 1) respiratory; 2) coagulation; 3) hepatic; 4) circulatory; 5) neurological; and 6) renal. Scores range from 0 to 4, with 0 being assigned when the system has not been reached, 1 and 2 when there is organ dysfunction, 3 and 4 when there is organ failure. The ECOG Scale of Performance Status scores between 0 and 4 according to the functional status of each subject. For example, a person who is considered fully active and able to perform all activities without restriction receives a score of 0.

---

[5] See a) https://www.youtube.com/watch?v=gSSvnV9ksUE; b) https://www.youtube.com/watch?v=qhxc7Y0P9ss; c) https://www.youtube.com/watch?v=_RbCfyv1Hvg (accessed 1 Apr. 2021).

[6] Ciara Nugente, 'Brazil's Bolsonaro denied COVID-19 was a problem. Now he's embracing vaccines. Here's what changed', *Time*, 10 March 2021, https://time.com/5946401/brazil-covid-19-vaccines-bolsonaro/ (accessed 28 Sept. 2021).

[7] Gustavo Ribeiro, 'Bolsonaro says only 60+ people should worry about COVID-19. That is, except for himself', *The Brazilian Report*, 24 March 2020, https://brazilian.report/liveblog/coronavirus/2020/03/24/bolsonaro-coronavirus-only-gets-60-people-except-for-himself/ (accessed 2 Oct. 2021).

[8] Alexandra Barrantes, 'COVID-19: are we all in the same boat?', *Development Pathways*, 16 April 2020, https://www.developmentpathways.co.uk/blog/COVIDVID-19-are-we-all-in-the-same-boat/ (accessed 2 Oct. 2021).

At the other end, scoring 4, are people assessed as "completely unable to perform basic self-care, totally confined to bed or chair". The assumption is that the worse the individual's performance, the lower his or her physiological reserve and the greater the chance of clinical failure, i.e. death. The scale considers the condition before COVID-19 acquisition and is not indicated for people with physical disabilities.

We do not intend to reproduce and analyse all the proposed protocols. It is sufficient to say that the Brazilian Society of Bioethics (SBB) fully supported the protocol proposed by AMIB. The Regional Council of Medicine of the State of Rio do Janeiro (CREMERJ), in turn, produced a similar recommendation, with the adoption of SOFA, the ECOG, and the verification of the existence and severity of incurable and progressive underlying diseases. For all these actors, the decision to distribute such emergency resources was seen as a prerogative of health professionals, more specifically, physicians. As a justification, the eminently technical character of the evaluation was appealed to.

In articles published in 2020, Dias and Gonçalves[9] analyse the main protocols suggested and identify four convergent aspects. Firstly, they all assume that (1) we are facing a scarcity situation, which therefore (2) makes it necessary to establish criteria for resource distribution. Then, they assume that (3) the medical-scientific criterion is the most appropriate for the organization of those who should receive emergency resources, (4) aiming, as the ultimate goal, to save the most significant number of people. Finally, analysing such premises from the standpoint of morality, Dias and Gonçalves point to the fallacious character of the first three and the dogmatic, unjustified way in which the principle of saving the most significant number of lives is assumed.

We want to return to some aspects highlighted by those authors. The first one concerns the argument regarding a scarcity situation. From the point of view of philosophical discussions on distributive justice, scarcity of resources is always a fact. Acknowledging it gives rise to different theories of distributive justice, each focusing on some aspect considered, by them, to be essential and, therefore, as having to be guaranteed for all. In this sense, theories that defend an egalitarian concept of justice, that is, that argue that at least some goods and/or resources should be equally distributed, would already assume as problematic an ordering of criteria for the distribution of essential goods. Thus, if the resources in question can be considered essential to guarantee any individual's life or basic functionings, how could we establish general criteria to determine who will access them? Moreover, in a society so marked by differences regarding access to resources due

⁹ Maria Clara Dias and Letícia Gonçalves, 'Escolha sobre quem deve viver: bioética e covid-19 no contexto brasileiro', *Brasil de Fato*, 28 April 2020, https://www.brasildefato.com.br/2020/04/28/artigo-escolha-sobre-quem-deve-viver-bioetica-e-covid-19-no-contexto-brasileiro (accessed 22 Nov. 2022).

to social determinants such as race, class, and sex/gender, how can we guarantee such factors will not intervene, once again, in the choice of those selected?

Furthermore, what about adopting a medical-scientific criterion as the most appropriate one for determining the fair distribution of an essential good? The adoption of criteria is not merely technical and morally neutral. The very process from which the criteria are defined determines who will be prioritized to a great extent. A decision-making forum that only includes physicians can clearly neglect important aspects to guarantee the essential functioning of specific population segments. To ensure the inclusion of all segments of society, giving more space for the debate would thus be the only legitimate way to validate any proposal on the criteria for resource distribution within a society committed to a concept of justice with universal aspirations.

The last shared assumption, namely that the purpose of establishing criteria for the distribution of scarce resources is to save as many lives as possible, requires a more robust moral discussion. What makes the ultimate duty to save the maximum number of lives seem so self-evident to the authors of all proposals? We could list some hypotheses, but the critical point is to highlight that none of the protocols sought to morally justify the endorsement of this objective. There is nothing evident in the objective that is dogmatically assumed by the protocols. From a philosophical point of view, we must demand that it be justifiable.

In Brazil, as in almost all parts of the world, doctors belong to a socioeconomic elite. Moreover, during their studies they go through a desensitization process that makes them even more distant from an integral perception of the other. How then can one not suspect that they would be biased when determining the survival probabilities of individuals who have long lived in conditions of total precariousness? What kind of comorbidities, or even characteristics, can amplify the vulnerability of individuals in the very society we live in? If we can identify these characteristics, would it not be reasonable to assume that they make them even more vulnerable in a pandemic context? In our view, this is when the issue stops being merely technical and starts requiring a political, historical, and social analysis of society itself. Therefore, we should deepen our analyses and reflections in dialogue with the available scientific data, to examine our assumptions and explore the hypotheses raised here, as we will now do.

15.3 Making Visible the Intersection of Vulnerabilities: the Effects of COVID-19 in Brazil and its Colonial Entanglements

Since May 2020, Brazil has been ranked among the ten countries with the highest death rate from COVID. From May to June of that same year, Brazil jumped to second place in the total number of deaths of victims of the pandemic. More than a year has passed and, since then, it has never left that position. In the face of this tragedy, all kinds of denialism continued to be manifested by agents of the current federal government, including the ministers of health—General Eduardo Pazuello[10] and Doctor Marcelo Queiroga.[11] A Parliamentary Commission in the Federal Senate was established to monitor and investigate the dissemination of fake news about COVID. These investigations found improper use of the so-called "early treatment", diversion of funds targeted to purchase vaccines, and even the involvement of a health operator in the use of the so-called "COVID kit", which included the use of drugs of proven ineffectiveness.[12]

At the time of writing this text, Brazil has exceeded 600,000 deaths from COVID-19,[13] with the greatest concentration in the most populous states: São Paulo (151,000 deaths), Rio de Janeiro (67,188), and Minas Gerais (55,008), all located in the south-east of the country. This total number of deaths makes Brazil, to date, the second country in the world to exceed 600,000 victims of COVID, behind only the United States of America, which already has lost 700,000 lives. It means that, proportionally, Brazil is the eighth country in rate of deaths from COVID, corresponding to 12.4% of the deaths by COVID in the world. Among the ten countries with the highest number of deaths per million inhabitants, three are Latin American: Peru (in first place), Brazil (eighth), and Argentina (tenth).[14]

Analysing the data and the geopolitical map of the deaths also allows us to outline the inequalities and social injustices that plague the country and collaborate to understand the most vulnerable and victimized people with COVID-19 in Brazil.

For the survey of updated and systematized data, we have based our findings on the following documents and reports: the socioepidemiological bulletin of COVID-19 in the favelas, developed by the COVID-19 Observatory bulletin of the Oswaldo Cruz Foundation (Fiocruz); the Platform for Monitoring the Indigenous Situation in the New Coronavirus Pandemic (COVID-19) in Brazil, developed by the Socio-environmental Institute; the Study of Avoidable Deaths by COVID in Brazil, developed by Movimento Alerta; the LGBTI+ Diagnosis in

---

[10] See https://brazilian.report/power/2021/05/19/official-health-ministry-minutes-denialism/ (accessed 20 Apr. 2022).

[11] See https://www.nexojornal.com.br/expresso/2021/09/19/Queiroga-o-ministro-médico-que-abraçou-o-negacionismo; https://brazilian.report/power/2021/05/19/official-health-ministry-minutes-denialism/; https://www.nexojornal.com.br/expresso/2021/09/19/Queiroga-o-ministro-médico-que-abraçou-o-negacionismo (accessed 20 Apr. 2022).

[12] 'Acompanhe a cobertura da CPI da Pandemia', *Senado Notícias*, 27 October [last update] 2021, https://www12.senado.leg.br/noticias/ao-vivo/cpi-da-pandemia (accessed 12 Oct. 2021).

[13] Stephen Eisenhammer, 'Brazil passes 600,000 COVID-19 deaths, Health Ministry says', *Reuters*, 8 October 2021, https://www.reuters.com/world/americas/brazil-passes-600000-COVIDVID-19-deaths-health-ministry-says-2021-10-08/ (accessed 10 Oct. 2021).

[14] 'COVID-19 Dashboard', *Center for Systems Science and Engineering (CSSE) at Johns Hopkins University (JHU)*, https://www.arcgis.com/apps/dashboards/bda7594740fd40299423467b48e9ecf6 (accessed 11 Oct. 2021).

the Pandemic, carried out by the #VoteLGBT Collective in partnership with Box1824.

The sources consulted were chosen because they (1) consider social inequality as a fundamental element to understand the dissemination of the new coronavirus (SARS-CoV-2) in some areas of the country; (2) recognize the impact of access to basic sanitation (access to drinking water) for the adoption of preventive sanitary measures; (3) recognize that precarious locations with a more significant number of people crowding together[15] are less likely to adopt social distancing; (4) realize that a large part of the impoverished population cannot follow the global call to "stay at home", because in their condition of being poor, salaried workers and, in significant part, informal workers, they had to continue making long journeys on precarious public transportation between their homes and workplaces.

In this way the documents under consideration expose structural racism as one of the sources of inequality in Brazil and reveal the health vulnerability in which the indigenous village population finds itself. In addition, the documents show an increase in domestic violence against women and violence against the LGBTI+ population. Adopting measures to prevent the spread of the virus, such as social isolation, prevented these populations from contacting their networks of friends and support. They were forced to remain confined side by side with their potential aggressors—family members who reject their orientation and gender identity.

In light of the documents mentioned above, we find and highlight some essential information.

15.4 Poverty as a Risk Factor: the Case of the Pandemic in Slums

When, in May 2020, Brazil appeared in the ranking of the ten countries with the highest rate of COVID deaths, the highest COVID-19 incidence rates were located in neighbourhoods considered marginal (see Fiocruz 2020a: 17). According to Fiocruz's Observatory Bulletin on Slums, this statement contrasted with the data provided by the Instituto Pereira Passos (IPP), the Brazilian Institute of Geography and Statistics (IBGE), and the Rio de Janeiro City Hall's COVID19 Panel. These latter sources stated that areas "without favelas" or with a "low concentration of favelas" had a higher rate of COVID infection and death. Fiocruz's Observatory Bulletin on Slums points out that these indicators were influenced by the availability of testing in places where this service was more widely

---

[15] 17.5 million people live in settlements in Brazil (see IBGE 2019).

available. The consequence was identifying and confirming cases in wealthy areas (see Fiocruz 2020a: 20).

The result of a lack of access to testing services was that the population of impoverished areas could be highly infected but without wide access to testing and, consequently, without a proper definition of the cause of death (see Fiocruz 2020a: 20). This statement can be proven when we analyse the lethality rate by COVID in areas with high and very high concentrations of slums. According to Fiocruz's Observatory Bulletin on Slums, an area without slums has a lethality rate of 9.23%, while in an area with a very high concentration of slums, it is 19.47%. It means that in impoverished areas with high concentrations of people, for every 100 people that get sick from COVID, 20 will die (see Fiocruz 2020a: 24).

These data reveal a further spectrum of people in situations of social vulnerability. Fiocruz's Observatory Bulletin on Slums revealed that the percentage of deaths is higher among the black population (see Fiocruz 2020a: 27). The research highlighted that in areas of very high, high, medium, and low concentration of people, the percentage of death by COVID of the black population was always higher than that of the white population.

The data were even more impressive in the second bulletin presented by Fiocruz's Observatory Bulletin on Slums. Analysing the second half of 2020, it was observed that 48% of deaths by COVID-19 were among black people and that, in impoverished areas, the risk of getting sick from COVID-19 increased after the age of 40 (see Fiocruz 2020b: 2). It should be noted that, according to the World Health Organization, the age category that indicates a subject falls in the so-called "risk group" is limited to people aged 60 years or older or with pre-existing conditions. This delineation had already been questioned by a study developed by the Artificial Intelligence Laboratory of the Federal University of Minas Gerais (LIA-UFMG). According to LIA-UFMG, however, there would be a reasonably major impact of deaths in people between 45 and 49 years old.[16] Although the study does not show the social reasons for this group having accumulated high numbers of deaths during the pandemic, we support the hypothesis that the pre-existing social environments and constraints magnify the vulnerability of groups in health crises, such as the pandemic we have been experiencing.

The report[17] published by UN Women in 2020 highlighted that, in cities such as São Paulo, black people are 62% more likely to die from homicide when compared to white people. This bulletin also presents data stating that people living in peripheral urban and rural regions were ten times more likely to die from COVID.

---

[16] See 'Inteligência Artificial sugere grupo de risco para COVID-19 a partir dos 45 anos', *Kunumi*, 9 April 2020, https://medium.com/kunumi/inteligência-artificial-sugere-grupo-de-risco-para-COVIDVID-19-a-partir-dos-45-anos-89dcc460b99c (accessed 14 Oct. 2021).

[17] See 'Incorporando mulheres e meninas na resposta à pandemia de COVID-19', *ONU Mulheres*, 15 October 2020, https://www.onumulheres.org.br/wp-content/uploads/2020/12/COVID19_2020_informe2.pdf (accessed 3 Oct. 2021).

This whole scenario must be understood through the lens of the economic impacts that affected the entire population, especially those whose disadvantage was already a reality before the pandemic. This data is important because it shows that Brazil was already going through a socioeconomic crisis before the pandemic. According to the UN Women report, in 2019, Brazil had an unemployment rate of 11%. It means that 12.6 million people were unemployed before COVID-19. The same report shows that in August 2020 the total number of unemployed people was 75.2 million, among whom the vast majority were women.

15.5 Racism and Sexism Aggravating Pandemic Risk: Unemployment, Hunger, and Domestic Violence

The economic impact has generated a significant increase in the homeless population. According to the census of the Municipal Secretariat of Social Assistance (SMAS) of Rio de Janeiro[18], 20% of the total number of homeless people declare that they have lost their homes since the beginning of the pandemic. The survey also revealed the predominant profile of homeless people: 40.1% of them are black men.

While, on the one hand, the COVID-19 mortality rate among men is still higher in Brazil, women were and still are socioeconomically vulnerable. They are susceptible to all sorts of domestic violence and food insecurity. On the other hand, when we add the effect of gender to this analysis, sexism becomes evident as a source of inequality fundamental to Brazil's social relations. Along with racism, sexism—and its intertwining with the effect of race—exposes nuances to be considered so that we can analyse the at-risk groups in the pandemic.

During the pandemic, starvation has become one of the most significant problems in Brazil.[19] Note that in 2014 Brazil stopped appearing on the hunger map, which meant that hunger was no longer considered a structural problem. According to the Brazilian Forum for Food Sovereignty and Food and Nutritional Security, this is no longer the case, as hunger in Brazil has again reached alarming numbers. The survey revealed that 43.4 million people in Brazil (20.5% of the population) do not have enough food, and 19.1 million people (9% of the population) are going hungry. The study "National Survey on Food Insecurity in the Context of the COVID-19 Pandemic in Brazil" also showed that households

---

[18] See 'Prefeitura do Rio inicia censo da população em situação de rua para formular políticas públicas e reinserir pessoas no mercado de trabalho', *Rio Prefeitura*, 26 October 2020, https://prefeitura.rio/noticias/prefeitura-do-rio-inicia-censo-da-populacao-em-situacao-de-rua-para-formular-politicas-publicas-e-reinserir-pessoas-no-mercado-de-trabalho/ (accessed 1 Oct. 2021).

[19] Tom Phillips, 'Outcry in Brazil over photos of people scavenging through animal carcasses', *The Guardian*, 3 October 2020, https://www.theguardian.com/world/2021/oct/03/outcry-in-brazil-over-photos-of-people-scavenging-through-animal-carcasses (accessed 10 Oct. 2021).

headed by women are 11.1% more likely to face hunger. The majority are black women (see RBPSSAN 2021). It is no coincidence that one can state that hunger has colour and gender in Brazil.

Hunger primarily affects racialized and sexualized bodies: black people, indigenous people, and women in the Global South. During the pandemic, newspaper and television headlines of impoverished and hungry people on the streets being arrested for stealing small amounts of food in large commercial establishments became frequent. The vast majority of these individuals are black people and women who risk their lives searching for food for their children. A recent and striking case depicts the arrest of a woman who stole an instant noodle and a drink mix from a commercial establishment because she claimed to be hungry. Mother of five children, unemployed, the woman was questioned by sensationalist television channels, and print and digital newspapers that profit from people's misery in extreme vulnerability.[20] When interviewed at the prison gate and asked about the reason for the theft, she said, "My biggest dream is to be a person!"

Still on the gender aspect, according to the survey "Visible and invisible: the victimisation of women in Brazil", published by DataFolha and the Brazilian Forum on Public Safety (FBSP), one in four Brazilian women (24.4%) over the age of 16 say they suffered some kind of violence or aggression in 2020 (the last twelve months), during the COVID-19 pandemic. According to this study—as with other research concerning recent epidemics such as the Zika virus (2015) and Ebola (2013)—it is evident that health crises exacerbate already existing inequalities, including those based on people's socioeconomic status, age, race, and gender (see FBSP 2021).

A survey by the Global Protection Cluster (GPC), a network led by the UN Refugee Agency (UNHCR), and international NGOs protecting people who are refugees and affected by humanitarian crises identified a 90% increase in cases of domestic violence worldwide, with an emphasis on impoverished countries. In this case, the GPC noted that this incidence could be even higher in countries living under humanitarian conflicts, such as Afghanistan, Syria, and Iraq.[21] For this reason, there was a global campaign to create digital forms of care for women. However, in socioeconomically deprived situations it was observed that internet access and even the question of "digital literacy" imposed difficulties in working with gender-based violence.

In some (mostly impoverished) countries, communication channels have been created in chat applications, such as WhatsApp, as a hotline to report aggression

---

[20] The Public Defender's Office of the State of São Paulo filed a writ of habeas corpus based on the "principle of insignificance", which guaranteed the woman's freedom.

[21] See 'Nearly 40 million at heightened risk of violence, discrimination and rights abuses as COVID spawns a "coping crisis"', *Global Protection Cluster*, https://www.globalprotectioncluster.org/2020/11/30/nearly-40-million-at-heightened-risk-of-violence-discrimination-and-rights-abuses-as-COVID-spawns-a-coping-crisis/ (accessed 2 Oct. 2021).

and ask for help. In Brazil, for example, the National Council of Justice (CNJ) created the "Red Light" campaign, the result of a Working Group to analyse the increase in cases of domestic violence during the pandemic. The central idea is that women can ask for help in pharmacies, public agencies, and bank branches with a red sign drawn on the palm of their hand. In these places attendants, on seeing the sign, immediately call the police authorities. Unofficial campaigns have also taken over social networks to promote a network of support, solidarity, and sorority among women.

The impoverishment of certain groups makes it essential that the pandemic not be seen only as a health crisis and that solutions be thought of not only in the short term to minimize current losses. Instead, they should be planned in the medium and long term so that new events do not increase the vulnerability of historically marginalized groups, making them "at-risk groups".

To summarize, we question the crude clinical terminology which frequently attributes to vulnerable groups the condition of "risk groups". We take a different approach to identify which groups and their functionings are being neglected, through an inadequate policy of confrontation, not only towards the pandemic but towards the wounds of a colonial past and its persistent structures of domination and exploitation.

15.6 LGBTI+ People in the Pandemic: Isolation and Insecurity

A research study conducted by the #VoteLGBT Collective and Box1824 presented national data on how the LGBTI+ community in Brazil was affected in the pandemic.[22] The research revealed three primary sources of aggravation: financial vulnerability, worsening mental health, and withdrawal from the support network. According to respondents, all of these impacts had some kind of relationship with the current government's intolerant policies towards LGBTQIA+ people, as seen in other countries such as Uganda and Panama (Oliveira et al. 2021). The survey showed that six out of ten LGBTI+ people have decreased or lost their income since the pandemic began.

Black people, women, transgender people, and the poor were even more economically vulnerable. The research also reported that the unemployment rate for the LGBTI+ community during the pandemic was 17.5%, while the overall rate for Brazil, according to IBGE, was 14.7%. The study has revealed two fundamental data: 41.53% of the LGBTI+ population live under food insecurity conditions. Furthermore, 55.19% of those interviewed reported harms to mental health,

---

[22] 'Diagnóstico LGBT+ na Pandemia', *#votelgbt*, June 2021, https://static1.squarespace.com/static/5b310b91af2096e89a5bc1f5/t/60db6a3e00bb0444cdf6e8b4/1624992334484/%5Bvote%2Blgbt%2B%2B%2Bbox1824%5D%2Bdiagnóstico%2BLGBT%2B2021+b+%281%29.pdf; <us>https://www.globalprotectioncluster.org/old/2020/11/30/nearly-40-million-at-heightened-risk-of-violence-discrimination-and-rights-abuses-as-COVID-spawns-a-coping-crisis/</us> (accessed 10 Oct. 2021).

among which 47.59% were diagnosed with anxiety. Among those interviewed, 98.7% expressed disapproval of the president, and 95% favoured impeachment. Such data seem to reflect that vulnerable populations are observing a close and necessary relationship between the spread of the pandemic in Brazil and the policies that have been (or have not been) applied to minimize its impact on their lives.

15.7 Indigenous Peoples: Socio-environmental and Ethnic-racial Risk in the Pandemic

This same political perception of the pandemic in Brazil has been denounced by part of the indigenous community. The "Our struggle is for life" report, developed by the Articulation of Indigenous Peoples of Brazil (Apib), shows how violence and persecution against indigenous peoples accelerated during the pandemic. There are 305 different indigenous peoples in the whole country, of which 162 were affected by the pandemic, leading to a total of 1,215 deaths by COVID. According to the report, in most cases the virus was carried to the indigenous tribes by the Special Secretariat for Indigenous Health—SESAI—staff, the department responsible for coordinating and executing the National Policy for the Health Care of Indigenous Peoples.

This was the case in Alto Rio Solimões, and Vale do Javari, in the state of Amazonas. It has the highest rate of infection among the indigenous population. The fact that these cases are concentrated primarily, although not exclusively, in the country's northern region creates a warning about what the report calls "complicity in destruction". According to Apib, large corporations have an interest in creating and deepening vulnerability among indigenous peoples. In this way, the violation of rights ends up following the flow of interests of international capital in exploiting the region. This statement is reflected in verifying the growth of illegal deforestation in and around indigenous territories since the start of the pandemic.

The Amazon, for example, recorded a 34.5% increase in deforestation in 2020; the Yanomami territory, in Roraima, 85%; and, in the state of Pará, the most devastated indigenous lands were the Munduruku, reaching 238%; the Kayapó IT, with 420%; and Trincheira-Bacajá, with an 827% increase. It is worth remembering that in May 2020 the Minister of the Environment, Ricardo Salles, said, "So for this, we need to make an effort to push through regulatory change and simplification of rules – while we have the advantage of less attention of the press because they are only talking about COVID."[23] For this reason, a platform was

---

[23] 'Ministro do Meio Ambiente defende passar "a boiada" e "mudar" regras enquanto atenção da mídia está voltada para a COVID-19', *G1*, 25 May, 2020, https://g1.globo.com/politica/noticia/2020/05/22/ministro-do-meio-ambiente-defende-passar-a-boiada-e-mudar-regramento-e-simplificar-normas.ghtml (accessed 14 Oct. 2021).

created to monitor the indigenous situation in the pandemic, based on data made available by Apib.

15.8 At-risk Groups: Colonial Vulnerability in Times of Pandemic

We observed that many efforts to combat the pandemic among vulnerable groups have been undertaken independently of the state itself. After all, one can see that such groups were and continue to be abandoned by the state when not directly victimized by it. In this way, we suggest that the term "risk groups", in and beyond the pandemic context, starts to be evaluated based on where the victimized subjects are located. This aspect seems fundamental to us. We can provide a more accurate diagnosis of the groups that remain victimized by the global pandemic crisis of COVID-19 and create more effective protective public policies.

For this reason, we call "at-risk groups" all those who, in the face of a system of structural violence and neglect, are exposed cruelly and disproportionately to the COVID-19 pandemic. Such exposure is nothing new for these groups. Long ago, even before the pandemic, they have already been (1) suffering from social isolation in the specific domain of global white privilege, which keeps incarcerating non-white bodies in the name of justice; (2) suffering moral and sexual violence from aggressors in domestic and public settings, including professional ones; (3) facing compulsory displacement—an ongoing political economy since colonialism that assigned the so-called "new world" the deculturated place where subhumanity lived; (4) being excluded from institutional processes that guarantee fundamental rights to live out their sexual orientations and gender identities.

All the processes that already nullify historically marginalized subjects were not taken into consideration. The risks imposed by the pandemic are being managed in a way that those who are privileged are protected from its worst impact while, simultaneously, at-risk groups are suffering. It is in this sense that we invoke a moral argument. It makes it possible to denounce and break with a historical process of colonial power relations, which generate oppression, subordination, and extermination of certain groups, and it also provides us with the theoretical basis necessary to suppress the hierarchical moral treatment between the various segments of society, broadening the scope of morality and justice.

In this way, we consider that analysing the impacts of the pandemic on specific populations and in some areas of the world, such as marginalized groups in Brazil, requires a deeper and more structural evaluation. For this, it is necessary to resort to a moral and justice perspective that addresses the structural problems sustaining the social inequalities that currently plague the marginalized population, but to consider the injustices committed in the past. Therefore, it seems essential to adopt a perspective that brings the decolonial turn.

By decolonial turn we understand the need to claim the adoption of a para-digm that allows analysing the colonial ghosts still sustaining the predominance of hegemonic epistemologies[24] to understand the world and its ills. In this sense, the decolonial turn is a call to denounce not only a kind of geopolitics of know-ledge but also its ethical collaboration with the persistent coloniality of power/knowledge and being in the "periphery of the world", the "edge of the planet", or the so-called "third world".

In this way we draw on decolonial inspirations to understand why the COVID-19 pandemic affects historically marginalized groups, i.e. groups that still bear the marks of a past of oppression and neglect. Among these theories we consider the Functionings Approach to be a theoretical proposal dedicated to the foundation of a more inclusive conception of morality and justice, which, from a practical point of view, seeks to identify, in each case, (1) which are the neglected basic functionings; (2) what factors contribute to this fact; and (3) what condi-tions need to be guaranteed so that they are fully realized.

This is a perspective built through the debate within the philosophical tradition,[25] but that aims, above all, to guide our empirical research in order to build public policies more adequate and compatible with the actual demands of the several segments of society—especially those who have always been on the margins.

15.9 Adopting a Decolonial Moral Paradigm

The Functionings Approach was conceived as a way to incorporate as the object of our moral consideration all human beings, non-human animals, and some inanimate objects, guaranteeing them a respectful, non-hierarchical, and egalitar-ian moral treatment, at least in what concerns the equal consideration of their basic functionings.

To this end, Dias (2014; 2020a; 2020b) proposes a form of minimalist identifi-cation of morality's focus, capable of breaking with a long process of identity determination, marked by a logic of exclusion—namely, individuals understood as functional systems. Such characterization will be called minimalist because it allows contemplation of all segments listed by traditional moral perspectives and also allows us to go a step further. According to the author, when characterized in this way, individuals can be identified both (1) as beings capable of feeling and responding to painful and/or pleasurable stimuli, therefore sentient beings, and

---

[24] According to Raymond Williams (1977: 109), hegemony is related to "dominant meanings and values". Then, epistemological hegemony represents a concern for the domination of one view of knowledge and the subordination of all other forms.

[25] For further information on the theoretical framework of the Functionings Approach and its debate with the philosophical tradition, see Dias (2014; 2020a; 2020b).

(2) as beings capable of apprehending information about their environment, relating it to a particular subjective universe of beliefs and desires and responding to them, acting in a manner consistent with the reflections made. These would be, then, individuals to whom we could attribute different degrees of what we ordinarily call rationality and freedom. Besides this, the characterization of the individual as a functional system also allows us to identify (3) objects such as books and glasses, and (4) complex systems such as an ecosystem and a geopolitical environment. Individuals belonging to group 3, inanimate objects, may or may not be the object of moral consideration, depending, contextually, on their relation to other systems or their position within a functional system. A mechanical leg can be understood as a coupled system that ensures an individual can move properly. Similarly, a pair of prescription glasses can be interpreted as a coupled system that ensures vision (Dias 2014; 2020a; 2020b).

The individuation of functional systems is not something fixed but something that concerns the particular circumstances of each individual. It means that we are all a complex of functional systems that transform themselves—incorporating or excluding other systems—and redefine their basic functionings in the course of our existence. As basic functionings, we will understand all those that make up the identity core of the individual in question: all the actions, functions, or capacities that guarantee the functional integrity of an individual. When impeded, those functionings violate the individual's perception of themselves or how they are understood in the social body. Such functionings may vary among different individuals and at the core of the same individual's existence.

FA rejects any attempt to essentialize or naturalize individual characteristics, hence the naturalization of the categories of race, sex/gender, and also species. In endorsing this perspective, we have no longer reasons to restrain the limits of morality to individuals who supposedly are similar to us or belong to our species. Non-human animals, forests, rivers, musical scores, monuments, and even cities are functional systems with which some of us are so identified that, without them, some of our essential functions would be lost forever. Therefore, actions or moral norms and principles of justice should ensure the basic functionings of the different functional systems. The neglect of the basic functionings of a system may put at risk the integrity of the various individuals or functional systems related to it.

Thus, if we return to the data presented previously, we conclude that the current pandemic has become yet another aggravating factor of systematic and structural violence. It violates the basic functionings of individuals/groups already historically marginalized and made vulnerable by a myopic moral and justice standard. Through the Functionings Approach, we can identify that coloniality is still present where there is denial, including institutional denial. Also, specific power/knowledge structures, institutional protocols, public policies, and recurrent social practices constitute violence and violation of the basic functionings of many segments of society. In this sense, the decolonial critique endorsed by the Functionings Approach is, above all, a denunciation of structural injustice.

Nevertheless, what exactly should we conclude? The denunciation raised by decolonial perspectives addresses the different ways in which the ghosts of the colonial past still persist today, in a kind of enduring phase with violence targeting vulnerable groups living in the most impoverished regions of the planet. These ghosts are not always visible. On the contrary, they are camouflaged and often become the very modus operandi that guarantees the permanence of some voices and epistemologies as those capable of unveiling problems and providing solutions. Other voices and forms of existence are hidden.

At the beginning of this chapter, we tried to show that the proposed protocols, developed at the start of the pandemic for the distribution of emergency health resources, are examples of this. They exclude from the debate the main interested parties, namely users of the public health system, leaving the decision up to physicians. Furthermore, they assume as a criterion of eligibility the patients with the lowest number of comorbidities, following protocols established in the Global North that perhaps cannot be simply assumed to accurately evaluate the chances of survival in countries, like ours, with a striking pre-existing adverse reality.

Similarly, we cannot fail to identify neglect and moral and political disrespect as the main reasons why, in the case of Brazil, the elderly, people with disabilities, women, black and indigenous populations, people living on the streets, residents of the peripheries, and the LGBTI+ population have been the segments most affected by the pandemic, even when not directly affected by the virus.

Furthermore, we highlight the following as factors that negatively affect already vulnerable groups: domestic violence against women and LGBTI+ people; social isolation and its resulting psychological and physical sequelae; inadequate socio-environmental conditions to keep oneself sanitized; and the increase in formal unemployment, hunger, and impoverishment. In this case, we insist: either the measures adopted to confront this pandemic and future ones should take into consideration the specific demands of different social groups and the fragilities to which they are exposed due to structural factors of Brazilian society; or, once again, we will only be facing the symptoms but not fighting the root of the problem, namely, an exploitative, colonial structure of social organization that, for centuries, has subjugated and victimized a large part of the population.

15.10 The Colonial Past and the Post-pandemic Future

Adopting a moral perspective that considers the diverse members of society as equal objects of moral respect or consideration, what measures can be taken to minimize the catastrophic effects of certain events, such as a pandemic, on the diverse beings of the planet? What analyses need to be made so that we understand the global effects coming from COVID-19 and how the pandemic settles differently in different regions? How does the future look for those who have always been left at the margins of legal and institutional safety nets?

Suppose we effectively assume a moral perspective that breaks with anthropocentric, ethnic-racial, socioeconomic, cultural, sex/gender, and sexual orientation hierarchies; our main effort, in that case, should be to promote a better distribution of resources and living conditions for the planet's various parts and diverse beings. Such a proposal seems unthinkable without adopting a decolonial turn that allows us to understand the colonialities that still haunt peoples and individuals and self-perpetuate, so that past and present injustices persist into the future.

Through the Functionings Approach, we seek to provide an instrument that, based on the investigation and identification of what can be considered a basic functioning for each individual and/or group, can contribute to the construction of public policies more appropriate to the genuine demands of all segments of society. To this end, FA invites us to let each individual and/or group express what is essential for them; that is, what makes their individual and/or collective integrity possible. We need to relearn to listen and see others more sensitively and the often subtle, almost imperceptible way their demands are expressed.

Adopting Brazil as a reference, we seek to show that certain social groups have had their essential functions neglected systemically and, thus, placed at constant risk, forming what we call "at-risk groups". The data generated by research carried out during the pandemic only point to how COVID-19 highlighted structural deficiencies in Brazilian society and disastrous policies of the current government, which potentiated the risks to which the segments in question are exposed. Beyond the pandemic, Brazil and the world, now and in the future, need to face a structural evil: a gap of socioeconomic inequality and an epistemic arrogance that silences and invisibilizes other ways of knowing and existing. For this, it seems essential to decolonize our view of the world and resort to voices that do not participate in the discussion posed by the hegemonic matrix that sustains the geopolitics of knowledge.

If the effects of colonialism on the periphery of the world were already quite visible, the pandemic has made the map of inequalities even more flagrant. Therefore, the protocol for confronting the COVID-19 pandemic, and other pandemics to come, cannot neglect the colonial flagellum: Brazil and the world need to break with hegemonic colonial power and knowledge structures and contribute to the construction of full democracies, with the reverberation of hitherto silenced voices.

The data presented in this article expose what has been hidden: we are not going through the same pandemic, despite living in the same space–time. We are, in fact, facing a social and moral paradigm crisis. We suspect that enriched nations and large corporations will offer new ways to overcome the so-called "health crisis". They will recreate new forms of subjugation and exploitation of at-risk groups, especially those living in the Global South, in impoverished regions, where the echo of the colonial past is still present, as in the case of Brazil. In this chapter, we have tried to point towards theoretical paths and practices that allow for creating sociopolitical spaces that enable voices, bodies, and accents—hitherto unnoticed, neglected, or persecuted—to effectively create another possible world and to build a more effective response to the next pandemic.

Bibliography

Arisi, B. M., Fernandes, E. R. (2017), *Gay Indians in Brazil: Untold Stories of the Colonization of Indigenous Sexualities* (Cham: Springer, 2017).

Costa, A. (2016), *Bem viver: uma oportunidade para imaginar outros mundos* (Rio de Janeiro: Autonomia Literária, 2016).

Dias, M. C. (ed.). (2014), *Functioning Approach: for a more inclusive moral point of view* (Amazon, 2014).

Dias, M. C. (2020a), *About us: expanding the frontiers of morality* (Editora Ape'Ku, 2020).

Dias, M. C. (ed.). (2020b), *Bioethics: theoretical foundations and applications* (Editora Ape'Ku, 2020).

Dias, M. C. (2020c), 'Feminismo e decolonialidade: contribuições de María Lugones para a promoção da justiça em sociedades periféricas', in M. C. Dias et al. (eds.), *Feminismos Decoloniais: Homenagem a María Lugones* (Editora Ape'Ku, 2020): 11–30.

Dias, M. C. (2020d), 'Caixa de Pandora', in M. C. Izidoro, S. Castro (eds.), *Políticas de Resistência: homenagem à María Lugones* (Fundação Fênix, 2020): 47–58.

FIOCRUZ (2020a), *Boletim socioepidemiológico da COVID-19 nas favelas: análise da frequência, incidência, mortalidade e letalidade por COVID-19 em favelas cariocas*. 01, Fundação Oswaldo Cruz, https://www.redalyc.org/journal/4063/406371825010/html/.

FIOCRUZ (2020b), *Boletim socioepidemiológico da COVID-19 nas favelas: análise da frequência, incidência, mortalidade e letalidade por COVID-19 em favelas cariocas*. 01. Fundação Oswaldo Cruz, https://portal.fiocruz.br/sites/portal.fiocruz.br/files/documentos/boletim_final.pdf.

Fórum Brasileiro de Segurança Pública, DataFolha Instituto de Pesquisa (2021), *Visível e invisível: a vitimização de mulheres no Brasil*. 3rd. https://dssbr.ensp.fiocruz.br/wp-content/uploads/2021/06/relatorio-visivel-e-invisivel-3ed-2021-v3.pdf.

IBGE (2019), '*O IBGE apoiando o combate à COVID-19. 01, Instituto Brasileiro de Geografia e Estatística*', https://covid19.ibge.gov.br/pnad-covid/.

Lugones, M. (2005), 'The coloniality of Gender. Worlds and Knowledge Otherwise', *Worlds & Knowledges Otherwise*: 1–17, https://globalstudies.trinity.duke.edu/sites/globalstudies.trinity.duke.edu/files/file-attachments/v2d2_Lugones.pdf.

Lugones, M. (2007), 'Heterosexualism and the colonial/modern gender system', *Hypatia* 22/1: 186–209.

Lugones, M. (2008), 'Colonialidad y género', *Tábula Rasa* 9: 73–101.

Lugones, M. (2010), 'Towards a decolonial feminism', *Hypatia* 25/4: 742–59.

Lugones, M. (2014), 'Rumo a um feminismo descolonial', *Revista Estudos Feministas* 22/3: 935–52.

Maldonado-Torres, N. (2007), 'Sobre la colonialidad del ser: contribuciones al desarrollo de un concepto', in C. Gómez, Santiago, and G. Ramon (eds.), *El giro decolonial: reflexiones para uma diversidad epistêmica más allá del capitalismo global* (Siglo del Hombre Editores, 2007).

Maldonado-Torres, N. (2017), 'On the coloniality of human rights', *Revista Crítica de Ciências Sociais* 114: 117–36.

Mignolo, W., and Walsh, C. (2018), *On decoloniality: concepts, analytics and praxis* (Durham, NC: Duke University Press, 2018).

Oliveira, F. A. G., et al. (2020), 'Locus Fraturado: resistências no Sul Global e práxis antiespecistas ecofeministas descoloniais', in M. C. Dias, et al. (eds.), *Feminismos Decoloniais: Homenagem a María Lugones* (Editora Ape'Ku, 2020).

Oliveira, F. A. G., et al. (2021), 'Grupos em risco: a transfobia e a patologização das identidades trans como categorias de análise político-pedagógica', *Revista Inclusiones* 8/3: 187–208.

Quijano, A. (2000), 'Coloniality of Power, Eurocentrism, and Latin America', in *Nepantla: Views from South* 1/3, Project MUSE: 533–80.

Rede Brasileira de Pesquisa em Soberania e Segurança Alimentar (2021), *Inquérito Nacional sobre Insegurança alimentar no contexto da pandemia da COVID-19 no Brasil*, http://olheparaafome.com.br/VIGISAN_Inseguranca_alimentar.pdf.

Restrepo, E. (2018), 'Coloniality of power', in *The international encyclopedia of anthropology* 1–6. 10.1002/9781118924396.wbiea2118, http://www.ram-wan.net/restrepo/documentos/coloniality.pdf.

Williams, R. (1977), *Marxism and literature* (London: New Left Books, 1977).

16

Fair Distribution of Burdens and Vulnerable Groups with Physical Distancing during a Pandemic

Eisuke Nakazawa and Akira Akabayashi

16.1 Introduction

Coronavirus disease 2019 (COVID-19) became a global pandemic on a scale far beyond anyone's expectations. While it is imperative to discuss the law and public health ethics relating to medical resource allocation and disaster triage during such a super-scale pandemic, it is also important to describe in detail the ongoing pandemic and the difficult situation of the citizens living in the midst of it.

An often-used indicator of wealth imbalance within a society is the relative poverty rate (usually referred to simply as the "poverty rate"). According to the Organization for Economic Cooperation and Development (OECD), this is defined as follows:

> The poverty rate is the ratio of the number of people (in a given age group) whose income falls below the poverty line; taken as half the median household income of the total population.   (OECD n.d.)

In 2018, the poverty rate in Japan was relatively high, at 15.4% (MHLW 2020a). It was the eighth highest among the thirty-eight countries in the OECD. Poverty among older people and single-adult households with children had become a social issue, while the reduction of economic inequality—more broadly, social inequality—had become a political issue. The COVID-19 pandemic resulted in an even higher poverty rate in Japan, a phenomenon that has become increasingly evident and distinct. One likely reason for this is that physical distancing as a policy to prevent the spread of COVID-19 infection has further isolated the poor and made them poorer, both socially and economically.

The COVID-19 pandemic has affected the livelihoods of many citizens, necessitating effective and aggressive public health interventions, some of which may not always be compatible with reducing social disparities. Some may argue that widening disparities during emergencies are acceptable to a certain extent.

Eisuke Nakazawa and Akira Akabayashi, *Fair Distribution of Burdens and Vulnerable Groups with Physical Distancing during a Pandemic* In: *Pandemic Ethics: From COVID-19 to Disease X.* Edited by: Dominic Wilkinson and Julian Savulescu, Oxford University Press. © Oxford University Press 2023. DOI: 10.1093/oso/9780192871688.003.0017

However, we believe that the reduction of social and economic disparities, even in times of emergency, can enhance the overall well-being of a society.

This chapter provides an empirically informed report on the social disparities that became apparent in Japan during the COVID-19 pandemic and evaluates the physical distancing policy which emerged as the main countermeasure against the COVID-19 pandemic in Japan.

We describe in detail the disproportionate burdens borne by two vulnerable groups—older people and foreigners in Japan during the COVID-19 pandemic, as these two relatively impoverished groups were some of the hardest hit by the pandemic. Specifically, we describe how Japan's physical distancing policy promoted the social isolation of older people and foreigners and expanded social and economic disparities. Second, we present preliminary recommendations for minimizing the scope of restrictions, as well as providing information and alternative communication tools to help reduce the disparity in physical distancing known to increase social isolation. These recommendations will have universal relevance as a guide for public health policymakers where justice is required. There is a trade-off between guaranteeing individual freedom of action and promoting the public good through the control of infectious diseases. Since this conflict is essential, it appears not only in COVID-19 but also in the unknown Disease X that we face somewhere in the future. In this chapter, we point out that public health policymakers are required to adjust the conflict in accordance with the principles of justice to protect the socially vulnerable.

16.2 Overview of COVID-19 Control Policies in Japan

By May 2022, the total number of COVID-19 cases in Japan was about 8.3 million, with about 30,000 deaths. The rate of 237.51 per million people (May 11, 2022) is low compared to those of the US and European countries, but much higher than those of China and Taiwan. On the other hand, South Korea experienced a massive outbreak from March to May 2022 (Figure 16.1). Japan has experienced six waves of SARS-CoV-2 infection spread. During each wave, the government has taken various measures to combat the spread, including restricting restaurant businesses, under the Act on Special Measures against Novel Influenza, which was amended in response to the COVID-19 pandemic. However, the medical and healthcare systems were exhausted during each wave and were on the verge of a crisis. This is because the shortage of hospital beds prevented many COVID-19 patients from being admitted to hospitals, even though they required admission. After the fourth wave, when the vaccine became widely available, social concern shifted to compatibility with economic activities rather than being shut down for COVID-19. However, Japan's real gross domestic product growth rate was −4.5% in 2020 and +1.7% in 2021, a slow recovery compared to that

Cumulative confirmed COVID-19 deaths per million people
Due to varying protocols and challenges in the attribution of the cause od death, the number of confirmed deaths
may not accurately represent the true number of deaths caused by COVID-19.

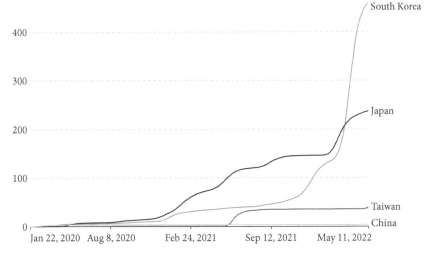

Figure 16.1 Cumulative confirmed COVID-19 deaths per million people in China, Japan, South Korea, and Taiwan. Data from Our World in Data (2022). Coronavirus (COVID-19) Deaths. Oxford, United Kingdom: Global Change Data Lab. https:// ourworldindata.org/covid-deaths.

of the world as a whole (−4.5% in 2020 and +5.2% in 2021) (International Monetary Fund 2022).

Along with vaccination and hand sanitization, physical distancing is an indispensable public health policy used to control the spread of COVID-19. It requires individuals to maintain a distance of at least 1 meter from one another and avoid crowded places or groups (WHO 2021). It also includes the practice of working from home instead of at the office, closing schools or switching to online classes, holding virtual instead of physical meetings, and cancelling or postponing conferences or other large gatherings (Maragakis 2020a). It is generally understood that physical distancing includes the donning of a face mask when outside and among strangers (Maragakis 2020b). The term "social distancing" has a similar meaning to the term "physical distancing." Globally, the phrase "social distancing" was used rather than "physical distancing" in the early stages of the COVID-19 pandemic in the spring of 2020. Subsequently, international organizations, such as the United Nations Children's Fund, advocated for the term "physical distancing" to be used (UNICEF 2020). To summarize the conceptual relationship between the two, physical distancing does not necessarily imply social separation; physically distanced persons may still be socially close.

During the COVID-19 pandemic, from 2020 to 2021, the status of social network services as social infrastructure increased dramatically. Simultaneously, the use of web-based telecommunications, such as Zoom, Webex, and Google Meet, became common in businesses, social communities, and educational institutions. Of course, this does not mean that internet technology is an absolute requirement for forming and maintaining a social community at an appropriate physical distance. It is certainly possible to maintain a social community using traditional media such as newspapers and newsletters, and in-person communities can still be maintained readily with strict infection control measures, even during a global pandemic.

In Japan, the term "social distancing" was commonly circulated through the media in 2020 when the government issued the first state of emergency in relation to COVID-19 (Cabinet Office Japan 2020).[1] For whatever reason, the Japanese gravitated toward the term "social distancing" over "physical distancing." Conversely, the word "San-Mitsu," which was coined in Japan, and its negative form were used instead of the phrase "physical distancing." "San-Mitsu" refers to the three situations that enhance the spread of COVID-19. In English, these are known as the "three Cs," and specifically refer to (1) closed spaces with poor ventilation, (2) crowded places with many people nearby, and (3) close-contact settings, such as close-range conversations (MHLW 2020b). "Avoid the San-Mitsu (= three Cs)" has become a government slogan to promote physical distancing in the Japanese social setting.

Along with physical distancing, infection control precautions such as hand sanitizing were recommended at a basic level in Japan. Alcohol disinfectant sprays became readily available at storefronts, not only in cafes and restaurants, where the risk of droplet infection is a concern, but also in supermarkets, convenience stores, drugstores, and even bookstores. Given that many people are diligently using them, it can be inferred that hand sanitizing is very thorough in Japan. The use of face masks is also quite common in Japan. As of the fall of 2021, the percentage of Japanese who wear face masks when going out is still very high. According to the OECD report, Japan and South Korea were the top countries for

---

[1] The declaration of a state of emergency in Japan is the implementation of public health policies to prevent the spread of a coronavirus pandemic in accordance with the provisions of Article 32, Paragraph 1, of the Act on Special Measures against Novel Influenza, etc. (Act No. 31 of 2012). The declaration of a state of emergency is made by the Prime Minister by recognizing the occurrence of a situation that is likely to cause extremely serious damage to the lives and health of the people and is likely to have an enormous impact on the lives of the people and the national economy due to nationwide and rapid spread, and designating the period and area where emergency measures will be taken. Under the Act on Special Measures against Novel Influenza, etc., prefectural governors may request residents not to go out of their residences or other places equivalent to their residences without permission, except when necessary to maintain their lives, and to cooperate in other ways necessary to prevent the spread of a new type of influenza (the Act on Special Measures against Novel Influenza, etc. Article 45, Paragraph 1, https://elaws.e-gov.go.jp/document?lawid=424AC0000000031). As far as the emergency declaration on COVID-19 is concerned, the first emergency declaration was issued on April 7, 2020, in seven prefectures: Tokyo, Kanagawa, Saitama, Chiba, Osaka, Hyogo, and Fukuoka. It was expanded to cover the entire country on April 16. Since then, a total of four emergency declarations have been issued intermittently as of October 2021.

mask usage throughout the pandemic, with a rate of over 90% (wearing of a mask all the time or most of the time when in public) (OECD 2021).

These basic infection control precautions such as hand sanitization and wearing face masks are less invasive than public health policies. In this context, invasiveness refers to the degree to which a public health policy restricts people's freedom of action. Although hand sanitization is not included in physical distancing, all physical distancing policies are invasive to some extent. Examples of such invasiveness include requests to restaurants and bars to stop serving alcoholic beverages; to restaurants, bars, cafes, and even department stores to reduce their operating hours; to theaters and cinemas to close; to restrict the number of spectators at large-scale events; to refrain from going out unnecessarily; to refrain from returning to one's hometown for holidays; to refrain from cross-town travel; and to work from home. These public health interventions are invasive in that they restrict the freedom of economic activity and freedom of movement.

Of course, this invasiveness has already been considered by the government. The Act on Special Measures against Novel Influenza, etc. stipulates that "in light of the fact that the freedoms and rights of the citizens should be respected, when implementing countermeasures against novel strains of influenza, etc., even if restrictions are imposed on the freedoms and rights of the citizens, such restrictions shall be the minimum necessary to implement such countermeasures" (Act on Special Measures against Novel Influenza 2012: Article 5).

However, to what extent can restrictions on freedom of economic activity and freedom of movement be deemed minimally necessary? Under what conditions are restrictions on freedom of economic activity and freedom of movement permissible? What kind of compensation would be justified for the social and economic losses caused by restrictions on freedom of economic activity or freedom of movement? In the next section, we consider older people and international students and foreign workers in Japan as examples of vulnerable groups, describe their experience of a severe situation in Japan during the pandemic, and discuss a fair distribution of burdens.

16.3 COVID-19: Older Individuals and Foreigners in Japan

16.3.1 Solitary Death and Social Isolation among Older People in Japan

Japan's population is aging rapidly and is often referred to as a super-aging society. In 2021, 29.1% of the total population will be older (65 years or older), the highest percentage globally, followed by Italy (23.6%) and Portugal (23.1%) (Statistics Bureau of Japan 2022). The number of older adults living apart from their children has been increasing yearly; in 1980, 69% of the older adults were living with their children, but by 2015 this percentage had dropped to 39% (Cabinet Office Japan 2017). Relatedly, the number of older adults living alone has also increased significantly; in 1980, 4.3% of older men and 11.2% of older women lived alone. By 2020, that number had increased to 15.5% for men and 22.4% for women (Cabinet Office Japan 2021).

The physical distancing policy dramatically reduced opportunities for older people to go out. Since COVID-19 tends to affect older people with greater severity, it can be assumed that older people have restricted their activities more readily. Stay-at-home policies for older people would naturally have helped to prevent the spread of COVID-19 and reduced the number of serious injuries. However, it also caused medical problems, such as exacerbation of chronic diseases and delayed detection of acute diseases due to a reduction in the number of hospital visits. For example, an analysis of medical fee claims data from 321 hospitals conducted using a medical database company shows that patients receiving motor rehabilitation declined by 27% in May 2020 compared to the pre-COVID-19 baseline, and declined still further by 4% in December 2021, with no recovery subsequently. In addition, prescriptions for dementia medications decreased by 22% in May 2020 and still remained at 11% lower in December 2021 (Nikkei 2022). Psychological damage caused by the loss of communication with family members living away from home must also be considered. For example, in a survey of 493 older adults, significant differences were found between the group with decreased frequency of going out and those with increased/unchanged frequency of going out, with respect to their pandemic-related psychological condition (Shimokihara et al. 2022: 439).

Physical distancing tends to cause social distancing, and this has become especially problematic for older people. In other words, restricted physical mobility may also limit the establishment and maintenance of social relationships. The main problem is the social isolation of older people due to COVID-19.

The most tragic consequence of social isolation among older people is the marked increase in solitary death. Solitary death, known as *kodokushi* or *koritsushi* in Japanese, has been recognized as a serious social issue. While many definitions of solitary death have been presented (Kanawaku 2018: 110–12; Ueda et al. 2010: 109–31), we have defined it as a death characterized by the following: (1) occurring at home, (2) involving someone living alone, (3) under conditions of social isolation (no care, no constant contact, lack of social connections), (4) where isolation is not the result of imprisonment, and (5) where death is not the result of the isolated person taking their own life (Nakazawa et al. 2021: 89). The core feature underlying the concept of solitary death is the separation from medical care and society (conditions 1–3) (Ueda et al. 2010). In this chapter, we focus on the form of solitary death occurring in a state of isolation that was not the result of coercion by another person, but rather arose spontaneously in society and was not intended by the individual. Accordingly, conditions 4 and 5 were added to the definition of solitary death.

Since March 2020, when restrictions were placed on citizens' lives, numerous cases of solitary death related to COVID-19 have been reported (Yomiuri 2021). Although data are lacking for Japan as a whole and only limited information is available, in Osaka, for example, the number of solitary deaths increased from 1,171 in 2019 to 1,314 in 2020, a 12.2% increase. A typical (fictional) case would be:

Mr. A was a 75-year-old man who lived alone in Tokyo. After losing his wife three years prior, he spent many of his days alone, watching TV in his room, and would leave every three days to go to a local convenience store to buy instant ramen for his meals. He had a 42-year-old son and a 40-year-old daughter, but both lived in different cities and were not close to their father. One day, Mr. A reached out to his daughter by phone, saying, "My chest hurts." After her father failed to answer the phone the next day, the daughter contacted the local police, who discovered that Mr. A had died at home. Subsequent inspection revealed that he had contracted the novel coronavirus.

Social isolation can negatively influence the health of older people. There is an undeniable risk that social isolation may lead to neglect of one's own health, and numerous examples have been reported of isolated people who eat excess junk food high in salt and fat, or of those who do not clean their rooms and let garbage accumulate in their rooms, which become increasingly less sanitary. Physical distancing as a countermeasure against the COVID-19 pandemic may further isolate these socially isolated older people. For one, older people may be more likely to refrain voluntarily from social activities. Additionally, physical distancing makes it difficult to provide support to those who are isolated.

Many solitary deaths end in above-ground decomposition due to delayed discovery; this is arguably one of the most tragic ways to die. Dying alone is bad enough, but delayed or non-discovery of the corpse is even worse. Intuitively, this represents a violation of human dignity.

The issue of solitary death is associated primarily with older people, but solitary death among COVID-19 patients has become a serious problem for the younger generation as well. Cases of solitary death during the pandemic included suspected COVID-19 patients with mild symptoms who died at home or in hotels after their conditions worsened rapidly during observation (Sato 2020; Iwamoto 2020). The scarcity of medical resources due to the COVID-19 pandemic was a key factor leading to such deaths.

Physical distancing should not hinder social support provision for older and other lonely people. In other words, physical distancing should not create more social distance. To achieve this, it is important to enhance social support that is feasible even with physical distancing, and to ensure the safety of in-person interactions through comprehensive PCR testing and vaccination recommendations.

16.3.2 International Students and Foreign Workers in Japan under the COVID-19 Pandemic

Older people are not the only isolated individuals in Japanese society. Foreign students residing in Japan, foreigners residing in Japan through the Program of Technical Intern Training for Foreign Nationals, and especially unauthorized immigrants constitute several of the vulnerable and marginalized groups in Japanese society. These socially vulnerable foreigners are the ones most likely to experience not only physical but also mental, social, and economic damage from the spread of COVID-19.

As of May 1, 2020, the number of international students staying in Japan was 2,795,597 (Ministry of Education, Culture, Sports, Science and Technology 2021).[2] Overall, this number represented a decrease by 32,617 (10.4%) compared to the previous year, which was attributed to COVID-19. The results of the 2021 survey have not yet been released, but the number of international students is expected to have decreased even further. The majority of foreign students studying in Japan are from Asia, with the largest number of students coming from China, Vietnam, Nepal, South Korea, Taiwan, Indonesia, Sri Lanka, Myanmar, Bangladesh, and Mongolia, in that order.

The Program of Technical Intern Training for Foreign Nationals in Japan was first established in 1993. The Technical Intern Training Program aims to transfer skills, technologies, or knowledge accumulated in Japan to developing and other regions, as well as promote international cooperation by contributing to the development of human resources that can fulfill roles in the economic development of those regions. According to the Japan International Trainee and Skilled Worker Cooperation Organization, Japanese law declares that "technical training should not be conducted as a means of adjusting labor supply and demand" (Japan International Trainee and Skilled Worker Cooperation Organization (n.d.)). Despite this philosophy, the Program of Technical Intern Training for Foreign Nationals merely serves as a means to acquire cheap foreign labor, with one deep-rooted criticism being its exploitation of foreigners. It has often been pointed out that there is insufficient social support for foreign technical intern trainees. By the end of 2020, there were 378,200 foreign technical intern trainees in Japan, down by 32,772 (8.0%) from the previous year (Immigration Services Agency in Japan 2021). The largest numbers of trainees in Japan are from Vietnam, China, and the Philippines, in that order.

The home countries of many international students and foreign technical intern trainees in Japan are not necessarily rich, and COVID-19 has made life

---

[2] The number of international students in this survey includes students who were unable to travel to Japan at the scheduled time due to the effects of COVID-19 and were forced to take online classes overseas.

difficult for them. Travel abroad is currently heavily restricted, and a significant number of international students and foreign technical intern trainees have reportedly been unable to return home temporarily, not just due to finances, but also because of challenges with transportation and quarantine. The poverty among these international students and foreign technical intern trainees is becoming increasingly and noticeably severe. This is an unprecedented phenomenon in Japan and was unheard of prior to the COVID-19 pandemic. One of the authors recently had the following experience:

> One Friday, toward the end of May 2021, I was suddenly approached by a young woman, presumably from Southeast Asia, in front of one of the terminal stations in Tokyo. She asked me to buy some sweets from her, as she was experiencing the deleterious effects of COVID-19. In the woman's hand was a bag of cookies and chocolates that she had probably purchased at the supermarket. The woman was selling them for 2,000 yen (a price much higher than the purchase price). Whenever she saw a Japanese businessman walking down the street, she would call out to him.

International students in Japan are restricted by law from working. Even international students with "Permission to Engage in Activity Other Than That Permitted Under the Status of Residence Previously Granted" may work up to twenty-eight hours per week to avoid interfering with their studies, which was the original purpose of their entry into Japan. They may not always be able to get appropriate jobs and are more likely to engage in manual labor. In addition, the Program of Technical Intern Training for Foreign Nationals in Japan has very strict restrictions on employment, and free economic activities are practically hindered.

Undocumented immigrants are foreigners for whom social support is more difficult to receive. They are foreigners and children of foreigners who have become unauthorized due to overstaying in the country. The Japanese government encourages unauthorized immigrants to return to their home countries, but special permission to stay has been established as a relief measure (Immigration Bureau 2009).[3]

According to the statistics compiled by the Ministry of Justice, as of January 2021 there were 82,868 unauthorized immigrants in Japan. After reaching a peak

---

[3] Special permission to stay involves normalizing the status of unauthorized immigrants under certain set conditions. Elements that contribute positively to the review process include a marital or parental relationship with someone with Japanese citizenship, having children in the public education system in Japan, or being a patient with a serious illness requiring treatment in Japan. The process also prioritizes cases "when the applicant has appeared in person at a regional Immigration Bureau to report that he or she is residing in the country without legal status" and "when there are humanitarian grounds or other special circumstances." In contrast, having a criminal record or staying in Japan after having entered it illegally are considered negative elements.

of 298,646 in 1993, this number began to decline because of promotional measures, such as the Special Permission to Stay. It then bottomed out in 2014 before rising again (Immigration Services Agency in Japan 2021; Solidarity Network with Migrants Japan 2020). If individuals whose data may have been excluded are considered, then there are even more people residing in Japan without authorization. In the United States, the number of unauthorized immigrants was estimated to be 10.5 million (23% of all immigrants) in 2017 (Pew Research Center 2020). In Europe, the number of unauthorized immigrants was estimated to have peaked at 4.1–5.3 million as of 2016 (Pew Research Center 2019). Although Japan's statistics may be an underestimation, it is still just a fraction of those residing in the United States and Europe. Nonetheless, the issue of unauthorized immigrants in Japan cannot be trivialized. By contrast, because unauthorized immigrants comprise a smaller population in Japan relative to that in the US and Europe, their rights as a minority might not be adequately protected.

The problems of poverty and restrictions on travel abroad during the COVID-19 pandemic are common to unauthorized immigrants in Japan. Unauthorized immigrants have the additional difficulty of accessing social support, such as the public health insurance system and primary care system. Primary care of patients infected with COVID-19 is very important not only for the prevention of serious illness in the patients themselves but also to prevent the spread of infection. In Japan, a primary care route has been established for the observation of COVID-19-related physical changes, such as fever, breathlessness, coughing, and abnormal taste. Individuals are encouraged first to contact their family doctor and the call center set up by the local government. Demand for the call centers is high because the system of family doctors in Japan is still inadequate. Call centers are available even for undocumented foreigners. As a universal principle, measures against infectious diseases are required not to discriminate between foreigners and Japanese, or between documented and undocumented immigrants. However, in reality, it is difficult for undocumented foreigners to have a family doctor or use call centers. Aside from the language barrier, another factor is the fear that medical institutions will report undocumented immigrants to the Immigration Service Agency of Japan, which controls immigration (Nakazawa and Akabayashi 2021). As a result, COVID-19 is considered to have worsened the lives of undocumented immigrants.

Normally, a patient with the Japanese national health insurance pays 30% of the medical costs incurred out of pocket (if aged less than 70 years). However, as COVID-19 is categorized as a designated infectious disease under the Infectious Disease Prevention Law, treatment is covered by public funds. Treatment is available even for unauthorized immigrants because participation in the public health insurance system is not required. This part of the current reality in Japan is consistent with justice.

16.3.3 A Short Summary: the Reality of Inequality in Japan

During the COVID-19 pandemic, physical distancing policies had social and economic ramifications, especially on socially vulnerable populations, such as the older generation, foreign students, and non-regular working foreigners. Surprisingly, social and economic disparities that had always existed became ever more apparent during COVID-19. For example, older people became deprived of opportunities for in-person communication because of the stay-at-home policy. Their avoidance of routine hospital visits and lack of exercise led to exacerbation of chronic illnesses, creating a health policy problem. The fear of dying alone also emerged as a considerable stress for isolated older people. The issue of social isolation of older people is a problem that Japanese society must now address. Foreign students, foreign technical intern trainees, and unauthorized immigrants lost much of their freedom of movement and economic activities due to the COVID-19 pandemic. Some vulnerable foreigners in Japan have experienced deterioration in their health conditions due to economic and linguistic restrictions. Providing the necessary social support for these individuals is yet another matter of concern, particularly with regard to Japan's international relations.

In light of the inequalities evident in Japanese society and based on the assumption that the reduction of social isolation will lead to the correction of social and economic disparities, we propose the implementation of the following policies to prevent the spread of a pandemic infection while also reducing social isolation and its negative repercussions.

16.4 Three Policy Measures to Improve the Welfare of Vulnerable Populations

In general, public health policies should be scrutinized in terms of the utility and risks posed by the implementation of the policy, the fairness of policy implementation, and the level to which citizen freedom and autonomy are ensured. This paper focuses on socioeconomic risks, provision of information to ensure that citizen rights and autonomy are upheld, and social support for public equality in the implementation of physical distancing as a measure against COVID-19.

Socially vulnerable individuals, such as socially isolated older people, foreign students, foreign technical intern trainees in Japan, and unauthorized immigrants are social groups that have experienced the deleterious effects of the physical distancing policy as a measure to contain the spread of COVID-19. While these individuals have been severely limited economically and socially by the physical distancing policy, others have not been as affected, and the disparity between these two groups is significant. In recent years, concerns have emerged about worsening social inequalities in Japan, and the COVID-19 pandemic has ultimately exacerbated these. Full-time employees of large corporations, civil servants, university professors, and the like are less likely to be affected by the economic impact of physical distancing, as they have little or no income loss due to the COVID-19 pandemic. However, older people, foreign students, foreign technical intern trainees, and unauthorized immigrants are forced to endure unstable employment as non-regular employees, even if they are able to work (presumably, some of the older people may be retired). The industry most affected by the physical distancing policy has been the food and beverage industry, which is supported primarily by these non-permanent employees. Therefore, these people suffer disproportionately through lost wages.

We introduce here three perspectives as policies to mitigate the burden on vulnerable populations. These are minimal restrictions, provision of appropriate information, and provision of context-sensitive communication tools. Of course, there are other ways to protect vulnerable populations. For example, coordination of consequential disadvantages through compensation. Such adjustments should be made by all means. However, before that, can we not provide the measures in advance to alleviate some of the burden on vulnerable populations? The three perspectives we present provide a starting framework for this discussion.

16.4.1 Minimize Restrictions

That the physical distancing policy has a significant effect in limiting the spread of COVID-19 infection must be emphasized. However, if physical distancing policies lead to increased social and economic disparities, physical distancing should be kept to a minimum. Preventing the spread of COVID-19 through physical distancing policies must be weighed against the deleterious effects of restricting the freedom of citizens. Notably, if the restriction of freedom affects the socially vulnerable the most, then the effectiveness of limiting the spread of COVID-19 and the disadvantages created by this restriction need to be re-evaluated as rigorously as possible. Based on the results of the re-evaluation, policies should be adjusted appropriately.

From the perspective of rigorous risk analysis, we argue that policymaking should avoid broad regulation via physical distancing requirements of all citizens subject to public health policy. In particular, what should be avoided are excessively precautionary public health interventions. What this means is that behavior B, which meets the following three conditions, should be regulated as an alternative to behavior A, which should be properly regulated:

(1) Behavior A is the direct cause of the spread of COVID-19 infection.

(2) Behavior B is an upstream of behavior A. This means that if a person does not exhibit behavior B, he will inevitably not manifest behavior A. However, manifesting behavior B does not imply that a person will inevitably exhibit behavior A.

(3) From a policy perspective, it is easier to restrict behavior B (a blanket policy) than to restrict behavior A (an ideally regulated policy).

For example, until October 24, 2021, bars and restaurants in Tokyo had to comply with the following three conditions in order to serve alcoholic beverages to customers: they had to (1) be certified by the Tokyo Metropolitan Government for infection control, (2) serve alcoholic beverages to groups of no more than four people, and (3) be open only until 8 p.m. These rules were established to curb preemptively the behavior of citizens who get drunk, remove their masks, and talk loudly and at close range, thus spreading droplets and increasing the risk of infection. However, these requirements are excessive, as groups of four or more people can still eat quietly and after 8 p.m., with minimal risk of infection. The only action that citizens need to take is to consider the existing medical and epidemiological information about SARS-CoV-2 (i.e. that it is transmitted by droplets), always be conscious that they themselves might be an infected carrier, and modify their behavior accordingly to minimize the spread of droplets. Of course, there may be some people who behave irresponsibly or act in ignorance. It may be in the public interest to regulate the behavior of such people through broad regulations. However, it is unfair because their possible emotional and cognitive development are not considered. What they need is education, and care that supports a flourishing social life. Such education and care will encourage those who behave irresponsibly or in ignorance to act as autonomously as possible. Similarly, calling for older people to stay home is too broad an application for infection control. As the main concern is to prevent droplet infection, forcing people to stay home in order to achieve this is not only paternalistic but may even cause mental and physical harm of older people. In a uniform, mutually monitored, society like Japan, people, especially older people, are very compliant with government demands, which can lead to problems of over-adaptation. In fact, lack of exercise due to the stay-at-home order has aggravated chronic diseases among older people. In addition, if people refrain from seeking out medical services at hospitals as a result of the stay-at-home order, this could delay the detection of diseases and thereby shorten their healthy lifespans. Naturally, it is expected that the broad regulation of social activities will prevent the spread of infectious diseases and thereby improve people's well-being. This is the very purpose of public health policy in general. However, as long as regulations undermine people's autonomous actions, the scope of application of such regulation must be well adjusted. Further, the government needs to make continuous efforts to adjust, while at the same time provide people with educational opportunities and care to improve their autonomy.

16.4.2 Provide Appropriate Information

It is important to provide information to the public in order to achieve an appropriate risk–benefit balance. However, when doing so, "easy to understand" is emphasized, often to a fault. Indeed, repeating a simple message can be very effective in severe emergencies, such as earthquakes or tsunamis. In the early stages, the provision of information about the COVID-19 pandemic was also not problematic, even if it was a simple repetition of the same message. However, the COVID-19 pandemic has now lasted for more than two years. Simple repetition of the same message is insufficient to provide useful information about such a long-lasting crisis situation. Crisis and emergency risk communications are conducted for different purposes and by different means than normal risk communications (CDC 2018). The COVID-19 pandemic, initially an emergency event, has gradually become a chronic social condition. Depending on its stage, a greater proportion of it should be treated thoughtfully within the scope of normal risk communications.

Information provided by the government and mass media regarding the prevention of the spread of COVID-19 must be rich in content, supported by scientific knowledge, while also being "easy to understand." Underestimating the learning capacity of citizens represents facile paternalism. Of course, the opposite problem of overestimating people's capacity, and providing overly complicated information, should also be avoided. Still, difficult information is better than paternalistic overestimation, since it may encourage higher levels of learning. Over the past two years since the pandemic began, the public has become very knowledgeable about COVID-19 and infectious disease control, as well as about vaccines and drugs to treat viral infections. Information must be provided in a way that aligns with the learning capacity of citizens, and a paternalistic emphasis on "easy to understand" should be avoided.

16.4.3 Alternative Communication Tools

During a pandemic, it is important to devise effective communication tools. As older people and foreigners can be difficult to reach with information, the provision of information during a pandemic must consider socially isolated groups such as these. Social web-based networks have become common, especially among young people. In addition, telecommunication software is an information technology tool, the rapid development of which symbolizes the era of COVID-19. These telecommunication tools and social networking services have penetrated deeply into the lives of the younger generation. However, there are many older people who cannot keep up with such technology-based communication tools, and the government has not developed any policies to accommodate this demographic. One possible solution for this would be for the government to promote actively the development of social networking services that are easily accessible to older people. Another possibility would be for the government and industry to work together to promote telecommunication using simple, easy-to-use devices. For example, hardware such as smartphones, for the older generation, with a large screen size and simple layout of applications, and the development of Social Network Service (SNS) software designed to include the older generation, would be promising.

Foreign students living in Japan, foreigners living in Japan through the Program of Technical Intern Training for Foreign Nationals in Japan, and unauthorized immigrants need a framework to support community building. Certainly, non-profit organizations (NPOs) and non-governmental organizations (NGOs) have supported foreign residents in Japan, and they have played an important role in the past. Such NPOs and NGOs play a wide range of roles, such as helping foreigners to work in Japan, supporting visa applications, and providing medical support. The physical distancing policy of COVID-19 has made it difficult for these NPOs and NGOs to operate, and there are probably many foreigners who have lost contact with Japanese society due to the stagnation of NPO and NGO activities. These foreign students living in Japan, foreigners living in Japan through the Program of Technical Intern Training for Foreign Nationals in Japan, and unauthorized immigrants need a network that would allow them to have contact with Japanese society in addition to the network in their home country.

16.5 Adjusting the Public Health Policy for a Future Disease X

Even if COVID-19 is successfully converged, our society will encounter another unknown infectious Disease X sometime in the future. We will then need to successfully apply the public health experience gained from COVID-19 to Disease X.

There can be no doubt that, with Disease X, the conflict of values inherent in public health policies, namely the conflict between respect for individual freedom of action and the public interest in containing a pandemic, will also be an issue. We do not insist on extremes. We oppose paternalistic policies that excessively restrict individual freedom. At the same time, we do not embrace an overly libertarian insistence on the absolute protection of individual freedom without regard to the public interest. Rather, we contrast the value of in-person communication with that of infection control by viewing it as a universal human value. Our strategy is a two-pronged justification. One is respect for the value of individual freedom of action, and the other is respect for the intrinsic value of in-person communication.

Opportunities for in-person communication have decreased markedly because of social distancing. In-person communication is defined as real face-to-face communication without the use of telecommunication through the internet. However, due to the COVID-19 pandemic, universities in Japan switched to online classes in April 2020. At the same time, the use of tools such as Zoom for business meetings has become common because of the drastic decrease in the opportunities for business trips by airplane. In-person communication is a means of achieving an arbitrary goal and is thought to increase learning efficiency in university classes and facilitate business meetings. One mechanism by which this happens may be the rich nonverbal content of in-person communication, which enhances the quality of communication. During the COVID-19 pandemic, we realized that in-person communication has not only instrumental but intrinsic value as well. Accordingly, the government should not underestimate citizens' desires for in-person communication.

As a policy to prevent the spread of COVID-19, large-scale public health policies targeting populations may not have ultimately faced the human beings themselves. Did policymakers overlook the specific nature of human beings, such as their diversity, growth, and ability to respond to situations? Was the policy not based on the premise of an extremely poor and uniform image of citizens, and was it implemented with a preset, broad, and blanket rigidity? Did such a uniform image of citizens include isolated older people and foreigners living in Japan? Assuming a very poor image of the target population of public health policy is not just a matter of overlooking the needs of minorities, and the ineptitude of policymakers should be called out.

With regard to Disease X, we will need to advance the public interest by controlling the pandemic while defending vulnerable populations and protecting the intrinsic value of in-person communication. That, of course, will not be an easy task. Here, we call for continued efforts by governments to adjust public health policies appropriately throughout time. Of course, finding effective policies to combat infectious diseases is an empirical matter. As with public health policies regarding COVID-19, it will be necessary to implement policies very cautiously (i.e. with a priority on saving lives) at the outset. However, governments and public health professionals need to adjust policies in a timely manner as academic knowledge accumulates and society changes. Furthermore, we would argue that this effort must not be neglected. Consideration for vulnerable populations in society is one such adjustment, which requires not only enhanced compensation but also the development of policies that reduce the burden on such populations in the first place. We propose three innovations in this context: minimal restrictions, providing appropriate information, and providing communication tools. These three need to be brought to bear on policies considered in the context of the sharp tension between respect for individual freedom of action, the intrinsic value of in-person communication, and the promotion of social good for the control of infectious diseases. Such ingenuity would be consistent with the principle of justice in protecting the livelihoods of vulnerable populations.

16.6 Conclusions

Physical distancing in COVID-19 has lowered the quality of life of older people living alone and socioeconomically disadvantaged foreign residents in Japan, effectively exacerbating the socioeconomic tension that was already present in these individuals in Japanese society. Given the intrinsic value of in-person communication, physical distancing as a public health policy to control the spread of COVID-19 should be acceptable, provided that substantial efforts are made to minimize the scope of restriction. To this end, public health policies that broadly apply blanket policies without considering the diversity of behaviors and social circumstances should be reconsidered. Ideally, information on public health policies provided to the public must be of higher quality and customized to accommodate the learning capabilities of the general populace. Furthermore, if in-person communication is to be restricted, it is essential to provide alternative communication tools, which will require additional consideration of populations that have difficulty using technology-based tools.

Bibliography

Act on Special Measures against Novel Influenza (2012) (Act No. 31 of 2012), https://elaws.e-gov.go.jp/document?lawid=424AC0000000031.

Cabinet Office Japan (2017), 'Annual Report on the Ageing Society', https://www8.cao.go.jp/kourei/whitepaper/w-2017/zenbun/29pdf_index.html.

Cabinet Office Japan (2020), 'Declaration of an emergency situation of new coronavirus infection', https://corona.go.jp/news/pdf/kinkyujitai_sengen_0407.pdf.

Cabinet Office Japan. (2021), 'Annual Report on the Ageing Society', https://www8.cao.go.jp/kourei/whitepaper/w-2021/zenbun/03pdf_index.html.

CDC (US Centers for Disease Control and Prevention) (2018), 'CERC: Introduction', https://emergency.cdc.gov/cerc/ppt/CERC_Introduction.pdf.

Immigration Bureau (Ministry of Justice) (2009), 'Guidelines on Special Permission to Stay in Japan', http://www.moj.go.jp/isa/content/930002562.pdf).

Immigration Services Agency in Japan. (2021), 'The number of foreign residents as of the end of 2020', https://www.moj.go.jp/isa/publications/press/13_00014.html.

International Monetary Fund (2022), 'Real GDP growth', https://www.imf.org/external/datamapper/NGDP_RPCH@WEO/OEMDC/ADVEC/WEOWORLD.

Iwamoto, S. (2020), 'Man with mild COVID-19 found in a state of cardiac arrest', *The Asahi Shimbun*, 12 December 2020, http://www.asahi.com/ajw/articles/14013991 (accessed 14 Dec. 2020).

Japan International Trainee and Skilled Worker Cooperation Organization (n.d.), 'What is the Technical Intern Training Program?' https://www.jitco.or.jp/en/regulation/index.html.

Kanawaku, Y. (2018). '*Koritsu-shi* (Solitary Death) and its actual situation', *Journal of Nippon Medical School* 14(3): 100–12.

Maragakis, L. L. (2020a), 'Coronavirus, Social and Physical Distancing and Self-Quarantine', https://www.hopkinsmedicine.org/health/conditions-and-diseases/coronavirus/coronavirus-social-distancing-and-self-quarantine.

Maragakis, L. L. (2020b), 'Coronavirus, Social and Physical Distancing and Self-Quarantine', https://www.hopkinsmedicine.org/health/conditions-and-diseases/coronavirus/coronavirus-social-distancing-and-self-quarantine.

MHLW (Ministry of Health, Labour and Welfare) (2020a), 'Overview of the 2019 National Survey on Living Standards 14', https://www.mhlw.go.jp/toukei/saikin/hw/k-tyosa/k-tyosa19/dl/03.pdf.

MHLW (Ministry of Health, Labour and Welfare) (2020b), 'Avoid the "Three Cs"', https://www.mhlw.go.jp/content/3CS.pdf.

Ministry of Education, Culture, Sports, Science and Technology (2021), 'Survey of International Student Enrollment' and 'Number of Japanese Students Studying Abroad', https://www.mext.go.jp/a_menu/koutou/ryugaku/1412692.htm.

Nakazawa, E., and Akabayashi, A. (2021), 'Unauthorized Immigrants in Japan Facing the COVID-19 Pandemic', *Journal of Seizon and Life Sciences* 32/1: 75–88.

Nakazawa, E., Yamamoto, K., London, A. J., and Akabayashi, A. (2021), 'Solitary death and new lifestyles during and after COVID-19: wearable devices and public health ethics', *BMC Medical Ethics* 22:89, https://doi.org/10.1186/s12910-021-00657-9.

Nikkei, A. (2022), 'COVID fears raise Japan's dementia risks as seniors shun hospitals: Doctors warn avoiding treatment could cut healthy life expectancy', https://asia.nikkei.com/Spotlight/Datawatch/COVID-fears-raise-Japan-s-dementia-risks-as-seniors-shun-hospitals

OECD (2021), 'Health for the People, by the People', 67–8, https://read.oecd.org/10.1787/c259e79a-en?format=pdf.

OECD (n.d.), 'Poverty rate', https://data.oecd.org/inequality/poverty-rate.htm.

Pew Research Center (2019), 'Europe's unauthorized immigrant total peaked in 2016 before leveling off', https://www.pewresearch.org/global/2019/11/13/europes-unauthorized-immigrant-population-peaks-in-2016-then-levels-off/pg_2019-11-13_eu-unauthorized_0-01/ (accessed November 24, 2022).

Pew Research Center (2020), 'Unauthorized immigrants are almost a quarter of U.S. foreign-born population', https://www.pewresearch.org/fact-tank/2020/08/20/key-findings-about-u-s-immigrants/ft_2020-08-20_immigrants_02/ (accessed November 24, 2022).

Sato, N. (2020), 'Shingata-corona, "nyuinfuyo" 83-sai shibo, tosho kensa kotowarare, yoseigo mo taiki, jitaku de kyuhen' [in Japanese] ['Novel Coronavirus—"No hospitalization necessary": 83-year-old patient dead. First denied testing, then told to standby following positive result, followed by rapid deterioration at home'], Tokyo Web, 1 May 2020, https://www.tokyo-np.co.jp/article/16976 (accessed 14 Dec., 2020).

Shimokihara, S., Maruta, M., Akasaki, Y., Ikeda, Y., Han, G., Kamasaki, T., Tokuda, K., Hidaka, Y., Akasaki, Y., and Tabira, T. (2022), 'Association between Frequency of Going Out and Psychological Condition among Community-Dwelling Older Adults after the COVID-19 Pandemic in Japan', *Healthcare* (Basel) 10/3: 439, doi:10.3390/healthcare10030439.

Solidarity Network with Migrants Japan (2020), '20 Proposals for Immigrant Society'. p. 58.

Statistics Bureau of Japan (2022), 'Koreisha no Jinko' ['Population of older adults'], https://www.stat.go.jp/data/topics/topi1291.html.

Ueda, T., Uehara, E., Kato, Y., Simizu, E., Ito, K., Mori, F., Kinosita, T., Fujihara, H., and Kawasumi, M. (2010), 'Kodokushi (Koritsushi) no teigi to kanrensuru yoin no kensho oyobi shisotekikokyu to kongo no kadai' [in Japanese] ['Definition, Factors Related to Solitary Death and Consideration on thought of dying alone'], *Nagoya keiei tanki daigaku kiyo* 51: 109–31.

UNICEF. (2020), 'Physical not social distancing', https://www.unicef.org/sudan/press-releases/physical-not-social-distancing#:~:text=Social%20distancing%2C%20which%20refers%20to,the%20spread%20of%20COVID%2D19.

WHO (2021), 'COVID-19: physical distancing', https://www.who.int/westernpacific/emergencies/covid-19/information/physical-distancing.

Yomiuri, S. (2021), 'A man who told his son not to come home because he was afraid of Corona was found dead two months after his death', June 16, 2021, https://www.yomiuri.co.jp/national/20210616-OYT1T50137/.

PART V
PANDEMIC X

17

Pondering the Next Pandemic

Liberty, Justice, and Democracy in the COVID-19 Pandemic

Nethanel Lipshitz, Jeffrey P. Kahn, and Ruth Faden

Policy decisions taken during the COVID-19 pandemic engaged difficult ethical questions. These decisions have proved to be challenging to implement as well as politically polarizing. The contributions in this volume address many of these questions, though not in one voice. They take different sides on some of the fundamental debates in the pandemic. One of the questions that arises from reading such a wide variety of views is how to move forward in the face of lingering and fundamental social and philosophical disagreements. Our aim in this chapter is to reflect on the contributions made to this collection, offer our own perspective on some of the debates they engage in, and identify some areas that will benefit from further attention by both scholars and policymakers.

The chapter is divided into three sections. The first concerns state interference with individual liberty in response to COVID-19. The second discusses global justice challenges in the context of responding to the pandemic. In the third section, we consider several issues that, though not much discussed in this volume, are important to pandemic preparedness, going forward.

17.1 Liberty-Restricting Measures

17.1.1 The Debate

In response to COVID-19, governments as well as private organizations issued various mandates and prohibitions, such as lockdowns, social distancing requirements, restrictions on gatherings, vaccine mandates, mask-wearing mandates, travel restrictions, border closures, mandates on factories to produce medical equipment, restrictions on the exportation of medical resources, and various restrictive regulations on businesses such as bars and restaurants.

These restrictions were undertaken as effective public health policies. However, they also interfere with people's freedom. These interferences deprive citizens of

Nethanel Lipshitz, Jeffrey P. Kahn, and Ruth Faden, *Pondering the Next Pandemic: Liberty, Justice, and Democracy in the COVID-19 Pandemic* In: *Pandemic Ethics: From COVID-19 to Disease X.* Edited by: Dominic Wilkinson and Julian Savulescu, Oxford University Press. © Oxford University Press 2023. DOI: 10.1093/oso/9780192871688.003.0018

the intrinsic value of freedom, and cause other harms, such as losses of income and education and other constitutive elements of well-being. How should we evaluate liberty-restricting measures in a time of a pandemic?

As an example of analysis of liberty-restricting measures, Kamm defends what might be regarded as the mainstream position in public health ethics, that liberty-restricting measures are often morally justified during a pandemic.[1] Kamm's preferred justification (and the one she recommends public health officials communicate to the public) is that some liberty-restricting measures prevent individuals from harming others. Kamm considers three significant risks of harm that individuals may pose to others if they do not wear masks, get vaccinated, or follow social distancing practices: 1) infecting others; 2) being a "host" for a virus to mutate, and 3) depleting health resources and overcrowding hospitals.[2]

According to Kamm, the risks individuals pose to others in terms of these harms justify certain restrictions on liberty. Since even libertarians recognize a duty to avoid harming others, Kamm argues that they should recognize the moral legitimacy of certain restrictions on liberty. This point is valid whether we think of posing a risk of harm as itself a kind of harm or we simply wish to reduce the probability of the occurrence of harm. A useful analogy in this respect is that of a neighbor shooting a rifle in their backyard.[3] It seems permissible, even from a libertarian perspective, to require the neighbor to stop. There can be no certainty that the neighbor's action will result in anyone being shot; yet restricting the neighbor's conduct is justified because there is a plausible risk of this happening if the neighbor persists in shooting a rifle in their backyard.

Other authors, however, are more hesitant. While no author in this collection categorically objects to liberty-restricting measures, several authors argue we should employ them less widely than has been done in the US and other countries during the COVID-19 pandemic. Blumenthal-Barby and Flanigan, for example, point out that we tolerate, as a society, many behaviors that have some non-negligible probability of seriously harming others, such as driving automobiles or drinking alcohol. Assuming that this level of toleration is justified, shouldn't we take a similar stance in tolerating behaviors that risk harming others during a pandemic? This question becomes more pressing once vaccines are widely available and individuals can take substantial steps to protect themselves from the more serious harms of being infected.

---

[1] Frances M. Kamm, 'Handling Future Pandemics: Harming, Not Aiding, and Liberty', Chapter 6 in this volume.

[2] Kamm, as we understand her, does not intend the list to be exhaustive. We could mention other harms that individuals who do not take certain measures may pose to others, such as harms to the well-being of healthcare workers in overcrowded hospitals. See, for example, Galanis et al. (2021) and Pappa et al. (2020).

[3] For this analogy, see the papers by Jennifer Blumenthal-Barby ('Bringing Nuance to Autonomy-Based Considerations in Vaccine Mandate Debates') and Jessica Flanigan ('The Risks of Prohibition during Pandemics'), Chapters 4 and 5 in this volume.

These disagreements notwithstanding, there is an element of philosophical agreement threading through this volume. Both sides appear to accept something like what has come to be called Mill's harm principle: it is sometimes justifiable to restrict freedom to prevent an agent from harming or posing a risk of harm to others. This broad agreement can be utilized in a conciliatory spirit in an attempt to devise policies in which both sides of the debate are asked to make some concessions. These policies will aim to give public expression to the shared idea that both harm reduction and freedom protection are important guiding values for public health decision-making. We will discuss two broad philosophical approaches for devising such policies, one suggested by several authors in this collection, and another not discussed in this volume and that we believe deserves further scholarly attention.

17.1.2 Selective Restrictions

The first approach is to introduce selective liberty-limiting policies, for example lockdowns for only older persons, as suggested by Savulescu,[4] or denying the unvaccinated access to public spaces, as suggested by Persad and Emanuel.[5] By restricting the liberties of only a subset of the population, selective policies sacrifice some freedom for the prevention of some significant harm and sacrifice some harm reduction for more freedom protection.

Liberty restriction for harm prevention or reduction can be justified on paternalistic or non-paternalistic grounds. Society may wish to restrict citizens' liberty at least in part for their own good, but there are non-paternalistic justifications as well. Kamm's argument is a case in point, as it centers on preventing individuals from harming others. The justification of selective restrictions may be paternalistic if it is intended to secure the health of older people or the unvaccinated. However, when defending selective restrictions, Savulescu as well as Persad and Emanuel do not compare them with a policy of no restrictions, but with a policy of universal restrictions, that is, restrictions applying to the great majority of society. When this is the comparison under discussion, paternalistic reasons cannot be invoked in favor of selective restrictions, since universal restrictions and selective restrictions would have similar health benefits for those whose liberty is restricted. What has to be assessed, then, is the non-paternalistic merit of these proposals.

---

[4] See Julian Savulescu, 'Ethics of Selective Restriction of Liberty in a Pandemic', Chapter 8 in this volume.

[5] See Govind Persad and Ezekiel Emanuel, 'Against Procrustean Public Health: Two Vignettes', Chapter 7 in this volume.

In the case of older persons, a non-paternalistic defense of selective restrictions rests on the disproportionate impact COVID-19 illness has in this population on healthcare capacity and healthcare staff, and on the possibility of improving societal functioning more generally for the rest of the population without causing much more harm. In the case of unvaccinated individuals, this sort of justification could be motivated if they pose greater risks of infecting others or of overcrowding hospitals compared to vaccinated individuals. Compared with universal restrictions, selective restrictions offer much more freedom and minimal increases in harm, and so offer a better balance of freedom protection and harm reduction. However, many of the benefits of these restrictions will redound to people other than those whose freedom will be restricted. If we wish to respect the *separateness* of persons, this feature of selective restrictions makes their justification difficult. Nonetheless, large enough benefits to society could possibly justify these selective measures, and Savulescu, as well as Persad and Emanuel, may be correct in taking the potential benefits of these measures to outweigh this kind of moral concern.

The separateness of persons, however, is not the only relevant ethical concern here. By definition, selective restrictions apply only to a particular subset of society, and thus appear to raise egalitarian concerns. However, Savulescu, as well as Persad and Emanuel, argue that selective restrictions raise no serious egalitarian concerns, as there are morally relevant differences between the groups whose liberty would be restricted and other groups.

We are skeptical that there is a morally relevant difference between the elderly and the young that could dispel egalitarian worries about selective restrictions. By contrast, in the case of the unvaccinated, the idea that selective restrictions do not violate an important precept of equality seems more plausible. Let us elaborate on these claims.

Liberals want people to have as much freedom as possible, consistent with certain constraints. They differ with regard to how these constraints should be specified. In Mill's case, people should have as much of certain freedoms as possible consistent with not harming others. Rawls (1971: 60), however, argues that people should have the most extensive basic liberty that is consistent with others having equal basic liberty.[6] Rawls's view implies an *egalitarian constraint* on the goal of providing people with as much basic liberty as possible. Any quarantine would restrict a basic liberty (assuming freedom of movement is a basic liberty), but a universal quarantine would equally restrict everyone's basic liberty and so would not violate the egalitarian constraint. In contrast, a selective lockdown for the

---

[6] Note that even when applied narrowly to basic liberties, Rawls's point may be relevant to various liberty-restricting measures enacted during the pandemic as well as certain selective liberty-restricting measures (such as selective lockdowns) that may be up for consideration.

elderly would restrict a basic liberty (freedom of movement) of some people but not others, and would thus violate the egalitarian constraint.

Perhaps an egalitarian *constraint* is too extreme. However, we think that at the very least there should be a strong *presumption* in favor of an equal distribution of basic liberties. If so, while a morally relevant difference could in principle justify the unequal distribution of even basic liberties, the threshold for what counts as a morally relevant difference should be quite high. It is against such a high threshold that we must assess the claim that there is a morally relevant difference between the elderly and the young, and it is in relation to a high threshold of justification that we are skeptical about the existence of a morally relevant difference between the elderly and the young that is significant enough to justify selective restrictions of the elderly.[7]

There is another egalitarian concern that is applicable to selective restrictions. To bring this concern into view, it is worthwhile bringing to mind the different ways in which the value of equality can be violated in selective and universal restrictions. Regarding universal restrictions, Nakazawa and Akabayashi point out that universal physical distancing policies in Japan disproportionately harm older people and foreigners.[8] Subramanian describes the special harms that universal lockdowns cause to women, people belonging to lower castes, and Muslims in India.[9] Dias and Oliveira offer similar observations about Brazil.[10] Indeed, a universal lockdown does not affect everyone equally, giving rise to a concern about disproportionate impact. Selective mandates, however, raise a set of egalitarian concerns in addition to disproportionate impact: unequal treatment by the state and inequality before the law. This should not be taken lightly. We need to be quite certain, then, that the difference we identify between groups is morally significant enough to dispel this egalitarian concern.

Older and younger persons clearly differ on various health-related measures, which explain why selective restrictions would be effective. Effectiveness,

---

[7] Advocates of selective restrictions may reject this egalitarian constraint or presumption for various reasons. For example, like other egalitarian principles, an egalitarian constraint or presumption would be vulnerable to the famous levelling-down argument (Savulescu and Cameron 2020). However, the levelling-down argument may not be generally decisive against egalitarian principles (Temkin 2002). Furthermore, selective restrictions may not be Pareto superior to universal restrictions. When everyone is in mandatory lockdown, restaurants, theaters, libraries, and resorts are also closed down. There is, generally, less to do outside. The point of selective restrictions is precisely to allow all such activities to resume. But then the burden (or the alternative cost) on the select groups being forced to stay at home also arguably increases. Finally, if we replace an egalitarian constraint with a strong egalitarian presumption, we can resist leveling down by arguing that it defeats the relevant presumption.

[8] See Eisuke Nakazawa and Akira Akabayashi, 'Fair Distribution of Burdens and Vulnerable Groups with Physical Distancing during a Pandemic', Chapter 16 in this volume.

[9] Sreenivasan Subramanian, 'COVID-19: An Unequal and Disequalizing Pandemic', Chapter 14 in this volume.

[10] Maria Clara Dias and Fabio A.G. Oliveira, 'Pandemic and Structural Comorbidity: Lasting Social Injustices in Brazil', Chapter 15 in this volume.

however, does not guarantee that the health-related differences are also morally relevant in the sense that they can dispel egalitarian concerns about selective restrictions. While effectiveness rationalizes a policy, it may not justify it morally.

This is not to deny that, for some decisions, health-related differences are morally relevant. However, we need to be careful not to take a difference that is morally relevant in one context (and, in that context, this difference dispels egalitarian concerns) and use it to justify unequal treatment in a different context, one for which the difference in question has less justificatory power. For example, the risks of becoming seriously ill and of dying increase exponentially after about age 60, and are most dramatic in those in their seventies, eighties, and nineties. For *distributive* purposes, this health-related difference is a reasonable basis for prioritizing older people in vaccination programs when supplies are constrained.[11] Prioritizing older people to receive vaccines also follows the ethical maxim of protecting the vulnerable (Goodin 1985). But it is more difficult to see how health-related differences between older and younger people could justify restricting basic liberties of some people but not others or violating some people's equality before the law.

One could argue that there is a reciprocity argument for a selective restriction: it is fair for those who benefit from a policy to be those who bear the burdens of the policy. The argument would be that it is unfair to burden younger people for the sake of older people, since younger people do not benefit as much as older people from a restriction.[12] But in a universal restriction younger people are not asked to restrict their liberty for the sake of older people. Rather, they are asked to restrict their liberty for the sake of equal distribution of basic liberties. Note also that the relevant comparison is between selective restriction and a universal restriction, and older people do not benefit from a selective restriction more than they would benefit from a universal restriction. Indeed, a selective restriction may be worse for older people. Restrictions on movement bring about harms of loneliness and isolation, which may be worse under a selective restriction. Since there is not added benefit to older people in a selective restriction, they should not be asked to carry *its* burden.

It may be argued that the elderly need certain freedoms less than younger people do, such as freedoms related to attending work and school. But these claims should be made with care, for the freedom of movement (which may be necessary for the young to work and to study) may also be necessary for the elderly to experience less social isolation and loneliness, and in these respects the elderly may even need these freedoms *more*.[13] It is questionable, then, whether

---

[11] As has been done in many countries. See Beaumont (2020).

[12] We thank Dominic Wilkinson for helpful comments on this section.

[13] For the effects of social isolation on older people in Japan, see the contribution of Nakazawa and Akabayashi (Chapter 16).

the differences that exist between the elderly and the young are sufficient to remove egalitarian concerns about placing legal restrictions on the basic liberties of one group that are not placed on the other.

The most compelling argument for a selective restriction would focus on the worry that older people, but not younger people, risk overwhelming health systems. But there are two ways to approach this difference. One is to count the special risk older people pose as part of a consequentialist calculation that could *override* the requirement to distribute liberties equally. Another is to regard the difference as morally relevant, so that there would be no requirement, in this case, to distribute basic liberties equally. We believe that the former approach is appropriate. For a fundamental liberty, what counts as a morally relevant difference should not be contingent and context-dependent. Suppose that country A and country B have the same proportion of young and old people, but country A has many more hospitals per capita, so it does not run a risk of its hospitals being overwhelmed. It would be odd to suggest that in country B there is a morally relevant difference between the young and the old in virtue of which they do not deserve the same basic liberties, but in country A there is no such difference.

To be clear, we do not wish to deny that restrictions imposed selectively on older people could be justified. But we need to be confident that the benefits to younger people and to society overall would be big enough to justify such restrictions. In calculating these benefits, we should also count the fact that older people, but not younger people, are likely to overwhelm hospitals. But even if there is a strong consequentialist argument in favor of selective restrictions, valid egalitarian concerns regarding such policies are likely to persist.[14] When assessing reasons for and against selective restrictions on the elderly, equality should weigh against them.

The case of selective restrictions for the unvaccinated is somewhat different, especially where vaccines are widely available and individuals who are unvaccinated exercise a choice. Unequal choices have been regarded by several egalitarians as a morally significant difference that justifies inequality.[15] And, arguably, one central function of law is to incentivize behavior by imposing burdens and conferring benefits on individuals who act or do not act in certain ways. Imposing sanctions that limit the liberty of those who do not abide by a certain policy is not typically seen as a violation of the ideal of equal treatment under the law. Indeed, we can regard a selective restriction on the unvaccinated not as a selective restriction at all, but as a universal conditional restriction, which says, "if you get vaccinated, you will enjoy certain liberties that otherwise you would not." The conditional form is apt here because it is in a person's power to make its

---

[14] The case for selective restrictions can be further strengthened if they also help society protect other vulnerable populations (for example, by allowing the opening of schools).

[15] See Arneson (1989), Cohen (1989), and Dworkin (1981).

antecedent true. The same cannot be said of the elderly and the young. If a state justifies a selective restriction by saying, "if you are young, you will enjoy certain liberties that otherwise you would not," the universality of this conditional formulation would ring hollow, because there is nothing an older person can do to be young. In justifying selective restrictions for the unvaccinated, then, perhaps we do not need to point to any morally relevant health-related, need-related, or even choice-related difference between them and the vaccinated. Even if unvaccinated people do not infect others at higher rates than vaccinated people, selective restrictions could be justified in their case if a state is justified in using public policy to encourage vaccination at the population level.[16]

To sum up, selective restrictions offer one approach to aligning freedom protection and harm prevention and reduction. They do so by distinguishing between *groups of people*, protecting certain freedoms for some while denying these freedoms to others. Our concern about this approach, at least when applied to some groups, is that it may not protect freedom in the *right way*, one that accepts an egalitarian presumption if not constraint, or a sufficiently robust ideal of equality before the law. There is, however, another approach, not explored in this volume: rather than distinguishing groups of people, we can distinguish between different kinds of freedom.

17.1.3 Different Freedoms

There is a common tendency in public debates to suppose that one should have some general view about liberty-restricting measures. An implication is that one must take a side: be either pro-mandates or anti-mandates. But if something like Mill's harm principle is appealed to as a shared normative commitment, a more nuanced approach is called for. Powers, Faden, and Saghai (2012), for example, reject the view that liberties of all kinds should enjoy an equal presumption in their favor in the formulation of public policies. They argue for an interpretation of Mill that emphasizes a distinction between three kinds of liberty interests: interests that are immune from state interference, interests that enjoy a presumption in favor of liberty, and interests that enjoy no such presumption.

The core insight for public health policy is that all liberties are not on a moral par and thus that the degree of justification required to support restrictive interventions turns not only on considerations of harm to others but also on the moral

---

[16] Another issue could be relevant here. Allen (2022: 89) argues that we need a response to the pandemic that fosters a sense of social solidarity. Burdening the elderly may be counterproductive in this respect, but burdening the unvaccinated may be supported. An argument can be made that people who *refuse* to get vaccinated fail to show the kind of solidarity we expect of citizens at a time of crisis, and that society is justified in asking them to bear the burdens of the failure to show this kind of solidarity.

importance of the specific kind of liberty at issue. Lockdowns, vaccine mandates, and mask-wearing mandates affect liberties of varying importance and should not be lumped together when thinking about the state's legitimacy to interfere. Thus, one may consistently object to lockdowns while supporting mask-wearing mandates. One can also object to lockdowns under certain risks of harm while allowing them under more serious risks of harm. What we need is a careful investigation of particular liberty-restricting measures and their expected harm-reducing effects. Disagreements will surely arise here too, but such inquiry may result in nuanced policies that restrict certain freedoms but not others, in certain circumstances but not others. These policies will have the virtue of being a compromise between extremes. If adopted, we would be asked to tolerate more harm and risk than some people might find acceptable, but less freedom than others think must be protected.

Note that this general proposal is not a version of weak paternalism. A weakly paternalistic justification of vaccine mandates could proceed from arguing that the choice to not get vaccinated is based on misinformation and so frustrates the agent's own ends. Blumenthal-Barby argues convincingly against such weakly paternalistic defenses of vaccine mandates (and other mandates). As a society, she points out, we often respect individual choices that are based on misinformation. Furthermore, some people refuse vaccination, say, for deep personal convictions. The proposal we outline here does not question people's decision-making processes, but, rather, distinguishes between different kinds of freedom. It concerns what is chosen, not how it is chosen. The idea is that the freedom to not wear a mask, even if some people take it very seriously, is a less important freedom than freedom of movement, even if some people do not attribute much importance to it.

That all freedoms are not on a moral par may already be presupposed in judgments people make about liberty-restricting measures.[17] The idea that a mask mandate and a lockdown violate freedoms of different importance may seem obvious, yet one hears little about it in public discussions or, for that matter, in this volume. Philosophers and bioethicists can contribute to public debates by offering a principled way of thinking about such distinctions, by encouraging their use in public decision-making, and by encouraging their use in communication between public health officials and the public.

In sum, moving forward in the face of disagreement may require some compromise. One option is to proceed with selective restrictions, as some authors propose. Another option is to assess the moral importance of different kinds of freedoms, as we propose. There may be other ways to construe the right balance

---

[17] One could argue, for example, that closing places of worship infringes on a more fundamental freedom compared with closing bars (say), and so requires a higher threshold of justification in terms of preventing harm to others.

between freedom protection and harm prevention and reduction. The right balance may require seeking concessions from people who tend to support liberty-restricting measures and people who tend to object to them. Such compromise is justified not only because of its consensus-building potential but also because it takes both freedom protection and harm prevention seriously. Ethically, that appears to be the right thing to do.

17.1.4 Taking Harm Prevention Seriously

At least two obstacles can derail us from striking the right balance between freedom protection and harm prevention and reduction. One is a misguided understanding of each of the values at stake. As mentioned, a correct understanding of the value of freedom protection may require some egalitarian constraint on the goal of offering people as much freedom as possible. This constraint may be integral to the value of freedom that we seek to promote, such that violations of it that increase aggregate freedom should not count as improvement in terms of freedom. The second is a failure to take one of these values seriously enough. It is our impression that some objections to liberty-restricting measures included in this volume do not take harm prevention and reduction seriously enough or do not have a rich enough understanding of the ethical requirement to prevent harm.

Flanigan, for example, objects to liberty restrictions partly because they are politically polarizing and because they erode public trust in institutions. Her claim requires more empirical substantiation, for it may well be the case that failure to enforce restrictions early on in a pandemic would cause great harm and would also erode trust in institutions. However, we would like to highlight a normative point made by Flanigan. She argues that authorities failed the public in different ways during the early days of the pandemic, so they lost the *standing* to issue coercive mandates later on. Flanigan argues that the tension between harm prevention and freedom protection should be resolved in favor of freedom protection because there is no one who may legitimately restrict the relevant freedoms.

We agree with Flanigan that a catastrophic, careless, or persistent failure to secure public health goods would erode the legitimacy of public health authorities. However, provided past failures were made in good faith and were reasonable at the time, we do not think that such failures alone are sufficient to undermine the legitimate authority of public health institutions. Moreover, although global and national public health authorities made numerous mistakes in their pandemic policy responses, any judgments about the implications of these mistakes for the legitimacy of these authorities during the course of the emergency must take account of the pressures to operate quickly in a rapidly evolving, ominous pandemic of a novel pathogen characterized by uncertainty. This does not mean that these authorities should not be held accountable for their failures, or that it is not critically important to understand how and why things went wrong. Our point is simply that we find the inference from the recognition that failures occurred to lack of present authority to be too harsh. In saying this we do not mean to imply that harm prevention is more important than freedom protection. Rather, we reject tilting policies too much in the freedom-protecting direction based on these kinds of considerations.

Flanigan allows liberty-restricting measures only where there is clear evidence that a less restrictive measure will not be effective in preventing serious harm. The problem, again, is that we often lack the relevant evidence and may have to make decisions in the face of uncertainty. In such cases, Flanigan advocates for a presumption of protecting rather than restricting liberty. This approach, we think, also fails to take harm prevention seriously enough. In the face of uncertainty, it may sometimes be extremely risky to *not* employ liberty restriction on a wide scale early on. In the case of COVID-19, it may have been sensible to begin with more restrictive measures even in the absence of solid evidence to the effect that no other measure would be less effective, and gradually loosen restrictions while continuing to monitor spikes in morbidity and mortality, health system functioning, and so on. Again, in saying this we do not prefer harm prevention to freedom protection. Rather, we take it to be a more reasonable balance between harm prevention and freedom protection under conditions of considerable uncertainty about both the magnitude and nature of the pandemic's harms and the likelihood that liberty-limiting interventions will contain these harms.

Flanigan and Blumenthal-Barby also argue that many liberty-restricting measures used during the pandemic are more like prohibiting a sober driver from driving than prohibiting a drunk driver from driving. In other words, the restrictions were excessive and society should have tolerated a greater level of risk to protect certain freedoms. In support of this claim, they argue that, once vaccines are available, the risk unvaccinated or unmasked individuals pose on others is low, as these other individuals can protect themselves through vaccination.

In one sense, this point is clearly right, and governments generally loosened liberty-restricting measures as the situation improved. That said, it is quite possible that, even in the presence of vaccine availability, rates of severe disease and death will remain high enough for a while, and will continue to overtax health workers and health systems. Until rates steadily decline, it may or may not be justified to maintain mask mandates or other liberty-restricting measures to contain these harms. This is just another instance of a policy judgment that requires an assessment of the moral importance of liberties at issue and the public health, justice, and other non-liberty interests that are at stake.

There is another important ethical issue here, concerning the special duty we have to protect the vulnerable in particular from being harmed.[18] Goodin (1985) has persuasively argued that we have a special ethical duty to protect those who are particularly vulnerable. In the case of this pandemic, the particularly vulnerable include persons with compromised immune systems who remain at significant risk of succumbing to severe COVID-19 disease even after vaccination, as well as elderly persons for whom waning of vaccine protection against severe outcomes over time is particularly worrisome. These individuals may remain vulnerable even when vaccinated. The elderly and individuals with compromised immune systems (and possibly healthcare workers) have a *special* claim on others to take measures not to infect them. This claim is more ethically weighty than garden-variety claims not to engage in behaviors that are risky to others, and it can arguably justify some restrictions on freedom that ordinarily will not be justified by considerations of harm prevention. Even when a driver is sober, her liberty to drive at the ordinary speed limit may be justifiably restricted when children are playing in the street. Assuming selective restrictions are not placed on vulnerable individuals, we should expect to interact with them in our daily lives. We may thus have a special duty to ensure that we do not impose health risks on them. We worry that, in generally siding with freedom protection, Flanigan (and perhaps Blumenthal-Barby) does not take possible harm to vulnerable populations seriously enough.

These comments help refine the general proposal made above to distinguish different kinds of freedom. When assessing any liberty-restricting measure, several considerations must be taken into account: 1) the value or importance of the liberty/freedom in question; 2) the probability and severity of the harm to others threatened by the liberty/freedom in question; 3) the likelihood that liberty-restricting measures will reduce this harm; 4) whether disadvantaged groups are disproportionately burdened by the liberty-restricting measures, and thus whether precepts of equality are respected; and 5) the extent to which vulnerable individuals will be affected by *not* implementing a certain liberty-restricting measure. Weighing these considerations in relation to particular liberty-restricting policies—and updating these assessments with the latest relevant empirical evidence as scientific knowledge accumulates—will allow public health officials to balance freedom protection and harm prevention in ways that may not appeal to everyone, but will offer a sound public justification for certain liberty-restricting measures.

---

[18] In several places, vulnerable populations expressed concerns about lifting restrictions. See, for example, BBC West (2022) and Mays et al. (2022).

17.2 Global Justice

Questions of justice loomed large over this pandemic. In many parts of the world, healthcare systems had to make difficult decisions to suspend services to some patients to make room for COVID patients. Available treatments for COVID patients were in short supply, as were diagnostic tests. These distributive dilemmas were largely addressed within countries. However, as Tasioulas and Wilkinson both point out, distributive principles formulated before the pandemic were often neglected during the pandemic by national public officials, and public officials did not want to be seen as practicing any form of explicit triage.[19] There is much to discuss regarding domestic distributive justice during COVID-19.[20] But as important as these domestic issues are, questions of global justice were more often taken up by the authors of this volume, so we concentrate on these issues in what follows.

It is the advent of COVID-19 vaccines that brought questions of global justice most dramatically into focus. Initial supplies of the vaccine were severely constrained. During this time, the wealthier nations of the world secured access for their populations through a series of pre- and post-market mechanisms that left poorer nations with limited to no vaccine (So and Woo 2020). Their conduct was completely in line with the global track record on access to medical countermeasures for epidemic threats; consider, for example, antiretroviral therapies for HIV-AIDS (Giuliano and Vella 2007). This conduct was also anticipated. In the early days of the COVID pandemic, an international consortium, ACT-A, and its vaccine arm, COVAX, were established expressly to bring about equitable global access to medical countermeasures this time around. And although COVAX did succeed in securing more doses of vaccine for LMICs compared to previous global experience, it failed to meet its overall objective, in part because of the conduct of HICs.[21]

Considerations of medical need should play an important role in assessing global distributions, and they point in a cosmopolitan direction, as ordinary citizens and national policy makers cannot assume that their co-nationals are the most needy. Following Schaefer, we can say that distributing medical resources by medical need realizes three ethical values: benefitting people and reducing harm, prioritizing the medically worse-off (as people with greater medical needs would have prior access to medical resources), and showing equal concern to

---

[19] See John Tasioulas 'The Uneasy Relationship Between Human Rights and Public Health: Lessons from COVID-19', Chapter 3, and Dominic Wilkinson 'Pluralism and Allocation of Limited Resources: Vaccines and Ventilators', Chapter 10 in this volume.

[20] See Kristina Orfali, 'Tragic Choices during the COVID-19 Pandemic: the Past and the Future', Chapter 12 in this volume.

[21] For discussion of COVAX, see Schaefer's and Gostin's contributions to this volume (Chapters 11 and 1).

individuals (as people with similar medical needs would have equal access to resources).[22] When vaccines first became available it was already clear that older persons were at far greater risk of succumbing to SARS Cov-2 infection than younger persons. That much of the world's population above the age of 60 live in high or middle income countries offers *some* justification for prioritizing these countries. However, even allowing for differential demography, initial global vaccine distributions were a far cry from any reasonable need-based distributive principle.

Could national partiality justify the distributive inequalities observed in the epidemic? Political philosophers disagree whether states are allowed to be partial to their own citizens and residents, or the extent to which they should be. Buchanan, who accepts the view that states may prioritize the interests of their own citizens and residents over those of foreigners, argues that there are limits to legitimate partiality, and that these limits were not respected during COVID-19.[23] We concur. Indeed, among the contributors to this collection, there appears to be consensus that governments of wealthy countries obtained and controlled more vaccines and other needed medical resources than they were justified to obtain and control. The medical needs of foreigners were excessively and unjustly discounted. Our view aligns with this broad consensus.

As several authors point out, it is not necessary to rely on any comprehensive *distributive* ideal or comprehensive account of global justice to defend the view that wealthier nations obtained and controlled more medical countermeasures than they were justified to obtain and control. Buchanan and Savulescu, for example, appeal to *a collective duty of easy rescue* to justify this charge: if wealthy countries can help poor countries to obtain life-saving medical resources with relatively little sacrifice to themselves, they morally ought to do so. According to Buchanan, wealthy countries could do much for poorer countries with little sacrifice to themselves, especially after the initial alarming phase of a pandemic has passed. Therefore, they are morally criticizable for not doing so.[24] We cannot always determine when a society is past its "alarming phase" because we cannot always know when the worst of a pandemic is indeed over, but the overall reasonableness of Buchanan's general position stands.

This way of arguing for a moral duty on the part of wealthy states to help poorer states is appealing because it invokes a widely held moral outlook that recognizes a moral duty of easy rescue. This duty does not presuppose further commitments to cosmopolitan egalitarian ideals or to distribution according to

[22] G. Owen Schaefer, 'Fairly and Pragmatically Prioritizing Global Allocation of Scarce Vaccines during a Pandemic', Chapter 11 in this volume.

[23] Allen Buchanan, 'Institutionalizing the Duty to Rescue in a Global Health Emergency', Chapter 2 in this volume.

[24] See also Larry Gostin, 'The Great Coronavirus Pandemic: An Unparalleled Collapse in Global Solidarity', Chapter 1 in this volume.

need. Moreover, it can be supported by both consequentialist and nonconsequentialist ethical theories. Its intuitive appeal can be teased out by considering a variation on the famous child-drowning-in-a-pond case.[25] If a collective effort is needed to save a drowning child with little sacrifice to the collective and its members, the collective has a moral duty to save the child. We believe that a duty of collective easy rescue (with its institutional implications) has a secure ethical footing.

However, the duty of collective easy rescue also has its limitations. Consider vaccines or PPE (personal protective equipment). These are not intended to rescue someone who is in danger, but to prevent one from getting into danger in the first place. If there is a pond in which children often drown, we may have a collective moral duty to build a fence around it, but that is not helpfully construed as a duty of *rescue*. The issue here may be merely semantic, but in thinking about global obligations, it may be useful to supplement the duty of easy rescue with other ethical perspectives while remaining neutral regarding comprehensive views of global justice.

One way of doing so is to appeal to human rights. Human rights are already recognized in international affairs as a source of political duties of states and international organizations. Canonical lists of human rights do not mention a human right to be rescued, so a human-rights perspective would presumably be distinct from a collective-duty-to-rescue perspective. Importantly, a human-rights perspective can be used to justify a duty to provide vaccines (say) to people living in LMICs. Suppose that wealthy countries enter bilateral agreements with pharmaceutical companies, "cornering" a large number of vaccine doses and raising their prices. This will put vaccines out of reach for poorer countries. How is that a human-rights violation? First, it risks putting people in poorer countries below a minimal level of well-being. Second, it puts people in poorer countries in a state of vulnerability and dependency. Third, the behaviors of wealthy countries during the pandemic suggests that they pose *standard threats* against which human rights are intended to protect.[26] Wealthy countries pose *threats* because they make much-needed medical resources less available to poorer countries, and they pose *standard* threats because, unless prevented, these aggressive marketplace practices by wealthier nations are to be expected in a global market economy with actors who hold unequal resources and bargaining power.

Powers and Faden (2019: 146–86) put forward another way to think about human rights and nationalism in global interactions that can be useful in this regard. Their view takes seriously both the moral responsibility of nation-states to secure human rights and structural justice domestically, *and* their responsibility to address impediments to human rights fulfillment elsewhere in the world that

---

[25] The thought experiment was popularized by Singer (1972).
[26] Following Shue (1996: 18, 29–32), these three points suggest a human-rights violation.

result from unfair differentials in interstate and global institutional power. Powers and Faden defend what they call the Principle of Interstate Reciprocity that establishes conditions under which the pursuit of national interests and global advantage is constrained. This principle prohibits a nation from pressing advantage for its own residents when this pursuit 1) undermines the human rights of residents of other nations and 2) foregoing the pursuit of advantage does not thereby put its own residents' basic human rights at substantial risk. Assuming a human-rights case for access to vaccines during a pandemic can be made, at minimum, the Principle of Interstate Reciprocity provides a foundation for a human-rights argument against leaving access to vaccines entirely to the global market economy.

We should note that neither the Principle of Interstate Reciprocity nor the duty of collective easy rescue requires a system of global vaccine allocation based solely on a moral principle like medical need, let alone cosmopolitan egalitarianism. A duty of easy rescue as well as a human-rights perspective allow nationalism to play some role in access to medical resources while providing justification for global restrictions on certain kinds of market practices, for example some kinds of bilateral agreements, as well as for global obligations to strengthen initiatives like COVAX.

17.3 Going Forward

Finally, we would like to flag three issues that have not been addressed much by the authors in this volume and which we believe deserve greater scholarly attention as we prepare for the next pandemic.

17.3.1 Democracy

The first set of issues concerns democracy and the particular challenges democracies have faced during this pandemic and that they are likely to face in future pandemics. Pandemics pose a legitimacy challenge to all political regimes, because all political regimes must work to secure the health of their populations (Allen 2022: 9–10). But pandemics like COVID-19 pose particular challenges to democracies, as democracies move slower than autocracies (Allen 2022: 101). Democratic deliberation takes time, and democracies tend to respect certain side-constraints on government action that limit their ability to implement some effective public health measures. When democratic governments implement such measures, they are accused of overreaching, and when they do not implement such measures, they are accused of not doing enough.

Disagreement has always been a virtue of democracy and a challenge to it. But the current epidemic exposes an acute epistemic concern that democracies face given their tendency to encourage epistemic tolerance. In liberal democracies, we value the free expression of different opinions and do not censor the media. The result is that citizens may be deeply divided on questions of fact, not just on questions of value. Furthermore, a society with free speech should expect not just reasonable disagreements about these matters but also a fair amount of epistemic confusion, from unsubstantiated rumors to full-out conspiracy theories. The ethical challenges this poses for pandemic preparedness and response, particularly when appealing to scientific evidence in justifying certain policies is seen as taking an ideological stance, need to be squarely confronted.

We have seen two concerning trends during the pandemic. One involves politicians who say they seek to simply "follow the science." This approach is misguided.[27] Scientists and other experts aim to tell us what the best available scientific evidence in their field is and may offer advice about the implications of that evidence for policy, but democracy is not the rule of experts. Politicians must make all-things-considered judgments (Allen 2022: 23). Politicians cannot evade making hard decisions about values and should not pretend to do so.

The second worrying trend is that of politicians with no scientific background who dismiss, ridicule, or simply ignore public health experts, including those who work for their government. While we certainly do not want political leaders or the citizenry to sheepishly and uncritically accept the views of experts, it would be impossible for democracies to effectively respond to pandemics without some reasonable regard for and reliance on the assessments of experts. The same normative point applies, of course, to experts in ethics and bioethics. They too should not be sheepishly followed in a democratic society. However, we know of no politician who declared to simply "follow the ethics." Indeed, as mentioned, in several countries certain principles of triage were formulated and endorsed before the pandemic, and then ignored during the pandemic.[28] Politicians did not want to be seen to be following any value-laden principle of triage and to engage in explicit ethical deliberation. *That* is worrying, and something for bioethicists to think about. Going forward, the fact that pandemics pose a predictable threat to democratic governance should be a central part of bioethical discourse.

17.3.2 Public Health and Government Overreach

Another democracy-related problem requires attention. In the past, public health authorities were criticized for not having enough "teeth." This criticism is in some contexts still valid, but in many countries public health authorities were able

---

[27] See John Tasioulas, 'The Uneasy Relationship between Human Rights and Public Health: Lessons from COVID-19', Chapter 3 in this volume.

[28] See also Wilkinson's and Tasioulas's contributions in this volume (Chapters 10 and 3).

during the pandemic to issue or influence significant liberty-restricting measures. That gives them a non-negligible amount of power. The problem, however, is that public health officials, like many officials in ministry-level positions, are not elected. Instead, they are appointed to their jobs by a democratically elected executive or by a ministry head whom the executive selected. Except for top public health leadership, elected bodies like parliaments or congresses play no role in these appointments, though they may have some oversight responsibility. When public health authorities are able to exercise significant power over the lives of the citizenry, they face a challenge to their legitimate authority that goes beyond the legitimacy of particular liberty-restricting measures.[29] In other words, the pandemic calls for a closer examination of the role public health authorities play in a democratic society. This issue is perhaps not unique to public health authorities; it applies to many agencies of government. But some aspects of this problem may be particularly problematic for public health authorities because of the kind of public good that they promote. Thinking about how best to prepare for the next pandemic, this is another area for bioethicists to examine.

17.3.3 Children

Finally, we note with concern the absence of specific attention to children in a volume devoted to the ethical dimensions of pandemic preparedness and response. Unlike with adults, ethical tensions between state intervention and individual liberty are not a central issue in the case of children. Instead, what matters most in the case of children is the impact of pandemic policies on their overall well-being. This point is underscored by the recognition that children have special justice claims, for two reasons. First, children are completely dependent on others and the social order to secure their well-being. Second, as a developmental matter, setbacks to interests in childhood not only harm children at the time they are experienced; these setbacks can reverberate over the whole of their lives, frustrating their interests well into adulthood (Powers and Faden 2006: 92–5). "Unlike a tainted sports event," Jonathan Kozol reminds us, "a childhood cannot be played again" (Kozol 1991: 217). If a childhood does not include the securing of critical milestones in knowledge and understanding, social and emotional development, and mental as well as physical health, prospects for a decent adult life can be profoundly undermined. We thus agree with Allen (2022: 46–9, 99) that we should think of schools somewhat like we think of hospitals. They should be the last to close and the first to reopen. However, we do not wish to downplay the health risks this may expose teachers to, and the other burdens that

---

[29] Although, in some places, elected officials can veto (or are needed to approve) certain measures.

teachers will face if they are deemed "essential workers." There are ethical dilemmas here, that is, material for bioethical discussion.

It is becoming increasingly clear that children across the globe have suffered significantly during the COVID-19 pandemic, and that children from poor or otherwise marginalized communities have suffered the most.[30] Although the full impact of disrupted schooling, in some cases for almost two years, is yet to be calculated, learning loss, developmental delay, and compromised mental health are already in evidence. Some of the world's most disadvantaged children will never return to school, erasing decades of advancements in education, especially for girls (Frohn 2021; Cameron et al. 2021).

Going forward, children must figure prominently in the ethics of pandemic preparedness. How the interests of children should be taken into account in pandemic planning raises questions about intergenerational justice that go beyond standard debates about whether lives saved or life-years saved is the correct measure in assessing the allocation of vaccines or ICU beds. Even when children are spared much of a pandemic's burden of disease, as is the case with SARS-CoV-2, other critical interests can be significantly harmed by policies designed to contain it (for example, schools closure). The global experience of the COVID-19 pandemic has been punctuated by a repeated failure to find morally acceptable trade-offs or alignments across different dimensions of well-being. Children in particular suffered from this failure, resulting in profound injustices to our youngest generation. How to prevent that from happening in the next pandemic will require careful integration of expertise in ethics with expertise in education, child development, and child health, and should be a top priority for pandemic planning.

17.4 Conclusion

A single chapter cannot do justice to all the intriguing and valuable contributions made in this volume. Our aim was more modest: to offer an (opinionated) presentation of some recurring themes and to begin a conversation about the various questions and answers discussed in this collection, with the hope that the conversation will continue beyond the pages of this book. We have also pointed out some areas for further consideration.

At the time of writing this chapter, the pandemic is still with us. We do not yet have a complete historical perspective on it or the full benefit of hindsight. But as the various contributions in this collection make all too clear, that does not mean we should wait. Valuable ethical lessons can already be learned from the

---

[30] For example, it has been estimated that, in low-income countries, lockdowns resulted in increased mortality among children. See Ma et al. (2021).

experience of the last two years. Democracies move slowly. To allow for proper democratic deliberation, time is needed. Somewhat paradoxically, the patience required for proper democratic decision-making makes the task of reflection more urgent. Both nationally and globally, after-action analyses and planning for the next pandemic are already well underway. These efforts must include a careful consideration of the ethics of pandemic preparedness and response. The global and national institutional reforms that follow should benefit from continued, on-point scholarship in political and moral philosophy responsive to the experience of this pandemic, as exemplified by the chapters in this volume.

Bibliography

Allen, D. (2022), *Democracy in the Time of Coronavirus* (Chicago: University of Chicago Press, 2022).

Arneson, R. J. (1989), 'Equality and Equal Opportunity for Welfare', *Philosophical Studies* 56/1: 77–93.

BBC West (2022), 'Covid: Medically vulnerable people fear end of rules', *BBC News*, 22 February 2022, https://www.bbc.com/news/uk-england-gloucestershire-60470880 (accessed 26 Apr. 2022).

Beaumont, P. (2020), 'Covid-19 vaccine: who are countries prioritising for first doses?', *The Guardian*, 18 November 2020, https://www.theguardian.com/world/2020/nov/18/covid-19-vaccine-who-are-countries-prioritising-for-first-doses (accessed 29 April 2020).

Cameron, E. C., et al. (2021), 'COVID-19 and Women', *International Perspectives in Psychology* 10/3: 138–46.

Cohen, G. A. (1989), 'On the Currency of Egalitarian Justice', *Ethics* 99/4: 906–44.

Dworkin, R. (1981), 'What Is Equality? Part 2: Equality of Resources', *Philosophy & Public Affairs* 10/4: 283–345.

Frohn, J. (2021), 'Troubled Schools in Troubled Times: How COVID-19 Affects Educational Inequalities and What Measures can be Taken', in *European Educational Research Journal* 20/5: 667–83.

Galanis, P., et al. (2021), 'Nurses' Burnout and Associated Risk Factors During the COVID-19 Pandemic: A Systematic Review and Meta-analysis', *Journal of Advanced Nursing* 77/8: 3286–302.

Giuliano, M., and Vella, S. (2007), 'Inequalities in health: access to treatment for HIV/AIDS.' *Annali-Istituto Superiore di Sanita*, 43/4: 313.

Goodin, R. E. (1985), *Protecting the Vulnerable* (Chicago: University of Chicago Press, 1985).

Kozol, J. (1991), *Savage Inequalities* (New York: Broadway Books, 1991).

Ma, L., et al. (2021), 'The Intergenerational Mortality Tradeoff of COVID-19 Lockdown Policies, Working Paper 28925', *Working Paper Series, National Bureau of Economic Research*.

Mays, J. C., et al. (2022), 'Covid News: Parents in Virginia Win Right to Mask Classmates of Their Vulnerable Children," *The New York Times*, March 24, 2022, https://www.nytimes.com/live/2022/03/24/world/covid-19-mandates-cases-vacc ine?action=click&module=coronavirus&variant=1_signup&state=default&pgtype =Article&region=body&context=storyline_push_signup&referringSource=articleS hare#a-virginia-judge-rules-that-12-families-can-enforce-mask-mandates-in-classrooms-for-their-vulnerable-children-despite-state-law (accessed 26 Apr. 2022).

Pappa, S., et al. (2020), 'Prevalence of Depression, Anxiety, and Insomnia among Healthcare Workers During the COVID-19 Pandemic: A Systematic Review and Meta-analysis', *Brain, Behavior, and Immunity* 88: 901–7.

Powers, M., and Faden, R. (2006), *Social Justice: The Moral Foundations of Public Health and Health Policy*. (Oxford: Oxford University Press, 2006).

Powers M., and Faden, R. (2019), *Structural Injustice: Power, Advantage and Human Rights* (Oxford, Oxford University Press, 2019).

Powers, M., Faden, R., and Saghai, Y. (2012), 'Liberty, Mill and the Framework of Public Health Ethics', *Public Health Ethics* 5/1: 6–25.

Rawls J. (1971), *A Theory of Justice* (Cambridge, MA: Harvard University Press, 1971).

Savulescu, J., and Cameron, J. (2020), 'Why Lockdown of the Elderly is not Ageist and why Levelling Down Equality is Wrong', *Journal of Medical Ethics* 46: 717–21.

Shue, H. (1996), *Basic Rights: Subsistence, Affluence, and U.S. Foreign Policy* (Princeton, NJ: Princeton University Press, 1996).

Singer, P. (1972), 'Famine, Affluence, and Morality', *Philosophy & Public Affairs* 1/3: 229–43.

So, A. D., and Woo, J. (2020), 'Reserving Coronavirus Disease 2019 Vaccines for Global Access: Cross Sectional Analysis', *BMJ* 371: 4750.

Temkin, L. (2002), 'Equality, Priority and the Levelling Down Objection', in Clayton, M., and Williams, A. (eds.), *The Ideal of Equality* (London: Palgrave Macmillan, 2002): 126–61.

Index

Note: Figures are indicated by an italic "*f*", following the page number.

For the benefit of digital users, indexed terms that span two pages (e.g., 52–53) may, on occasion, appear on only one of those pages.